PEGAN DIET COOKBOOK

600 Tasty Recipes for Your Whole Family –
Embrace the Pegan Lifestyle and Improve Your
Wellbeing Through Healthy Foods

SHEILA J. BAKER

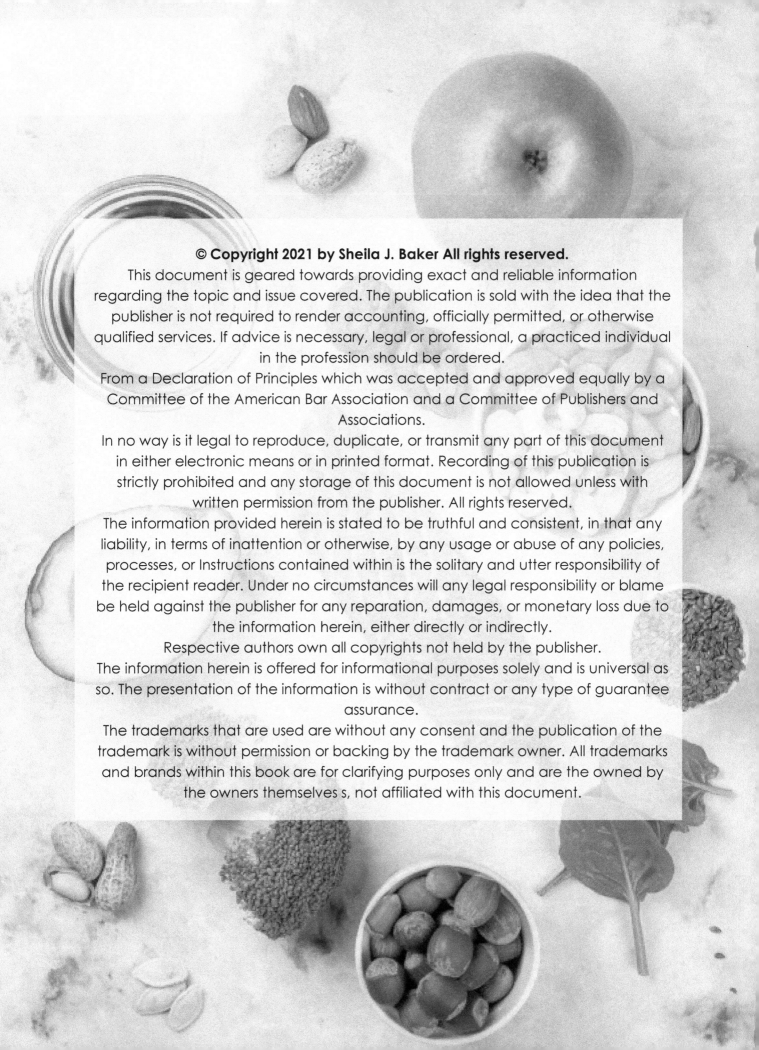

Table of Contents

Introduction

The foundation of our diet in America, as well as increasingly across the globe, consists of ultra-processed industrial food produced in ways that harm the environment, climate, and human health. It's a trend that will have disastrous implications for mankind and the environment.

Six out of ten Americans suffer from a chronic ailment linked to our ultra-processed diet—heart disease, diabetes, dementia, cancer, you name it. We are metabolically unwell in around 88% of the population, which means almost 9 out of 10 of us are diabetes. The financial cost of this is enormous: Health care consumes one out of every 5 dollars in our economy. And almost all of it goes toward treating chronic diseases that are virtually completely caused by diet.

The environmental implications are disastrous. In the name of producing vast expanses of maize, wheat, and soy, we've exhausted our fresh water supplies, harmed our aquatic & terrestrial ecosystems, & wiped-out pollinator, livestock, and edible plant species.

The global economy is being fed on a diet of fossil fuels, water, and soil. This diet has led to the great destabilization of our climate.

We urgently need to replace our current food system with an environmentally sustainable model that can deliver healthy diets abundant in fruits, vegetables, nuts and seeds, legumes, and grass-fed meats.

The way we feed ourselves has repercussions for ourselves as well as for the planet. It is not too late to begin to fix this broken system.

Pegan, a name derived from Paleo and Vegan diets, is specifically designed to solve both health and environmental problems. The Pegan diet provides all of the nutritional benefits of a Paleo diet while cutting out any animal products.

There are many specific benefits to this diet:

-Weight loss: This diet is specifically designed to allow for weight loss, something that is not common with vegan diets.

-Digestive benefits: With fewer animal products in your system, your digestive tract will operate more smoothly.

-Environmental impact: Animal agriculture is extremely harmful to our environment and natural resources. Pegan diets limit the amount of products that come from animals anymore.

The Pegan Diet is also environmentally friendly. There are much less animal products in our diet, so less damage is being done to our earth. Peganism is not a new concept; it's been around for thousands of years.

In this book, you'll not only learn the basics of the Pegan diet, but you'll also find a ton of easy-to-follow recipes that will make it easy to customize the diet for everyone in the family.

You'll kick off each day with a breakfast of whole grains or fruit and healthy fat, and lunch will typically be a lean meat, vegetable, and salad. Dinner is often a lot like lunch as well with more salads to keep you satiated. You'll find a ton of delicious recipes for virtually every meal in this book, including snacks and desserts that taste great while fitting into your new Pegan diet lifestyle.

In this book, you'll find everything you need to know about the Pegan diet and get your family on board with the diet. What you'll learn is a healthy, whole food plant-based diet that's low in protein and fat that can be modified for everyone from the picky kid who won't eat anything except meatballs to the parents looking to bring their children into a healthy lifestyle.

The Pegan Diet

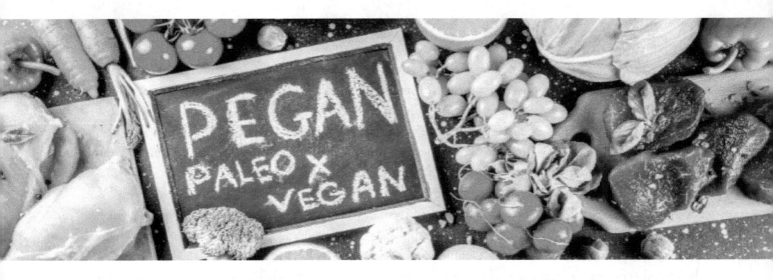

Pegan Diet is a worldwide trending diet that originated from a mysterious combination of Paleo and Vegan diets that didn't make sense on paper. The term Pegan was coined by Dr. Mark Hyman, director of the Cleveland Clinic Centre for Functional Medicine, who says the Pegan way of eating is not only the most sensible diet designed for the human race, but also the healthiest one.

Dr. Mark Hyman's Pegan Diet is a hybrid of the paleo and vegan diets, with the premise that both paleo and vegan eating (when done correctly) prioritize whole, new plant foods.

Dr. Hyman has helped countless men and women around the world lose weight, establish healthy relationships with food, heal their digestive systems, treat tough conditions like depression or anxiety, and even reverse severe diseases like type 2 diabetes, high blood pressure, or cancer.

To understand the convergence, primary focus has to be laid on the individual aspects involved.

Vegan Diet

A Vegan diet is built on a certain set of strict rules, with the primary rule prohibiting consumption of all animal products and giving most importance to plant-based foods. This diet lacks meat and other rich sources of bio-molecules like dairy and eggs. Most vegans are extremely careful about what they consume. Apart from the restrictions mentioned above, they also avoid processed animal products like gelatin, which is often added to foods, even those that seem vegan.

The resulting diet is essentially one low in calories, cholesterol, and saturated fat. It is also being good for those with heart conditions, as it assists in cholesterol and blood pressure regulation. Vegan as a diet is getting increasingly accepted due to its many health benefits.

The vegan diet is very advantageous as it reduces the risk of developing obesity, certain cancers, and type II diabetes. However, the diet falls short of certain amino acids that are the building blocks for proteins, which can only be achieved through diet. Moreover, it is deficient in iron, calcium, zinc, and vitamin B12.

Paleo Diet

Its followers were the ancient people of the Stone Age. As a predecessor, the Paleo diet uses only food available to our ancestors and eliminates or restricts the modern foods. The paleo diet involves higher level consumption of meat and vegetables with a very light sprinkling of fruits and nuts. Additions and alternatives like grains, beans, added sugar, dairy and several kinds of oils are to be avoided.

By way of comparison, the founders of the paleo diet, the cave people, consumed foods that were hunted by our hunter ancestors and included grass-fed meat, fish, eggs, nuts, fruit, and organic low-starch vegetables. Although the fat content isn't restricted, foods like grains, legumes, refined sugar, potatoes, most dairy products, and certain oils are prohibited.

Most Paleo dieters have small portions of meat included with every meal. This means that approximately 30-50% of a person's daily energy is obtained through meat. These levels are twice the number when compared to current nutrition guidelines that fluctuate around 15% to 25% of a day's energy obtained through meat.

Pegan Diet

Designing a dietary plan involves following a certain set of guidelines so we know what to eat and how much. What makes the Pegan diet easy to follow is that the rules are so much more adaptable.

For some individuals, a strict Paleo diet is too heavy and expensive to follow. It is also problematic when you consider the health issues. Veganism, on the other hand, is equally restrictive and quite a challenge for people to stick to. Hence the integration of these two highly opposing diets, the Pegan diet, a perfect mixture of health benefits and few limitations makes a lot of sense for those of us who want to follow a healthy lifestyle and agree add a limited number of animal-based proteins in their diet.

The Pegan Diet is a diet that incorporates the best parts of veganism and paleo. It encourages people to remove gluten, dairy, soy, corn, potatoes, rice and sugar from their diet. The Pegan Diet also encourages an increased consumption of vegetables and fruit and regards animal products as an occasional indulgence rather than a staple food source.

Most diets are designed to control your weight through calorie restriction which reduces hunger. The Pegan Diet helps you control your hunger entirely through eating more nutrient dense foods such as high-quality vegetables while reducing total calories by natural caloric reduction or exercise/activity. This has been shown to have a far greater effect on satiety, allowing individuals to feel fuller for longer and resist cravings

The Pegan Diet emphasizes the importance of flexibility. Flexibility allows Pegan's to fit the diet around their lifestyle and vice versa, without rules or rigid structures, so they can enjoy food as long as it fits into the 13 Pillars of the Pegan Diet. This also means that if you go out for dinner or a friend for dinner, you can still enjoy your meal knowing that the next day you will be eating plenty of fruit and vegies.

The 13 Pillars of the Pegan Diet:

1. **Sugar should be avoided at all costs**. That includes avoiding sugar, flour, and processed carbs, all of which induce an increase in insulin production. Consider sugar in all its forms as a once-in-a-while indulgence, something we consume in moderation. People should think of it as a recreational drug. It's something you do for pleasure now and again, but it's not something you eat every day.

2. **Plants make up most of your diet.** Vegetables should fill more than half of your plate, as we taught previously. The greater the color, the deeper it is. The more the diversity, the better. Veggies that are mainly non-starchy should be used. In moderation (12 cup per day), winter squashes & sweet potatoes are acceptable, but don't overdo it! Even though French fries are America's most popular vegetable, they don't qualify.

3. **Beware of fruit.** This is where there may be some misunderstanding. Some Paleo supporters advise eating mainly low-sugar fruits like berries, whereas vegan activists advise eating all fruit. Most of the Pegan supporters seem to feel better whenever they stick to low-glycemic fruits and treat themselves to the rest like a pleasure. Stick to berries, kiwis, watermelon, grapes, melons, and other similar fruits. Consider dried fruit to be sweets and use it sparingly.

4. **Pesticides, antibiotics, hormones, & GMO foods should all be avoided.** Additionally, there is no space for chemicals, preservatives, additives, colors, artificial sweeteners, or other potentially harmful substances. You should not consume an ingredient if you do not have it in your kitchen for cooking.

5. **Consume meals that are high in healthful fats.** I'm talking about omega-3 fatty acids and other healthy fats found in nuts, seeds, olive oil, and avocados, to name a few. Yes, saturated fat from fish, whole eggs, grass-fed or sustainably produced beef, grass-fed butter or ghee, plus organic virgin coconut oil and coconut butter are all acceptable sources of saturated fat.

6. **Most vegetable, nut, & seed oils,** like canola, sunflower, maize, grapeseed, and particularly soybean oil, which currently accounts for about 10% of our calories, **should be avoided.** Small quantities of expeller or cold-pressed nut & seed oils, such as sesame, macadamia, and walnut, may be used as condiments or flavorings. Avocado oil is ideal for cooking at higher temperatures.

7. **Dairy should be avoided or limited.** Dairy isn't good for most people; therefore, we suggest avoiding it, except for yogurt, kefir, ghee, grass-fed butter, and even cheese if it doesn't bother you. Instead of cow dairy, try goat or sheep dairy. Also, choose organic and grass-fed wherever possible.

8. **Consider meat & animal products as a side dish**, or as we like to call them, "Condi-meat," rather than a main meal. Meat should be a side dish, with vegetables taking center stage. Per meal, servings should be no more than 4 to 6 ounces. We usually prepare three or four veggie side dishes at a time.

9. **Consume low-mercury seafood** that has been responsibly grown or harvested. Choose low-mercury and low-toxin fish such as sardines, herring, anchovies, & wild-caught salmon. They should also be collected or cultivated in a sustainable manner.

10. **Gluten should be avoided.** Because "Franken wheat" is the main source of gluten, seek for wheat types like einkorn. Wheat should only be consumed if you are not gluten-intolerant, and even then, only on rare occasions. Dr. Alessio Fasano of Harvard, the world's leading gluten specialist, has conducted research that shows gluten damages the gut, even in individuals who aren't gluten-sensitive and have no symptoms.

11. **Consume gluten-free whole grains in moderation.** They still increase blood sugar and have the potential to cause autoimmunity. All grains have the potential to raise blood sugar levels. Low-glycemic grains such as black rice, teff, buckwheat, quinoa, and amaranth should be eaten in modest amounts (1/2 cup each meal). A grain- and bean-free diet may be crucial for type 2 diabetics, as well as individuals with autoimmune disease or digestive problems, in managing and even curing their condition. Stick to the 10-Day Detox Diet or a diabetic ketogenic diet.

12. **Beans should only be consumed occasionally.** The best legume is lentils. Large, starchy beans should be avoided. Beans have a high fiber, protein, & mineral content. However, for some people, they create digestive issues, and the lectins and phytates in them may impede mineral absorption. If you have diabetes, a high-bean diet may cause blood sugar increases. Moderate quantities (up to 1 cup per day) are OK.

13. **To customize your strategy**, get tested. What is effective for one individual may not be effective for another. This is what we mean when we say that everyone should ultimately work with a professionally trained nutritionist to customize their diet even further with the appropriate testing.

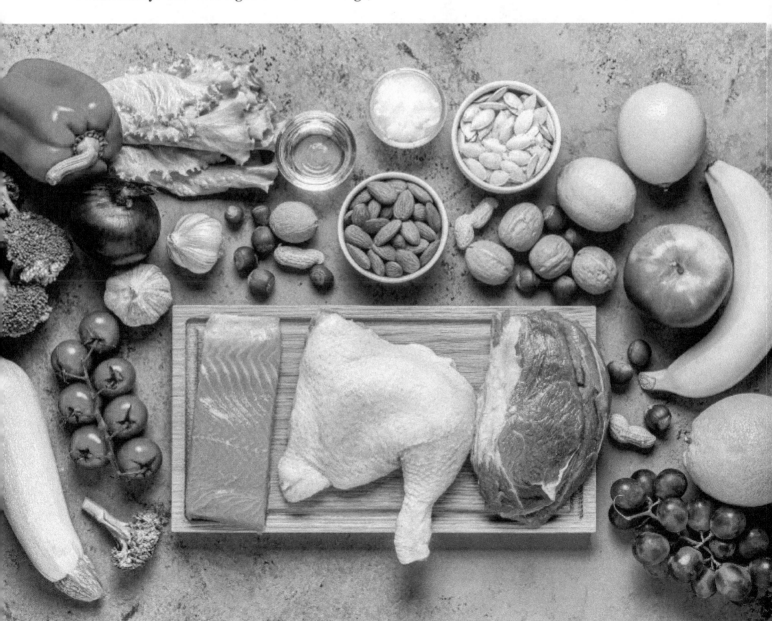

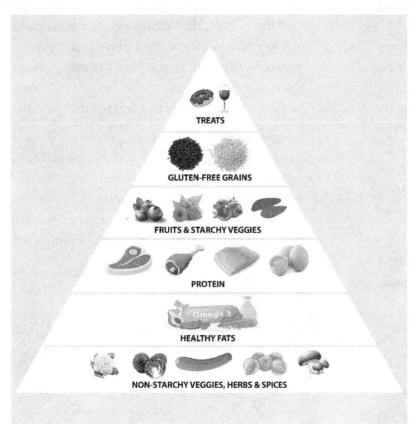

Non-Starchy Vegetables, Herbs & Spices: Unlimited Colorful, non-starchy vegetables, herbs, and spices are at the bottom of the pyramid. The more color, the better.

Blue and purple vegetables can help prevent aging because they contain anthocyanins, or antioxidants, according to Mark. Green veggies like broccoli and artichokes are also good choices. As he says, "Artichokes contain powerful detoxifying compounds and have prebiotics that help fertilize all the good bacteria in your gut. Gut bacteria are crucial to your health."

Healthy Fats: Three to five servings, says the doctor While many people blame fat for their health problems, there's such a thing as "good fat."

The Pegan diet does not mean that you will never be able to eat pasta. "Most diets are exclusive. The Pegan food pyramid includes everything, just focusing on quality," the doctor says of his diet.

Protein: 4 to 6 ounces of animal protein, up to a cup of legumes

The Pegan diet is not high in protein, but Mark says it is important to incorporate quality animal protein: grass-fed beef & dairy products, wild-caught seafood (or sustainably raised if you must eat farmed fish), and pasture-raised meats.

It doesn't need to be costly, yet like Rach says, "You truly need to know where your food comes from."

The top notch, thick proteins and supplements like B12 that you get from lean meats and fish are extremely hard to get from a simply vegetarian diet, the doc says.

Fruit And Starchy Veggies: 1 cup of low-glycemic natural product, ½ cup of dull veggies

Blueberries, raspberries, strawberries and pomegranates are instances of organic products with a low glycemic record, which is the thing that you should focus on the Pegan diet, Mark says.

Winter squash and yams are instances of dull veggies with useful for-your carotenoids and cancer prevention agents.

Gluten-Free Grains: ½ to 1 cup

You can have grains, however search for "great" grains that are low starch, low glycemic and don't have a ton of gluten — like quinoa and wild rice, the doc says.

Treats: Sparing

Benefit

The Pegan diet is a diet that focuses on healthy, natural foods. It tries to eliminate processed foods and most animal-based products, instead eating more vegetables and fruit. There are no specific rules for what is or isn't allowed, so the focus is on making good choices within one's own lifestyle. The Pegan diet also eschews gluten, a main source of many nutrients, including antioxidants, fiber, vitamins and minerals.

And it's not just the foods that you have to worry about; the Pegan diet is packed with supplements and powders that are meant to replace food. While it's true that many of us are deficient in nutrients, it's best to get your nutrients from food.

If you're a vegan or vegetarian, there is no doubt that this diet gives you the opportunity to eat a large variety of fruits and vegetables, but it can be very challenging to get your daily requirements of protein from the diet. And it's not just protein; manganese, zinc, vitamin B6 and many other essential minerals are lacking in this diet.

Benefits of Pegan Diet:

1) Healthier Manipulation - You can have foods that are packaged and processed if you choose, but they should be avoided for the most part. By removing processed foods from the diet it allows the body to become more in tune with its natural balance and will allow it to heal from any health issues.

2) Disease prevention - by focusing on whole foods and avoiding food additives and preservatives, you reduce diabetes, heart disease, high blood pressure, chronic pain and dementia. By focusing on healthy natural foods you reduce your risk of these diseases and slow the aging process.

3) Losing weight - by avoiding processed and highly processed foods you can reduce your weight by following the Pegan diet. This is one of its main focuses and it allows for a healthy way of losing weight without having to do much work. The focus is on making healthy choices that appeal to you so that you may lose weight naturally.

4) Heart health - not only does the Pegan diet focus on healthy natural foods but it also includes a lot of healthy spices. It encourages you to add more spices to your meals and to your dishes, which can be beneficial for your heart. This is because spices such as cinnamon, cloves, cumin, nutmeg and black pepper have been shown to reduce LDL cholesterol and triglyceride levels in the blood.

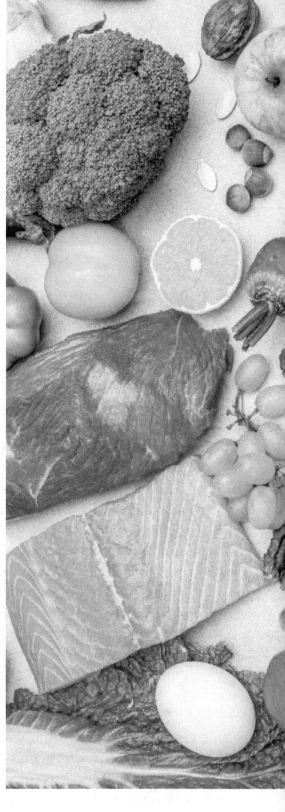

5) Cancer prevention - the Pegan diet includes a lot of foods that are beneficial for your health. It promotes foods such as vegetables, grains, fruits and it also encourages you to add more spices to your diet. Spices including cinnamon, cloves, cumin, nutmeg and black pepper have been shown to reduce LDL cholesterol and triglyceride levels in the blood. Foods such as cinnamon, cloves, cumin and black pepper has been shown to prevent cancer by slowing the growth of cancer cells.

6) Improving brain function - the Pegan diet promotes health and helping your body to use all of its energy wisely. It encourages you to add more spices to your diet which is important for your brain's function. The already mentioned spices have been proven to improve memory and learning ability.

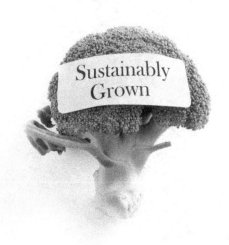

Sustainably Grown

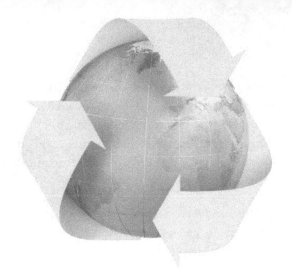

10 Tips to Eat Sustainable Food on a Budget

1. Grow your own

You needn't bother with a nursery, and it requires little exertion to grow a couple of pots of your number one spices and vegetables and it's so fulfilling. You can develop anyplace, on windowsills, on the patio, or on the carport. Start with spices as they can be so costly to purchase and occupy little space. Attempt up-cycling your unfilled egg encloses to grower for seedlings and utilizing old bean jars and milk bottles for plant pots. A single pot of fresh herbs will only cost you about $10 and will last for up to 3 months. The big pots contain everything from thyme, rosemary, parsley and basil with a variety of flavors and fragrances. They are so easy to grow, just put them in a year-round sunny spot, water regularly and snip the leaves as needed. Now you can have fresh herbs to garnish your meals for very little money.

2. Eat less meat

Meat is at the highest point of my need list with regards to purchasing natural. Natural affirmation from the Soil Association guarantees that the meat is natural as well as that it is high government assistance. Meat is costly, purchase less and make vegetables the focal point of consideration. At the point when you do purchase meat purchase less expensive cuts like shoulder and stomach, they take longer cooking yet are frequently more delicious than the excellent cuts. One of the best ways to save organic food is to eat less meat. Meat has a high saturated fat content and it is a leading contributor to heart disease and cancer. This

is one of the simplest ways to eat organic and cut down your carbon emissions. Meat is a high carbon intensive food source and if you eat less of it, you will be reducing your food miles. Try buying free range meat and even organic chicken. You always get what you pay for. If you buy the cheapest meat, you are paying for the feed it has consumed and is probably fed on cheap, rubbish food.

3. Reduce waste

The normal family squanders between 20-30% of their food, through fumbling the larder, over purchasing, and helpless stockpiling. I consider this to be a financial plan for purchasing better quality and natural food. Ensure you
utilize your most seasoned meat and vegetables first and construct your dinner plan around those fixings. I save an attract my refrigerator for the most established create and turn the produce into it before it gets cooked.

4. Buy in bulk

Purchasing food in bulk can help you save money over time. Bulk purchases are frequently less expensive. Stick to long-lasting foods like pastas, legumes, dried foods, and veggies like potatoes and onions. You can also get complete butchered animals at a fair price. Freeze them in individual parts, then cut and defrost as needed.

5. Buy seasonal

When produce is in season, it is less expensive. For starters, it won't have to be shipped halfway around the world, and it will be more plentiful. There are applications that can help you figure out what's in season right now and where you can buy the freshest produce for your meals.

6. Cook from scratch

Comfort food varieties are more costly than cooking raw ingredient from scratch, as long as you take care of your fixings and use them sparingly. I like to prepare additional parts of food that I can have for lunch the following day or freeze for use later.

7. Know the 'Clean fifteen'

The Environmental Working gathering have delivered a rundown called the 'clean fifteen' naming the least pesticide ridden vegetables. On the off chance that you can't stand to purchase all natural, these leafy foods are the best non-natural produce to purchase – avocados, sweet corn, pineapples, cabbage, frozen peas, onions, asparagus, mangoes, papayas, kiwis, eggplant, grapefruit, melon, cauliflower and yams.

These are the awesome keep away from: apples, strawberries, grapes, celery, peaches, spinach, sweet chime peppers, imported nectarines, cucumbers, cherry tomatoes, imported snap peas and potatoes.

8. Join a local organic box scheme

Neighborhood box plans are not generally the least expensive alternative but rather they will ordinarily contend with the costs of natural grocery store produce. They will give a decent base of elements for the week, save you time shopping and backing neighborhood ranches. On the off chance that they give you an alternative to, purchase a veg box without potatoes. This will give you a bigger assortment of fixings.

Imported natural produce costs significantly more so keep away from boxes that utilization imported produce. Local produce is organically grown where it is grown. The chances of a chemical being used in the soil or by the chemicals being sprayed on plants are less than other products because it isn't transported very far. However, organic foods are not always located near each other or on an island, so you will have to search for them. Although local food is more expensive, it is a better quality. Purchasing food from local farms also supports the local economy because people get to spend their money where they live, instead of sending it elsewhere.

9. Create an organic buying group or co-op

Club along with others keen on purchasing natural produce and set up a center. This will give you purchasing power, as you will have a bigger spend. It will likewise permit you to purchase from co-usable wholesalers, for example, Essential-exchanging and Suma center. Communities are a truly strong model for business and cooperating that can likewise set aside you cash as a person.

In the event that purchasing naturally is beyond the realm of imagination, ensure that the produce is liberated from pesticides by washing it prior to eating it.

10. Shop wisely and avoid supermarkets

Natural food is seen as an excellent thing and can be over expensive subsequently. General stores are at risk of this, so it is ideal to avoid them. General stores regularly have their costs available on the web, note down the cost of the things you normally buy and compare them to online natural products stores, farmers market and greengrocers to find who has the best groceries.

Simple 7-Day Meal Plan

THE FOUR THINGS YOU NEED TO REMEMBER ARE:

1) Your plate should be filled with veggie superstars

2) Include 1-2 servings of healthy fats

3) Most meals should include at least a portion of protein the size of a condiment

4) Inflammatory foods should be avoided as much as possible (most grains, foods that cause gassiness or constipation, processed and packaged foods).

DAY 1
B: Egg White Scramble with Cherry Tomatoes & Spinach
L: Indonesian-Style Spicy Fried Tempeh Strips
D: Classic Chicken Cooking with Tomatoes & Tapenade

DAY 2
B: Mini Pegan Pancakes with Blueberry Syrup
L: Rainbow Chickpea Salad
D: Pasta with Lemon and Artichokes

DAY 3
B: Lime and Cucumber Electrolyte Drink
L: Pegan Cauliflower and Squash Salad
D: Black Bean Burgers

DAY 4
B: Breakfast "Burritos" with Avocado and Pico de Gallo
L: Summer Rolls
D: Spicy Tomato-Lentil Stew

DAY 5
B: Veggie-Eggy Muffins
L: Cauliflower Caesar Salad with Chickpea Croutons
D: Smoky Red Beans and Rice / Herb Roasted Chicken

DAY 6
B: Zucchini and Scallion Pancakes
L: Kale Apple Roasted Root Vegetable Salad
D: Greek Meatballs

DAY 7
B: Egg Breakfast Muffins
L: Grilled Carrots with Chickpea Salad
D: Pork with Pinto beans & Potatoes

BREAKFAST RECIPES

1. Grain-Free Nutty Granola

Preparation Time: 7 Minutes
Cooking Time: 25 Minutes
Servings: 6
Ingredients:

- 11/2 cups chopped raw walnuts or pecans
- 1 cup raw almonds, sliced
- 1/2 cup seeds, toasted or roasted unsalted sunflower, sesame, or shelled pumpkin
- 1/4 cup unsweetened coconut flakes
- 1/2 cup coconut oil or unsalted grass-fed butter, melted
- 1 tablespoon maple syrup
- 1 teaspoon alcohol-free vanilla extract
- 1 teaspoon ground cinnamon, or to taste
- 1/4 teaspoon sea salt or Himalayan salt

Directions:

1. Preheat oven to 300F.
2. Set a rimmed baking sheet with parchment paper or foil.
3. Add the walnuts, almonds, seeds, and coconut flakes to a large bowl. In a separate bowl, mix the oil with the maple syrup, vanilla, cinnamon, and salt. Pour over the nut mixture, tossing to coat.
4. Scatter the mixture evenly on the prepared baking sheet and bake until golden brown, about 25 minutes, stirring once halfway through. Cool completely.

Nutrition: Calories 248 Fat: 25g Carbs: 6g Fiber: 3g Sugar: 2g Protein: 4g Sodium: 40mg

2. Overnight Chia Seed Pudding

Preparation Time: 5 Minutes
Cooking Time: 0 Minutes
Servings: 1
Ingredients:

- 3 tablespoons chia seeds
- 1 cup coconut milk or unsweetened nut milk
- 1 teaspoon alcohol-free vanilla extract
- 1 teaspoon maple syrup (optional)

Directions:

1. In a large jar or bowl, merge all the ingredients, stirring to mix. Close or cover and refrigerate overnight.
2. The next day, add your preferred toppings and enjoy.

Nutrition: Calories 293 Fat: 19g Carbs: 21g Fiber: 17g Sugar: 1g Protein: 10g Sodium: 367mg

3. Mini Pegan Pancakes with Blueberry Syrup

Preparation Time: 5 Minutes
Cooking Time: 15 Minutes
Servings: 4
Ingredients:

- 1 very ripe banana
- 2 large eggs
- 1 tablespoon alcohol-free vanilla extract
- 1 teaspoon ground cinnamon
- Pinch sea salt or Himalayan salt
- 1/4 cup coconut oil, divided
- 2 cups fresh or frozen blueberries

Directions:

1. In a medium bowl, press the banana until softened. Add the eggs and continue to mash until smooth and most of the chunks are blended. Stir in the vanilla, cinnamon, and salt.
2. Warmth 1 tablespoon of the coconut oil in a large skillet or flat cast iron pan over medium heat. Set in 2 to 3 tablespoons of the batter to form 3-inch rounds. Cook the pancakes four at a time until set and golden brown, 2 to 4 minutes total, flipping once. Transfer to a plate to cool. Repeat until the remaining batter is used up, adding 1 tablespoon coconut oil in between each batch.
3. In a separate, small saucepan, add the blueberries and remaining 1 tablespoon coconut oil. Cook over medium heat, constantly mashing berries with a wooden spoon, until juices reduce to a syrup-like consistency, 3 to 5 minutes. Set aside to cool.
4. Serve pancakes with the blueberry syrup on the side.

Nutrition: Calories 224 Fat: 17g Carbs: 18g Fiber: 3g Sugar: 12g Protein: 4g Sodium: 48mg

4. Easy Avocado-Baked Eggs

Preparation Time: 5 Minutes
Cooking Time: 15 Minutes
Servings: 4
Ingredients:

- 2 medium or large avocados, halved and pitted
- 4 large eggs
- 1/4 teaspoon freshly ground black pepper

Directions:

1. Preheat the oven to 425F.
2. Set out some of the pulp from the avocado halves, leaving enough space to fit an egg, reserving the pulp for Easy Guacamole (see the recipe Ceviche Fish Tacos with Easy Guacamole).
3. Line an 8-by-8-inch baking pan with foil. Place the avocado halves in the pan to fit snugly in a single layer, folding the foil around the outer avocados to prevent tipping.
4. Set 1 egg into each avocado half; season with pepper. Bake, uncovered, until the whites are set and the egg yolks are cooked to your desired doneness, 12 to 15 minutes. Detach from the oven and let rest for 5 minutes before serving.

Nutrition: Calories 433 Fat: 37g Carbs: 16g Fiber: 12g Sugar: 1g Protein: 16g Sodium: 154mg

5. Veggie-Eggy Muffins

Preparation Time: 10 Minutes
Cooking Time: 20 Minutes
Servings: 6
Ingredients:

- Extra-virgin olive oil, coconut oil, or clarified butter, for greasing (optional)
- 12 large eggs
- 2 teaspoons sea salt or Himalayan salt
- 2 teaspoons freshly ground black pepper
- 1 medium red bell pepper
- 1 medium orange, yellow, or green bell pepper, seeded and diced
- 1 cup packed baby spinach, finely chopped
- 1/2 cup thinly sliced scallions
- 1 small jalapeño pepper, seeded and minced (optional)

Directions:

1. Preheat the oven to 350F. Grease a 12-hole muffin pan or use paper muffin liners.
2. In a large bowl, place the eggs, salt, and pepper and beat until fluffy. Add the peppers, spinach, scallions, and jalapeño, stirring to combine.
3. Ladle the egg mixture evenly into the prepared muffin pan.
4. Bake until a toothpick or paring knife comes out clean when inserted, about 20 minutes. Let the muffins cool before serving.

Nutrition: Calories 83 Fat: 5g Carbs: 3g Fiber: 1g Sugar: 1g Protein: 7g Sodium: 385mg

6. Meat-Free Eggs Benedict with Lemon Hollandaise Sauce

Preparation Time: 12 Minutes
Cooking Time: 6 Minutes
Servings: 2
Ingredients:
Hollandaise Sauce:

- 3 large egg yolks (save whites for other use)
- 1/2 cup extra-virgin olive oil, ghee, or clarified butter
- 1 tablespoon lemon juice (from about 1/2 lemon)
- Pinch salt
- Pinch cayenne pepper

Eggs:

- 2 teaspoons apple cider vinegar
- 4 large eggs
- 1 large ripe beefsteak or heirloom tomato, ends removed, cut into 4 thick slices
- 1 cup baby spinach
- Freshly ground black pepper

Directions:

1. For the hollandaise sauce, bring a pot of water, filled to about 4 inches up the sides, to a boil. Set aside 2 tablespoons of the hot water. In a medium metal bowl, whisk the egg yolks. Add in the olive oil, hot water, lemon juice, salt, and cayenne and continue whisking. However, the bowl over the pot of boiling water. Whisk constantly until the sauce thickens, 1 to 2 minutes, keeping the bowl from touching the boiling water, to prevent the eggs from curdling. Remove the bowl of hollandaise sauce from the pot of water, and set it aside on another part of the stovetop.
2. To poach the eggs, reduce the heat under the pot of boiling water to a simmer and add the vinegar. Prepare a paper-towel lined plate. One at a time, gently crack the eggs into a small bowl, and then use the bowl to slowly slide 2 of the eggs into the water. Simmer for 2 minutes. Using a slotted spoon, transfer the eggs to the paper towel-lined plate. Repeat the process with the remaining 2 eggs.
3. To serve, divide the tomato slices between two plates. Top each tomato with a few spinach leaves, 1 poached egg, and 2 heaping tablespoons of the warm hollandaise. Season with black pepper and serve immediately.

Nutrition: Calories 423 Fat: 39g Carbs: 6g Fiber: 2g Sugar: 4g Protein: 16g Sodium: 242mg

7. Zucchini and Scallion Pancakes

Preparation Time: 5 Minutes
Cooking Time: 5 Minutes
Servings: 4
Ingredients:

- 1/3 cup filtered water
- 2 tablespoons ground flax seeds
- 1 teaspoon coconut oil
- 3 large zucchinis, grated
- Salt and freshly ground black pepper, to flavor
- 1/4 cup scallion, chopped finely

Directions:

1. In a bowl, mix together ground flax seeds and water and set aside.
2. In a large skillet, warmth oil on medium heat.
3. Attach zucchini and cook, stirring occasionally.
4. Set in salt and black pepper and immediately, detach from heat.
5. Set the zucchini into a large bowl and let it cool slightly.
6. Attach flax seed mixture and scallion and mix till well combined.
7. Warmth a griddle and grease it.
8. Add 1/4 of the zucchini mixture into preheated griddle.
9. Cook for 2-3 minutes. Carefully set the side and cook for 1-2 minutes further.
10. Repeat with the remaining mixture.

Nutrition: Calories: 69 Fat: 2.7g Sodium: 27mg Carbs: 9.6g Fiber: 3.8g Sugar: 4.4g Protein: 3.7g

8. Blueberry Pancakes

Preparation Time: 5 Minutes
Cooking Time: 10 Minutes
Servings: 4
Ingredients:

- 1/2 cup coconut flour
- 1 teaspoon baking soda
- 2 drops liquid stevia
- Pinch of salt
- 4 organic eggs
- 1 cup unsweetened almond milk
- 1 teaspoon organic vanilla extract
- 2 tablespoons fresh blueberries
- 2 tablespoons coconut oil

- 2 tablespoons maple syrup

Directions:

1. In a large bowl, merge together flour, baking soda and salt.
2. In another bowl, add egg, milk and vanilla extract and beat till well combined.
3. Attach egg mixture into flour mixture and mix till well combined.
4. Gently, fold in blueberries.
5. In a large skillet, warmth oil on medium heat.
6. Attach desired amount of mixture in the skillet. With the back of wooden spoon, spread the mixture in skillet evenly.
7. Cook for about 2-3 minutes. Carefully, change the side and cook for 1-2 minutes further.
8. Repeat with remaining mixture.
9. Serve with the drizzling of maple syrup.

Nutrition: Calories: 233 Fat: 14.6g Sodium: 491mg Carbs: 17.3g Fiber: 6.4g Sugar: 7.9g Protein: 8.8g

9. Garlicky Zucchini with Poached Eggs

Preparation Time: 10 Minutes
Cooking Time: 10 Minutes
Servings: 2

Ingredients:

- 1 tablespoon olive oil
- 2 small garlic cloves, minced
- 2 large zucchinis, spiralized with blade C
- Salt and freshly ground black pepper, to flavor
- 2 organic eggs

Directions:

1. In a large skillet, armth oil on medium heat.
2. Attach garlic and sauté for about 1 minute.
3. Attach zucchini, salt and black pepper and cook for about 3-4 minutes.
4. Set the zucchini mixture into 2 large serving plates.
5. Meanwhile in a large pan, set 2-3-inches water to a simmer on high heat.
6. Carefully, crack the eggs in water one by one. Secure the pan and turn off the heat.
7. Keep, sealed for about 4 minutes or till desired cooking of the egg is reached.
8. Place the eggs over zucchini.
9. Whisk the eggs with salt and black pepper and serve.

Nutrition: Calories: 179 Fat: 12g Sodium: 94mg Carbs: 12.2g Fiber: 3.6g Protein: 9.6g

10. Chia Seed Pudding

Preparation Time: 15 Minutes
Cooking Time: 0 Minutes
Servings: 2

Ingredients:

- 1 cup unsweetened almond milk
- 2 tablespoons maple syrup
- 1/4 cup chia seeds
- 1/4 teaspoon organic vanilla extract
- 1/2 of small apple, cored and sliced
- 2 tablespoons almonds, chopped

Directions:

1. In a large bowl, merge all ingredients except apple and almonds and stir to combine well.
2. Cover and refrigerate for at least 30-40 minutes.
3. Top with apple and almonds and serve.

Nutrition: Calories: 185 Fat: 9.8g Sodium: 92mg Carbs: 26.9g Fiber: 7.1g Sugar: 16.1g] Protein: 4.9g

11. Zucchini and Banana Bread

Preparation Time: 10 Minutes
Cooking Time: 45 Minutes
Servings: 6

Ingredients:

- 1/2 cup coconut flour
- 11/2 teaspoons baking soda
- Pinch of salt
- 1/4 cup coconut oil, softened
- 2 teaspoons vanilla extract
- 11/2 cups ripe bananas, peeled and mashed
- 1 cup zucchini, grated and squeezed
- 1 teaspoon orange zest, grated freshly

Directions:

1. Preheat the oven to 350 degrees F.
2. Grease a loaf pan.
3. In a large bowl, merge together flour, baking soda and salt.
4. In another bowl, add oil and vanilla and beat well.
5. Add banana and beat till well combined.
6. Mix oil mixture into flour mixture.
7. Fold in zucchini and orange zest. Set the mixture into prepared loaf pan evenly.
8. Bake for about 40-45 minutes or till a toothpick nested in the center comes out clean.

Nutrition: Calories: 166 Fat: 10.9g Sodium: 364mg Carbs: 15.5g Fiber: 5.2g Sugar: 5.8g Protein: 2.6g

12. Egg Breakfast Muffins

Preparation Time: 5 Minutes
Cooking Time: 20 Minutes
Servings: 6

Ingredients:

- 1 cup of diced broccoli
- Salt and pepper {to taste}
- 8 eggs
- 1 cup of diced onion
- 1 cup of diced mushrooms

Directions

1. Meanwhile, heat oven to 350 degrees F.
2. After which you dice all vegetables.
3. After that, in a large mixing bowl, set together eggs, salt, vegetables, and pepper.
4. Then pour mixture into a greased muffin pan, the mixture should evenly fill 8 muffin cups.
5. At this point, bake 18-20 minutes, or until a toothpick inserted in the middle comes out clean.
6. Finally, you serve and enjoy!

Nutrition: Calories 83 Fat: 5g Carbs: 3g Fiber: 1g Sugar: 1g

13. Simple Blueberry Muffins

Preparation Time: 5 Minutes
Cooking Time: 15 Minutes
Servings: 8-10
Ingredients:

- 1 cup of almond meal/almond flour
- 1/2 cup of raw honey
- 1/3 cup of coconut oil {melted}
- 1/2 teaspoon of baking powder
- 1/2 cup of fresh blueberries
- 1 cup of almond butter
- 3 eggs {whisked}
- 1/3 cup of unsweetened shredded coconut
- 1/2 teaspoon of baking soda
- 1/4 teaspoon of sea salt
- A pinch of cinnamon

Directions:

1. Meanwhile, heat your oven to 350 degrees.
2. After which you mix all ingredients together in a bowl. If you're good at baking, you'll know to mix the dry then the wet ingredients then mix together, but I do all the ingredients together and it works perfectly
3. After that, place ingredients into 8-10 silicone muffin cups in a muffin tin. Or better still you can use muffin tin paper liners.
4. Then, bake for 15-20 minutes. Remember to keep an eye on it, they will puff up and look adorable.
5. Enjoy.

Nutrition: Calories: 179 Fat: 12g Sodium: 94mg Carbs: 12.2g

14. Paleo Almond Zucchini Bread

Preparation Time: 5 Minutes
Cooking Time: 15 Minutes
Servings: 6
Ingredients:

- 1 1/2 cups of almond flour (or better still a combination of almond and cashew flour)
- 1 1/2 teaspoons of baking soda
- 1/2 teaspoon of salt
- 1 teaspoon of cinnamon
- 1 cup of grated zucchini, squeezed of excess water then measured to 1 cup
- 3 eggs
- 3 tablespoons of maple syrup
- 1 large banana mashed
- 1 tablespoon of melted coconut oil

Directions:

1. Meanwhile, heat oven to 350 degrees and line a loaf pan with parchment paper.
2. After which you whisk together dry ingredients in a large bowl.
3. After that, add wet ingredients except zucchini and whisk until thoroughly combined.
4. Then, add zucchini and stir until combined.
5. At this point, pour batter into parchment lined loaf pan.
6. Furthermore, bake for about 35 minutes until top is browned and center of the bread is set.
7. After that, detach from oven and let cool in the pan on a wire rack for 5 minutes.

8. Finally, remove bread from loaf pan by pulling on the sides of the parchment paper and set back on the wire rack before slicing.

Nutrition: Calories: 166 Fat: 10.9g Sodium: 364mg Carbs: 15.5g Fiber: 5.2g

15. Paleo Strawberry Donuts

Preparation Time: 30 Minutes
Cooking Time: 20 Minutes
Servings: 12
Ingredients:

- 3 tablespoons of coconut oil or ghee
- 1/4 cup of honey
- 1 teaspoon of pure vanilla extract
- 1/4 cup of freeze dried strawberries, ground to a powder
- 1/4 teaspoon of sea salt
- 4 large eggs {room temperature}
- 1/2 cup of coconut milk, warm
- 1 teaspoon of apple cider vinegar
- 1/2 cup of coconut flour
- 1/2 teaspoon of baking soda

Topping

- 2 tablespoons of coconut butter
- 1/4 cup of freeze dried strawberries {coarsely ground}
- 1-ounce raw cacao butter {melted}
- 1 teaspoon of honey

Direction for the donuts:

1. Meanwhile, heat a doughnut maker. Remember, if using a doughnut pan, preheat the oven to 350F and grease the pan liberally with butter.
2. After that, using a stand mixer or electric hand mixer, beat the eggs with the coconut oil on medium-high speed until creamy.
3. After which you add the vinegar, milk, honey, and vanilla and beat again until combined.
4. Furthermore, using a fine mesh sieve or sifter, sift the remaining dry ingredients into the bowl.
5. At this point, beat on high until smooth.
6. This is when you scoop the batter into a large Ziploc bag, seal the top, and snip one of the bottom corners.
7. Then, pipe the batter into the doughnut mold, filling it completely.
8. Finally, cook until the doughnut machine indicator light goes off. NOTE: for the oven, bake for 17 minutes.
9. After which you remove the doughnuts and cool on a wire rack.
10. Feel free to trim if necessary.

Directions for topping:

1. First, mix the coconut butter, cacao butter, and honey in a shallow bowl.
2. After which you place in the freezer for 5 minutes to thicken.
3. Then, once the donuts are completely cooled, dip them in the glaze then dip the tops in the ground up strawberries.
4. Finally, place in the refrigerator for 20 minutes to allow the glaze to set.

Nutrition: Calories: 179 Fat: 12g Sodium: 94mg Carbs: 12.2g

16.   Pumpkin spice muffins with maple butter frosting

Preparation Time: 15 Minutes
Cooking Time: 30 Minutes
Servings: 6-8
Ingredients:
For the muffins

- 3/4 cup of full-fat coconut milk or better still heavy cream
- 1 1/2 teaspoons of vanilla extract
- 1/2 cup of coconut flour (preferably from Tropical Traditions)
- 1 teaspoon of pumpkin pie spice
- 4 eggs {lightly beaten}
- 1/4 cup of canned pumpkin purée
- 1/2 cup of blanched almond flour (preferably from nuts.com)
- 1/2 teaspoon of baking soda
- 1/4 teaspoon of sea salt (I prefer Redmond)

For the maple butter frosting

- 1/4 cup of coconut butter, softened in the microwave or a bath of warm water on the stove
- 1 Tablespoon of maple syrup

Directions for the muffins

1. Meanwhile, heat oven to 350
2. After which you combine the wet ingredients (coconut milk, eggs, pumpkin purée, and vanilla) in one bowl. Mix thoroughly.
3. After that you combine the dry ingredients (coconut flour, almond flour, baking soda, salt and spices) in another bowl. Mix thoroughly.
4. At this point, add the wet ingredients to the dry and mix until a wet dough forms.
5. This is when you drop the dough into muffin cups to approximately two-thirds full.
6. Then, place a ramekin half-filled with water in the oven before adding the muffins
7. Finally, bake for 30 minutes and remove from oven.
8. This is when you allow them to cool before adding frosting.

Direction for the frosting

1. First, combine softened coconut butter and maple syrup.
2. Then, once muffins are cooled, top with frosting and shaved chocolate, if you want.
3. Finally, to shave chocolate, just take some of the chocolate you definitely stockpile in your freezer and run it across a cheese grater.

Nutrition: Calories: 265 Fat: 7.7g Sodium: 19mg Carbs: 48.3g Fiber: 5.4g

17.   Strawberry Paleo Pancake

Preparation Time: 15 Minutes
Cooking Time: 30 Minutes
Servings: 6
Ingredients:

- 2 eggs
- 1/2 teaspoon of nutmeg
- 1/4 teaspoon of baking powder
- Coconut oil for frying
- 1 1/2 cups of ground almond meal flour
- 1/2 teaspoon of cinnamon
- 1/2 cup of pureed strawberries
- 1/4 cup of coconut or better still almond milk

Directions:

1. First, mix all the ingredients except the coconut oil for frying.
2. After which you add the coconut oil to a frying pan and heat till melted.
3. After that, use 1/4 cup batter to make each pancake.
4. Then, fry until golden brown.
5. Finally, top with more pureed strawberries or real Vermont maple syrup.

Nutrition: Calories 248 Fat: 25g   Carbs: 6g Fiber: 3g Sugar: 2g

18.   Jumbo Chickpea Pancake

Preparation Time: 10 Minutes
Cooking Time: 10 Minutes
Servings: 6
Ingredients:

- 1/4 cup of chopped red pepper
- 1/4 teaspoon of garlic powder
- 1/8 teaspoon of ground black pepper
- 1/2 cup + 2 tablespoons water
- 1 green onion, chopped (about 1/4 cup)
- 1/2 cup of chickpea flour (AKA garbanzo flour or besan)
- 1/4 teaspoon of fine grain sea salt
- 1/4 teaspoon of baking powder
- A pinch of red pepper flakes (it is optional)
- For serving: avocado, hummus, salsa, cashew cream (optional)

Directions

1. First, prepare the vegetables and set aside.
2. Meanwhile, warmth a 10-inch skillet over medium heat.
3. After that, in a small bowl whisk together the garlic powder, salt, chickpea flour, baking powder, peppers, and optional red pepper flakes.
4. After which you add the water and whisk well until no clumps remain.
5. Then you stir in the chopped vegetables.
6. Furthermore, when the skillet is pre-heated
7. At this point, pour on all of the batter (if making 1 large pancake) and quickly spread it out all over the pan.
8. This is when you cook for 5-6 minutes on one side
9. Remember, flip pancake carefully and cook for another 5 minutes, until lightly golden.
10. Finally, serve on a large plate and top with your desired toppings.
11. Remember, leftovers can be wrapped up and placed in the fridge.
12. Feel free to reheat on a skillet until warmed throughout.

Nutrition: Calories: 233 Fat: 9g Sodium: 321 mg Carbs: 11g Fiber: 4 g

19.   Egg White Scramble with Cherry Tomatoes & Spinach

Preparation Time: 5 minutes
Cooking Time: 8-10 minutes
Servings: 4
INGREDIENTS:

- 1 tbsp. Olive oil
- 1 whole Egg
- 10 Egg whites
- ¼ tsp. Black pepper

- ½ tsp. Salt
- 1 garlic clove, minced
- 2 cups cherry tomatoes, halved
- 2 cups packed fresh baby spinach
- ½ cup Light cream or Half & Half

DIRECTIONS:

1. Whisk the eggs, pepper, salt, and milk. Prepare a skillet using the med-high temperature setting. Toss in the garlic when the pan is hot to sauté for approximately 30 seconds.
2. Pour in the tomatoes and spinach and continue to sauté it for one additional minute. The tomatoes should be softened, and the spinach wilted.
3. Add the egg mixture into the pan using the medium heat setting. Fold the egg gently as it cooks for about two to three minutes. Remove from the burner.

NUTRITION: Calories 142 Protein: 15g Fat: 2g Carbs 4g

20. Greek Yogurt with Fresh Berries, Honey and Nuts

Preparation time: 5 minutes
Cooking time: 0 minutes
Servings: 1
INGREDIENTS:

- 6 oz. nonfat plain Greek yogurt
- 1/2 cup fresh berries of your choice
- 1 tbsp .25 oz crushed walnuts
- 1 tbsp honey

DIRECTIONS:

1. In a jar with a lid, add the yogurt. Top with berries and a drizzle of honey. Top with the lid and store in the fridge for 2-3 days.

NUTRITION: Calories: 250 Carbs: 35 Fat: 4g Protein: 19g

21. Quinoa Bake with Banana

Preparation time: 15 minutes
Cooking time: 1 hour & 10 minutes
Servings: 8
INGREDIENTS:

- 3 cups medium over-ripe Bananas, mashed
- 1/4 cup molasses
- 1/4 cup pure maple syrup
- 1 tbsp cinnamon
- 2 tsp raw vanilla extract
- 1 tsp ground ginger
- 1 tsp ground cloves
- 1/2 tsp ground allspice
- 1/2 tsp salt
- 1 cup quinoa, uncooked
- 2 1/2 cups unsweetened vanilla almond milk
- 1/4 cup slivered almonds

DIRECTIONS:

1. In the bottom of a 2 1/2-3-quart casserole dish, mix together the mashed banana, maple syrup, cinnamon, vanilla extract, ginger, cloves, allspice, molasses, and salt until well mixed.
2. Add in the quinoa, stir until the quinoa is evenly in the banana mixture. Whisk in the almond milk, mix until well combined, cover and refrigerate overnight or bake immediately.

3. Heat oven to 350 degrees F. Whisk the quinoa mixture making sure it doesn't settle to the bottom.
4. Cover the pan with tinfoil and bake until the liquid is absorbed, and the top of the quinoa is set, about 1 hour to 1 hour and 15 minutes.
5. Turn the oven to high broil, uncover the pan, sprinkle with sliced almonds, and lightly press them into the quinoa.
6. Broil until the almonds just turn golden brown, about 2-4 minutes, watching closely, as they burn quickly. Allow to cool for 10 minutes then slice the quinoa bake
7. Distribute the quinoa bake among the containers, store in the fridge for 3-4 days.

NUTRITION: Calories: 213 Carbs: 41g Fat: 4g Protein: 5g

22. Sun Dried Tomatoes, Dill and Feta Omelet Casserole

Preparation time: 15 minutes
Cooking time: 40 minutes
Servings: 6
INGREDIENTS:

- 12 large eggs
- 2 cups whole milk
- 8 oz fresh spinach
- 2 cloves garlic, minced
- 12 oz artichoke salad with olives and peppers, drained and chopped
- 5 oz sun dried tomato feta cheese, crumbled
- 1 tbsp fresh chopped dill or 1 tsp dried dill
- 1 tsp dried oregano
- 1 tsp lemon pepper
- 1 tsp salt
- 4 tsp olive oil, divided

DIRECTIONS:

1. Preheat oven to 375 degrees F. Chop the fresh herbs and artichoke salad. In a skillet over medium heat, add 1 tbsp olive oil.
2. Sauté the spinach and garlic until wilted, about 3 minutes. Oil a 9x13 inch baking dish, layer the spinach and artichoke salad evenly in the dish
3. In a medium bowl, whisk together the eggs, milk, herbs, salt and lemon pepper. Pour the egg mixture over vegetables, sprinkle with feta cheese.
4. Bake in the center of the oven for 35-40 minutes until firm in the center. Allow to cool, slice an and distribute among the storage containers. Store for 2-3 days or freeze for 3 months

NUTRITION: Calories: 196 Carbs: 5g Fat: 12g Protein: 10g

23. Mediterranean Breakfast Egg White Sandwich

Preparation time: 15 minutes
Cooking time: 30 minutes
Servings: 1
INGREDIENTS:

- 1 tsp vegan butter
- ¼ cup egg whites
- 1 tsp chopped fresh herbs such as parsley, basil, rosemary
- 1 whole grain seeded ciabatta roll

- 1 tbsp pesto
- 1-2 slices muenster cheese (or other cheese such as provolone, Monterey Jack, etc.)
- About ½ cup roasted tomatoes
- Salt, to taste
- Pepper, to taste

Roasted Tomatoes:
- 10 oz grape tomatoes
- 1 tbsp extra virgin olive oil
- Kosher salt, to taste
- Coarse black pepper, to taste

DIRECTIONS:

1. In a small nonstick skillet over medium heat, melt the vegan butter. Pour in egg whites, season with salt and pepper, sprinkle with fresh herbs, cook for 3-4 minutes or until egg is done, flip once.
2. In the meantime, toast the ciabatta bread in toaster. Once done, spread both halves with pesto.
3. Place the egg on the bottom half of sandwich roll, folding if necessary, top with cheese, add the roasted tomatoes and top half of roll sandwich.
4. For the roasted tomatoes, preheat oven to 400 degrees F. Slice tomatoes in half lengthwise. Then place them onto a baking sheet and drizzle with the olive oil, toss to coat.
5. Season with salt and pepper and roast in oven for about 20 minutes, until the skin appears wrinkled

NUTRITION: Calories: 458 Carbs: 51g Fat: 0g Protein: 21g

24. Breakfast Taco Scramble

Preparation time: 15 minutes
Cooking time: 1 hour & 25 minutes
Servings: 4
INGREDIENTS:
- 8 large eggs, beaten
- 1/4 tsp seasoning salt
- 1 lb. 99% lean ground turkey
- 2 tbsp Greek seasoning
- 1/2 small onion, minced
- 2 tbsp bell pepper, minced
- 4 oz. Can tomato sauce
- 1/4 cup water
- 1/4 cup chopped scallions or cilantro, for topping

For the potatoes:
- 12 (1 lb.) Baby gold or red potatoes, quartered
- 4 tsp olive oil
- 3/4 tsp salt
- 1/2 tsp garlic powder
- Fresh black pepper, to taste

DIRECTIONS:

1. In a large bowl, beat the eggs, season with seasoning salt. Preheat the oven to 425 degrees F. Spray a 9x12 or large oval casserole dish with cooking oil.
2. Add the potatoes 1 tbsp oil, 3/4 teaspoon salt, garlic powder and black pepper and toss to coat. Bake for 45 minutes to 1 hour, tossing every 15 minutes.

3. In the meantime, brown the turkey in a large skillet over medium heat, breaking it up while it cooks. Once no longer pink, add in the Greek seasoning.
4. Add in the bell pepper, onion, tomato sauce and water, stir and cover, simmer on low for about 20 minutes. Spray a different skillet with nonstick spray over medium heat.
5. Once heated, add in the eggs seasoned with 1/4 tsp of salt and scramble for 2–3 minutes, or cook until it sets.
6. Distribute 3/4 cup turkey and 2/3 cup eggs and divide the potatoes in each storage container, store for 3-4 days.

NUTRITION: Calories: 450 Fat: 19g Carbs: 24.5g Protein: 46g

25. Blueberry Greek Yogurt Pancakes

Preparation time: 15 minutes
Cooking time: 15 minutes
Servings: 6
INGREDIENTS:
- 1 1/4 cup all-purpose flour
- 2 tsp baking powder
- 1 tsp baking soda
- 1/4 tsp salt
- 1/4 cup sugar
- 3 eggs
- 3 tbsp vegan butter unsalted, melted
- 1/2 cup milk
- 1 1/2 cups Greek yogurt plain, non-fat
- 1/2 cup blueberries optional
- Toppings:
- Greek yogurt
- Mixed berries – blueberries, raspberries and blackberries

DIRECTIONS:

1. In a large bowl, whisk together the flour, salt, baking powder and baking soda. In a separate bowl, whisk together butter, sugar, eggs, Greek yogurt, and milk until the mixture is smooth.
2. Then add in the Greek yogurt mixture from step to the dry mixture in step 1, mix to combine, allow the patter to sit for 20 minutes to get a smooth texture – if using blueberries fold them into the pancake batter.
3. Heat the pancake griddle, spray with non-stick butter spray or just brush with butter. Pour the batter, in 1/4 cupful's, onto the griddle.
4. Cook until the bubbles on top burst and create small holes, lift up the corners of the pancake to see if they're golden browned on the bottom
5. With a wide spatula, flip the pancake and cook on the other side until lightly browned. Serve.

NUTRITION: Calories: 258 Carbs: 33g Fat: 8g Protein: 11g

26. Cauliflower Fritters with Hummus

Preparation time: 15 minutes
Cooking time: 15 minutes
Servings: 4
INGREDIENTS:
- 2 (15 oz) cans chickpeas, divided
- 2 1/2 tbsp olive oil, divided, plus more for frying
- 1 cup onion, chopped, about 1/2 a small onion
- 2 tbsp garlic, minced
- 2 cups cauliflower, cut into small pieces, about 1/2 a large head

- 1/2 tsp salt
- Black pepper
- Topping:
- Hummus, of choice
- Green onion, diced

DIRECTIONS:

1. Preheat oven to 400°F. Rinse and drain 1 can of the chickpeas, place them on a paper towel to dry off well.
2. Then place the chickpeas into a large bowl, removing the loose skins that come off, and toss with 1 tbsp of olive oil, spread the chickpeas onto a large pan and sprinkle with salt and pepper.
3. Bake for 20 minutes, then stir, and then bake an additional 5-10 minutes until very crispy.
4. Once the chickpeas are roasted, transfer them to a large food processor and process until broken down and crumble - Don't over process them and turn it into flour, as you need to have some texture. Place the mixture into a small bowl, set aside.
5. In a large pan over medium-high heat, add the remaining 1 1/2 tbsp of olive oil. Once heated, add in the onion and garlic, cook until lightly golden brown, about 2 minutes.
6. Then add in the chopped cauliflower, cook for an additional 2 minutes, until the cauliflower is golden.
7. Turn the heat down to low and cover the pan, cook until the cauliflower is fork tender and the onions are golden brown and caramelized, stirring often, about 3-5 minutes.
8. Transfer the cauliflower mixture to the food processor, drain and rinse the remaining can of chickpeas and add them into the food processor, along with the salt and a pinch of pepper.
9. Blend until smooth, and the mixture starts to ball, stop to scrape down the sides as needed
10. Transfer the cauliflower mixture into a large bowl and add in 1/2 cup of the roasted chickpea crumbs, stir until well combined.
11. In a large bowl over medium heat, add in enough oil to lightly cover the bottom of a large pan. Working in batches, cook the patties until golden brown, about 2-3 minutes, flip and cook again. Serve.

NUTRITION: Calories: 333 Carbs: 45g Fat: 13g Protein: 14g

27. Overnight Berry Chia Oats

Preparation time: 15 minutes
Cooking time: 5 minutes
Servings: 1

INGREDIENTS:

- 1/2 cup Quaker Oats rolled oats
- 1/4 cup chia seeds
- 1 cup milk or water
- Pinch of salt and cinnamon
- Maple syrup, or a different sweetener, to taste
- 1 cup frozen berries of choice or smoothie leftovers
- Toppings:
- Yogurt
- Berries

DIRECTIONS:

1. In a jar with a lid, add the oats, seeds, milk, salt, and cinnamon, refrigerate overnight. On serving day, puree the berries in a blender.

2. Stir the oats, add in the berry puree and top with yogurt and more berries, nuts, honey, or garnish of your choice. Enjoy!

NUTRITION: Calories: 405 Carbs: 65g Fat: 11g Protein: 17g

28. Feta & Quinoa Egg Muffins

Preparation Time: 20 minutes
Cooking Time: 45-50 minutes
Servings: 12

INGREDIENTS:

- 1 cup cooked quinoa
- 2 cups baby spinach, chopped
- ½ cup Kalamata olives
- 1 cup tomatoes
- ½ cup white onion
- 1 tbsp. Fresh oregano
- ½ tsp. Salt
- 2 tsp.+ more for coating pans olive oil
- 8 eggs
- 1 cup crumbled feta cheese
- Also Needed: 12-cup muffin tin

DIRECTIONS:

1. Heat the oven to reach 350° F. Lightly grease the muffin tray cups with a spritz of cooking oil.
2. Prepare a skillet using the medium temperature setting and add the oil. When it's hot, toss in the onions to sauté for two minutes.
3. Dump the tomatoes into the skillet and sauté for one minute. Fold in the spinach and continue cooking until the leaves have wilted (1 min.).
4. Transfer the pot to the countertop and add the oregano and olives. Set it aside.
5. Crack the eggs into a mixing bowl, using an immersion stick blender to mix them thoroughly. Add the cooked veggies in with the rest of the fixings.
6. Stir until it's combined and scoop the mixture into the greased muffin cups. Set the timer to bake the muffins for 30 minutes until browned, and the muffins are set. Cool for about ten minutes. Serve.

NUTRITION: Calories: 295 Carbs: 3g Fat: 23g Protein: 19g

29. 5-Minute Heirloom Tomato & Cucumber Toast

Preparation Time: 10 minutes
Cooking Time: 6-10 minutes
Servings: 1

INGREDIENTS:

- 1 small Heirloom tomato
- 1 Persian cucumber
- 1 tsp. Olive oil
- 1 pinch Oregano
- Kosher salt and pepper as desired
- 2 tsp. Low-fat whipped cream cheese
- 2 pieces Trader Joe's Whole Grain Crispbread or your choice
- 1 tsp. Balsamic glaze

DIRECTIONS:

1. Dice the cucumber and tomato. Combine all the fixings except for the cream cheese. Smear the cheese on the bread and add the mixture. Top it off with the balsamic glaze and serve.

NUTRITION: Calories: 239 Carbs: 32g Fat: 11g Protein: 7g

30. Greek Yogurt with Walnuts and Honey

Preparation Time: 5 Minutes
Cooking Time: 0 minutes
Servings: 4

INGREDIENTS:

- 4 cups Greek yogurt, fat-free, plain or vanilla
- ½ cup California walnuts, toasted, chopped
- 3 tbsps. Honey or agave nectar
- Fresh fruit, chopped or granola, low-fat (both optional)

DIRECTIONS:

1. Spoon yogurt into 4 individual cups. Sprinkle 2 tbsps. Of walnuts over each and drizzle 2 tsps. Of honey over each. Top with fruit or granola, whichever is preferred.

NUTRITION: Calories 300 Fat: 10g Carbs: 25g Protein: 29g

31. Tahini Pine Nuts Toast

Preparation Time: 5 minutes
Cooking Time: 0 minutes
Servings: 2

INGREDIENTS:

- 2 whole-wheat bread slices, toasted
- 1 tsp. Water
- 1 tbsp. Tahini paste
- 2 tsps. Feta cheese, crumbled
- Juice of ½ lemon
- 2 tsps. Pine nuts
- A pinch of black pepper

DIRECTIONS:

1. In a bowl, mix the tahini with the water and the lemon juice, whisk well, and spread over the toasted bread slices. Top each serving with the remaining ingredients and serve for breakfast.

NUTRITION: Calories 142 Fat: 7.6g Carbs: 13.7g Protein: 5.8g

32. Feta – Avocado & Mashed Chickpea Toast

Preparation Time: 10 minutes
Cooking Time: 15 minutes
Servings: 4

INGREDIENTS:

- 15 oz. Can Chickpeas
- 2 oz. - ½ cup Diced feta cheese
- 1 Pitted avocado
- Fresh juice:
- 2 tsp. Lemon (or 1 tbsp. Orange)
- ½ tsp. Black pepper
- 2 tsp. Honey
- 4 slices Multigrain toast

DIRECTIONS:

1. Toast the bread. Drain the chickpeas in a colander. Scoop the avocado flesh into the bowl. Use a large fork/potato masher to mash them until the mix is spreadable.
2. Pour in the lemon juice, pepper, and feta. Combine and divide onto the four slices of toast. Drizzle using the honey and serve.

NUTRITION: Calories: 337 Carbs: 43g Fat: 13g Protein: 13g

33. Feta Frittata

Preparation Time: 15 minutes
Cooking Time: 25 minutes
Servings: 2

INGREDIENTS:

- 1 small clove Garlic
- 1 Green onion
- 2 Large eggs
- ½ cup Egg substitute
- 4 tbsp. Crumbled feta cheese - divided
- 1/3 cup Plum tomato
- 4 thin Avocado slices
- 2 tbsp. Reduced-fat sour cream
- Also Needed: 6-inch skillet

DIRECTIONS:

1. Thinly slice/mince the onion, garlic, and tomato. Peel the avocado before slicing. Heat the pan using the medium temperature setting and spritz it with cooking oil.
2. Whisk the egg substitute, eggs, and the feta cheese. Add the egg mixture into the pan. Cover and simmer for four to six minutes.
3. Sprinkle it using the rest of the feta cheese and tomato. Cover and continue cooking until the eggs are set or about two to three more minutes.
4. Wait for about five minutes before cutting it into halves. Serve with the avocado and sour cream.

NUTRITION: Calories: 460 Carbs: 8g Fat: 37g Protein: 24g

34. Smoked Salmon and Poached Eggs on Toast

Preparation Time: 10 minutes
Cooking Time: 4 minutes
Servings: 4

INGREDIENTS:

- 2 oz avocado smashed
- 2 slices of bread toasted
- Pinch of kosher salt and cracked black pepper
- 1/4 tsp freshly squeezed lemon juice
- 2 eggs see notes, poached
- 3,5 oz smoked wild salmon
- 1 TBSP. Thinly sliced scallions
- Splash of Kikkoman soy sauce optional
- Microgreens are optional

DIRECTIONS:

1. Take a small bowl and then smash the avocado into it. Then, add the lemon juice and also a pinch of salt into the mixture. Then, mix it well and set aside.
2. After that, poach the eggs and toast the bread for some time. Once the bread is toasted, you will have to spread the avocado

on both slices and after that, add the smoked salmon to each slice.

3. Thereafter, carefully transfer the poached eggs to the respective toasts. Add a splash of Kikkoman soy sauce and some cracked pepper; then, just garnish with scallions and microgreens.

NUTRITION: Calories: 459 Protein: 31 g Fat: 22 g Carbs: 33 g

35. Honey Almond Ricotta Spread with Peaches

Preparation Time: 5 minutes
Cooking Time: 8 minutes
Servings: 4
INGREDIENTS:
- 1/2 cup Fisher Sliced Almonds
- 1 cup whole milk ricotta
- 1/4 teaspoon almond extract
- Zest from an orange, optional
- 1 teaspoon honey
- Hearty whole-grain toast
- English muffin or bagel
- Extra Fisher sliced almonds
- Sliced peaches
- Extra honey for drizzling

DIRECTIONS:
1. Cut peaches into a proper shape and then brush them with olive oil. After that, set it aside. Take a bowl; combine the ingredients for the filling. Set aside.
2. Then just pre-heat grill to medium. Place peaches cut side down onto the greased grill. Close lid cover and then just grill until the peaches have softened, approximately 6-10 minutes, depending on the size of the peaches.
3. Then you will have to place peach halves onto a serving plate. Put a spoon of about 1 tablespoon of ricotta mixture into the cavity (you are also allowed to use a small scooper).
4. Sprinkle it with slivered almonds, crushed amaretti cookies, and honey. Decorate with the mint leaves.

NUTRITION: Calories: 187 Protein: 7 g Fat: 9 g Carbs: 18 g

36. Mediterranean Eggs Cups

Preparation Time: 10 minutes
Cooking Time: 20 minutes
Servings: 8
INGREDIENTS:
- 1 cup spinach, finely diced
- 1/2 yellow onion, finely diced
- 1/2 cup sliced sun-dried tomatoes
- 4 large basil leaves, finely diced
- Pepper and salt to taste
- 1/3 cup feta cheese crumbles
- 8 large eggs
- 1/4 cup milk (any kind)

DIRECTIONS:
1. Warm the oven to 375°F. Then, roll the dough sheet into a 12x8-inch rectangle. Then, cut in half lengthwise.
2. After that, you will have to cut each half crosswise into 4 pieces, forming 8 (4x3-inch) pieces dough. Then, press each into the bottom and up sides of the ungreased muffin cup.

3. Trim dough to keep the dough from touching, if essential. Set aside. Then, you will have to combine the eggs, salt, pepper in the bowl and beat it with a whisk until well mixed. Set aside.
4. Melt the butter in 12-inch skillet over medium heat until sizzling; add bell peppers. You will have to cook it, stirring occasionally, 2-3 minutes or until crisply tender.
5. After that, add spinach leaves; continue cooking until spinach is wilted. Then just add egg mixture and prosciutto.
6. Divide the mixture evenly among prepared muffin cups. Finally, bake it for 14-17 minutes or until the crust is golden brown.

NUTRITION: Calories: 240 Protein: 9 g Fat: 16 g Carbs: 13 g

37. Low-Carb Baked Eggs with Avocado and Feta

Preparation Time: 10 minutes
Cooking Time: 15 minutes
Servings: 2
INGREDIENTS:
- 1 avocado
- 4 eggs
- 2-3 tbsp. Crumbled feta cheese
- Nonstick cooking spray
- Pepper and salt to taste

DIRECTIONS:
1. First, you will have to preheat the oven to 400 degrees F. After that, when the oven is on the proper temperature, you will have to put the gratin dishes right on the baking sheet.
2. Then, leave the dishes to heat in the oven for almost 10 minutes After that process, you need to break the eggs into individual ramekins.
3. Then, let the avocado and eggs come to room temperature for at least 10 minutes. Then, peel the avocado properly and cut it each half into 6-8 slices.
4. You will have to remove the dishes from the oven and spray them with the non-stick spray. Then, you will have to arrange all the sliced avocados in the dishes and tip two eggs into each dish. Sprinkle with feta, add pepper and salt to taste, serve.

NUTRITION: Calories: 280 Protein: 11 g Fat: 23 g Carbs: 10 g

38. Mediterranean Eggs White Breakfast Sandwich with Roasted Tomatoes

Preparation Time: 15 minutes
Cooking Time: 10 minutes
Servings: 2
INGREDIENTS:
- Salt and pepper to taste
- ¼ cup egg whites
- 1 teaspoon chopped fresh herbs like rosemary, basil, parsley,
- 1 whole-grain seeded ciabatta roll
- 1 teaspoon butter
- 1-2 slices Muenster cheese
- 1 tablespoon pesto
- About ½ cup roasted tomatoes
- 10 ounces' grape tomatoes
- 1 tablespoon extra-virgin olive oil
- Black pepper and salt to taste

DIRECTIONS:

1. First, you will have to melt the butter over medium heat in the small nonstick skillet. Then, mix the egg whites with pepper and salt.
2. Then, sprinkle it with the fresh herbs. After that cook it for almost 3-4 minutes or until the eggs are done, then flip it carefully.
3. Meanwhile, toast ciabatta bread in the toaster. Place the egg on the bottom half of the sandwich rolls, then top with cheese
4. Add roasted tomatoes and the top half of roll. To make a roasted tomato, preheat the oven to 400 degrees. Then, slice the tomatoes in half lengthwise.
5. Place on the baking sheet and drizzle with olive oil. Season it with pepper and salt and then roast in the oven for about 20 minutes. Skins will appear wrinkled when done.

NUTRITION: Calories: 458 Protein: 21 g Fat: 24 g Carbs: 51 g

39. Greek Yogurt Pancakes

Preparation Time: 10 minutes
Cooking Time: 5 minutes
Servings: 2
INGREDIENTS:

- 1 cup all-purpose flour
- 1 cup whole-wheat flour
- 1/4 teaspoon salt
- 4 teaspoons baking powder
- 1 tablespoon sugar
- 1 1/2 cups unsweetened almond milk
- 2 teaspoons vanilla extract
- 2 large eggs
- 1/2 cup plain 2% Greek yogurt
- Fruit, for serving
- Maple syrup, for serving

DIRECTIONS:

1. First, you will have to pour the curds into the bowl and mix them well until creamy. After that, you will have to add egg whites and mix them well until combined.
2. Then take a separate bowl, pour the wet mixture into the dry mixture. Stir to combine. The batter will be extremely thick.
3. Then, simply spoon the batter onto the sprayed pan heated too medium-high. The batter must make 4 large pancakes.
4. Then, you will have to flip the pancakes once when they start to bubble a bit on the surface. Cook until golden brown on both sides.

NUTRITION: Calories: 166 Protein: 14 g Fat: 5 g Carbs: 52g

40. Mediterranean Feta and Quinoa Egg Muffins

Preparation Time: 15 minutes
Cooking Time: 15 minutes
Servings: 12
INGREDIENTS:

- 2 cups baby spinach finely chopped
- 1 cup chopped or sliced cherry tomatoes
- 1/2 cup finely chopped onion
- 1 tablespoon chopped fresh oregano
- 1 cup crumbled feta cheese
- 1/2 cup chopped {pitted} kalamata olives
- 2 teaspoons vegetable oil
- 1 cup cooked quinoa
- 8 eggs
- 1/4 teaspoon salt

DIRECTIONS:

1. Pre-heat oven to 350 degrees Fahrenheit, and then prepare 12 silicone muffin holders on the baking sheet, or just grease a 12-cup muffin tin with oil and set aside.
2. Finely chop the vegetables and then heat the skillet to medium. After that, add the vegetable oil and onions and sauté for 2 minutes.
3. Then, add tomatoes and sauté for another minute, then add spinach and sauté until wilted, about 1 minute.
4. Place the beaten egg into a bowl and then add lots of vegetables like feta cheese, quinoa, veggie mixture as well as salt, and then stir well until everything is properly combined.
5. Pour the ready mixture into greased muffin tins or silicone cups, dividing the mixture equally. Then, bake it in an oven for 30 minutes or so.

NUTRITION: Calories: 113 Protein: 6 g Fat: 7 g Carbs: 5 g

41. Mediterranean Eggs

Preparation Time: 15 minutes
Cooking Time: 20 minutes
Servings: 2
INGREDIENTS:

- 5 tbsp. Of divided olive oil
- 2 diced medium-sized Spanish onions
- 2 diced red bell peppers
- 2 minced cloves garlic
- 1 teaspoon cumin seeds
- 4 diced large ripe tomatoes
- 1 tablespoon of honey
- Salt
- Freshly ground black pepper
- 1/3 cup crumbled feta
- 4 eggs
- 1 teaspoon zaatar spice
- Grilled pita during serving

DIRECTIONS:

1. Add 3 tablespoons of olive oil into a pan and heat it over medium heat. Along with the oil, sauté the cumin seeds, onions, garlic, and red pepper for a few minutes.
2. After that, add the diced tomatoes and salt and pepper to taste and cook them for about 10 minutes till they come together and form a light sauce.
3. With that, half the preparation is already done. Now you just have to break the eggs directly into the sauce and poach them.
4. However, you must keep in mind to cook the egg whites but keep the yolks still runny. This takes about 8 to 10 minutes.
5. While plating adds some feta and olive oil with zaatar spice to further enhance the flavors. Once done, serve with grilled pita.

NUTRITION: Calories: 304 Protein: 12 g Fat: 16 g Carbs: 28 g

42. Pastry-Less Spanakopita

Preparation Time: 5 minutes
Cooking Time: 20 minutes
Servings: 4

INGREDIENTS:

- 1/8 teaspoons black pepper, add as per taste
- 1/3 cup of Extra virgin olive oil
- 4 lightly beaten eggs
- 7 cups of Lettuce, preferably a spring mix (mesclun)
- 1/2 cup of crumbled Feta cheese
- 1/8 teaspoon of Sea salt, add to taste
- 1 finely chopped medium Yellow onion

DIRECTIONS:

1. Warm the oven to 180C and grease the flan dish. Once done, pour the extra virgin olive oil into a large saucepan and heat it over medium heat with the onions, until they are translucent.
2. Add greens and keep stirring until all the ingredients are wilted. Season it with salt and pepper and transfer the greens to the prepared dish and sprinkle on some feta cheese.
3. Pour the eggs and bake it for 20 minutes till it is cooked through and slightly brown.

NUTRITION: Calories: 325 Protein: 11.2 g Fat: 27.9 g Carbs: 7.3 g

43. Date and Walnut Overnight Oats

Preparation Time: 5 minutes
Cooking Time: 20 minutes
Servings: 2

INGREDIENTS:

- ¼ Cup Greek Yogurt, Plain
- 1/3 cup of yogurt
- 2/3 cup of oats
- 1 cup of milk
- 2 tsp date syrup or you can also use maple syrup or honey
- 1 mashed banana
- ¼ tsp cinnamon
- ¼ cup walnuts
- Pinch of salt (approx.1/8 tsp)

DIRECTIONS:

1. Firstly, get a mason jar or a small bowl and add all the ingredients. After that stir and mix all the ingredients well. Cover it securely, and cool it in a refrigerator overnight.
2. After that, take it out the next morning, add more liquid or cinnamon if required, and serve cold. (However, you can also microwave it for people with a warmer palate.)

NUTRITION: Calories: 350 Protein: 14 g Fat: 12 g Carbs: 49 g

44. Pear and Mango Smoothie

Preparation time: 5 minutes
Cooking time: 0 minutes
Servings: 1

INGREDIENTS:

- 1 ripe mango, cored and chopped
- ½ mango, peeled, pitted and chopped
- 1 cup kale, chopped
- ½ cup plain Greek yogurt
- 2 ice cubes

DIRECTIONS:

1. Add pear, mango, yogurt, kale, and mango to a blender and puree. Add ice and blend until you have a smooth texture. Serve and enjoy!

NUTRITION: Calories: 293 Fat: 8g Carbs: 53g Protein: 8g

45. Eggplant Salad

Preparation time: 20 minutes
Cooking time: 15 minutes
Servings: 8

INGREDIENTS:

- 1 large eggplant, washed and cubed
- 1 tomato, seeded and chopped
- 1 small onion, diced
- 2 tablespoons parsley, chopped
- 2 tablespoons extra virgin olive oil
- 2 tablespoons distilled white vinegar
- ½ cup feta cheese, crumbled
- Salt as needed

DIRECTIONS:

1. Pre-heat your outdoor grill to medium-high. Pierce the eggplant a few times using a knife/fork. Cook the eggplants on your grill for about 15 minutes until they are charred.
2. Keep it on the side and allow them to cool. Remove the skin from the eggplant and dice the pulp. Transfer the pulp to a mixing bowl and add parsley, onion, tomato, olive oil, feta cheese and vinegar.
3. Mix well and chill for 1 hour. Season with salt and enjoy!

NUTRITION: Calories: 99 Fat: 7g Carbs: 7g Protein: 3.4g

46. Artichoke Frittata

Preparation time: 5 minutes
Cooking time: 10 minutes
Servings: 4

INGREDIENTS:

- 8 large eggs
- ¼ cup Asiago cheese, grated
- 1 tablespoon fresh basil, chopped
- 1 teaspoon fresh oregano, chopped
- Pinch of salt
- 1 teaspoon extra virgin olive oil
- 1 teaspoon garlic, minced
- 1 cup canned artichokes, drained
- 1 tomato, chopped

DIRECTIONS:

1. Pre-heat your oven to broil. Take a medium bowl and whisk in eggs, Asiago cheese, oregano, basil, sea salt and pepper. Blend in a bowl.
2. Place a large ovenproof skillet over medium-high heat and add olive oil. Add garlic and sauté for 1 minute. Remove skillet from heat and pour in egg mix.
3. Return skillet to heat and sprinkle artichoke hearts and tomato over eggs. Cook frittata without stirring for 8 minutes.
4. Place skillet under the broiler for 1 minute until the top is lightly browned. Cut frittata into 4 pieces and serve. Enjoy!

NUTRITION: Calories: 199 Fat: 13g Carbs: 5g Protein: 16g

47. Full Eggs in a Squash

Preparation time: 15 minutes
Cooking time: 20 minutes
Servings: 5

INGREDIENTS:

- 2 acorn squash
- 6 whole eggs
- 2 tablespoons extra virgin olive oil
- Salt and pepper as needed
- 5-6 pitted dates
- 8 walnut halves
- A fresh bunch of parsley

DIRECTIONS:

1. Pre-heat your oven to 375 degrees Fahrenheit. Slice squash crosswise and prepare 3 slices with holes. While slicing the squash, make sure that each slice has a measurement of ¾ inch thickness.
2. Remove the seeds from the slices. Take a baking sheet and line it with parchment paper. Transfer the slices to your baking sheet and season them with salt and pepper.
3. Bake in your oven for 20 minutes. Chop the walnuts and dates on your cutting board. Take the baking dish out of the oven and drizzle slices with olive oil.
4. Crack an egg into each of the holes in the slices and season with pepper and salt. Sprinkle the chopped walnuts on top. Bake for 10 minutes more. Garnish with parsley and add maple syrup.

NUTRITION: Calories: 198 Fat: 12g Carbs: 17g Protein: 8g

48. Barley Porridge

Preparation time: 5 minutes
Cooking time: 25 minutes
Servings: 4

INGREDIENTS:

- 1 cup barley
- 1 cup wheat berries
- 2 cups unsweetened almond milk
- 2 cups water
- ½ cup blueberries
- ½ cup pomegranate seeds
- ½ cup hazelnuts, toasted and chopped
- ¼ cup honey

DIRECTIONS:

1. Take a medium saucepan and place it over medium-high heat. Place barley, almond milk, wheat berries, water and bring to a boil. Reduce the heat to low and simmer for 25 minutes.
2. Divide amongst serving bowls and top each serving with 2 tablespoons blueberries, 2 tablespoons pomegranate seeds, 2 tablespoons hazelnuts, 1 tablespoon honey. Serve and enjoy!

NUTRITION: Calories: 295 Fat: 8g Carbs: 56g Protein: 6g

49. Tomato and Dill Frittata

Preparation time: 5 minutes
Cooking time: 10 minutes
Servings: 4

INGREDIENTS:

- 2 tablespoons olive oil
- 1 medium onion, chopped
- 1 teaspoon garlic, minced
- 2 medium tomatoes, chopped
- 6 large eggs
- ½ cup half and half
- ½ cup feta cheese, crumbled
- ¼ cup dill weed
- Salt as needed
- Ground black pepper as needed

DIRECTIONS:

1. Pre-heat your oven to a temperature of 400 degrees Fahrenheit. Take a large sized ovenproof pan and heat up your olive oil over medium-high heat. Toss in the onion, garlic, tomatoes and stir fry them for 4 minutes.
2. While they are being cooked, take a bowl and beat together your eggs, half and half cream and season the mix with some pepper and salt.
3. Pour the mixture into the pan with your vegetables and top it with crumbled feta cheese and dill weed. Cover it with the lid and let it cook for 3 minutes.
4. Place the pan inside your oven and let it bake for 10 minutes. Serve hot.

NUTRITION: Calories: 191 Fat: 15g Carbs: 6g Protein: 9g

50. Strawberry and Rhubarb Smoothie

Preparation time: 5 minutes
Cooking time: 3 minutes
Servings: 1

INGREDIENTS:

- 1 rhubarb stalk, chopped
- 1 cup fresh strawberries, sliced
- ½ cup plain Greek strawberries
- Pinch of ground cinnamon
- 3 ice cubes

DIRECTIONS:

1. Take a small saucepan and fill with water over high heat. Bring to boil and add rhubarb, boil for 3 minutes. Drain and transfer to blender.
2. Add strawberries, honey, yogurt, cinnamon and pulse mixture until smooth. Add ice cubes and blend until thick with no lumps. Pour into glass and enjoy chilled.

NUTRITION: Calories: 295 Fat: 8g Carbs: 56g Protein: 6g

51. Bacon and Brie Omelet Wedges

Preparation time: 10 minutes
Cooking time: 10 minutes
Servings: 6

INGREDIENTS:

- 2 tablespoons olive oil
- 7 ounces smoked bacon
- 6 beaten eggs
- Small bunch chives, snipped
- 3 ½ ounces brie, sliced
- 1 teaspoon red wine vinegar
- 1 teaspoon Dijon mustard
- 1 cucumber, halved, deseeded and sliced diagonally
- 7 ounces' radish, quartered

DIRECTIONS:

1. Turn your grill on and set it to high. Take a small-sized pan and add 1 teaspoon of oil, allow the oil to heat up. Add lardons and fry until crisp. Drain the lardon on kitchen paper.
2. Take another non-sticky cast iron frying pan and place it over grill, heat 2 teaspoons of oil. Add lardons, eggs, chives, ground pepper to the frying pan. Cook on low until they are semi-set.
3. Carefully lay brie on top and grill until the Brie sets and is a golden texture. Remove it from the pan and cut up into wedges.
4. Take a small bowl and create dressing by mixing olive oil, mustard, vinegar and seasoning. Add cucumber to the bowl and mix, serve alongside the omelet wedges.

NUTRITION: Calories: 35 Fat: 31g Carbs: 3g Protein: 25g

52. Pearl Couscous Salad

Preparation time: 15 minutes
Cooking time: 0 minutes
Servings: 6

INGREDIENTS:

- For Lemon Dill Vinaigrette:
- Juice of 1 large sized lemon
- 1/3 cup of extra virgin olive oil
- 1 teaspoon of dill weed
- 1 teaspoon of garlic powder
- Salt as needed
- Pepper
- For Israeli Couscous:
- 2 cups of Pearl Couscous
- Extra virgin olive oil
- 2 cups of halved grape tomatoes
- Water as needed
- 1/3 cup of finely chopped red onions
- ½ of a finely chopped English cucumber
- 15 ounces of chickpeas
- 14 ounces can of artichoke hearts (roughly chopped up)
- ½ cup of pitted Kalamata olives
- 15-20 pieces of fresh basil leaves, roughly torn and chopped up
- 3 ounces of fresh baby mozzarella

DIRECTIONS:

1. Prepare the vinaigrette by taking a bowl and add the ingredients listed under vinaigrette. Mix them well and keep aside. Take a medium-sized heavy pot and place it over medium heat.
2. Add 2 tablespoons of olive oil and allow it to heat up. Add couscous and keep cooking until golden brown. Add 3 cups of boiling water and cook the couscous according to the package instructions.
3. Once done, drain in a colander and keep aside. Take another large-sized mixing bowl and add the remaining ingredients except the cheese and basil.
4. Add the cooked couscous and basil to the mix and mix everything well. Give the vinaigrette a nice stir and whisk it into the couscous salad. Mix well.
5. Adjust the seasoning as required. Add mozzarella cheese. Garnish with some basil. Enjoy!

NUTRITION: Calories: 393 Fat: 13g Carbs: 57g Protein: 13g

53. Coconut Porridge

Preparation time: 15 minutes
Cooking time: 0 minutes
Servings: 6

INGREDIENTS:

- Powdered erythritol as needed
- 1 ½ cups almond milk, unsweetened
- 2 tablespoons vanilla protein powder
- 3 tablespoons Golden Flaxseed meal
- 2 tablespoons coconut flour

DIRECTIONS:

1. Take a bowl and mix in flaxseed meal, protein powder, coconut flour and mix well. Add mix to saucepan (placed over medium heat).
2. Add almond milk and stir, let the mixture thicken. Add your desired amount of sweetener and serve. Enjoy!

NUTRITION: Calories: 259 Fat: 13g Carbs: 5g Protein: 16g

54. Crumbled Feta and Scallions

Preparation time: 5 minutes
Cooking time: 15 minutes
Servings: 12

INGREDIENTS:

- 2 tablespoons of unsalted butter
- ½ cup of chopped up scallions
- 1 cup of crumbled feta cheese
- 8 large sized eggs
- 2/3 cup of milk
- ½ teaspoon of dried Italian seasoning
- Salt as needed
- Freshly ground black pepper as needed
- Cooking oil spray

DIRECTIONS:

1. Pre-heat your oven to 400 degrees Fahrenheit. Take a 3-4-ounce muffin pan and grease with cooking oil. Take a non-stick pan and place it over medium heat.
2. Add butter and allow the butter to melt. Add half of the scallions and stir fry. Keep them to the side. Take a medium-sized bowl and add eggs, Italian seasoning and milk and whisk well.

3. Add the stir fried scallions and feta cheese and mix. Season with pepper and salt. Pour the mix into the muffin tin. Transfer the muffin tin to your oven and bake for 15 minutes. Serve with a sprinkle of scallions.

NUTRITION: Calories: 106 Fat: 8g Carbs: 2g Protein: 7g

55.   *Quinoa Chicken Salad*

Preparation time: 15 minutes
Cooking time: 20 minutes
Servings: 8
INGREDIENTS:
- 2 cups of water
- 2 cubes of chicken bouillon
- 1 smashed garlic clove
- 1 cup of uncooked quinoa
- 2 large sized chicken breasts cut up into bite-sized portions and cooked
- 1 large sized diced red onion
- 1 large sized green bell pepper
- ½ cup of Kalamata olives
- ½ cup of crumbled feta cheese
- ¼ cup of chopped up parsley
- ¼ cup of chopped up fresh chives
- ½ teaspoon of salt
- 1 tablespoon of balsamic vinegar
- ¼ cup of olive oil

DIRECTIONS:
1. Take a saucepan and bring your water, garlic and bouillon cubes to a boil. Stir in quinoa and reduce the heat to medium low.
2. Simmer for about 15-20 minutes until the quinoa has absorbed all the water and is tender. Discard your garlic cloves and scrape the quinoa into a large sized bowl.
3. Gently stir in the cooked chicken breast, bell pepper, onion, feta cheese, chives, salt and parsley into your quinoa.
4. Drizzle some lemon juice, olive oil and balsamic vinegar. Stir everything until mixed well. Serve warm and enjoy!

NUTRITION: Calories: 99 Fat: 7g Carbs: 7g Protein: 3.4g

56.   *Spicy Early Morning Seafood Risotto*

Preparation time: 5 minutes
Cooking time: 15 minutes
Servings: 4
INGREDIENTS:
- 3 cups of clam juice
- 2 cups of water
- 2 tablespoons of olive oil
- 1 medium-sized chopped up onion
- 2 minced cloves of garlic
- 1 ½ cups of Arborio Rice
- ½ cup of dry white wine
- 1 teaspoon of Saffron
- ½ teaspoon of ground cumin
- ½ teaspoon of paprika
- 1 pound of marinara seafood mix
- Salt as needed
- Ground pepper as needed

DIRECTIONS:
1. Place a saucepan over high heat and pour in your clam juice with water and bring the mixture to a boil. Remove the heat.
2. Take a heavy bottomed saucepan and stir fry your garlic and onion in oil over medium heat until a nice fragrance comes off.
3. Add in the rice and keep stirring for 2-3 minutes until the rice has been fully covered with the oil. Pour the wine and then add the saffron.
4. Keep stirring constantly until it is fully absorbed. Add in the cumin, clam juice, paprika mixture 1 cup at a time, making sure to keep stirring it from time to time.
5. Cook the rice for 20 minutes until perfect. Finally, add the seafood marinara mix and cook for another 5-7 minutes.
6. Season with some pepper and salt. Transfer the meal to a serving dish. Serve hot.

NUTRITION: Calories: 386 Fat: 7g Carbs: 55g Protein: 21g

57.   *Rocket Tomatoes and Mushroom Frittata*

Preparation time: 5 minutes
Cooking time: 15 minutes
Servings: 4
INGREDIENTS:
- 2 tablespoons of butter
- 1 chopped up medium-sized onion
- 2 minced cloves of garlic
- 1 cup of coarsely chopped baby rocket tomato
- 1 cup of sliced button mushrooms
- 6 large pieces of eggs
- ½ cup of skim milk
- 1 teaspoon of dried rosemary
- Salt as needed
- Ground black pepper as needed

DIRECTIONS:
1. Pre-heat your oven to 400 degrees Fahrenheit. Take a large oven-proof pan and place it over medium-heat. Heat up some oil.
2. Stir fry your garlic, onion for about 2 minutes. Add the mushroom, rosemary and rockets and cook for 3 minutes. Take a medium-sized bowl and beat your eggs alongside the milk.
3. Season it with some salt and pepper. Pour the egg mixture into your pan with the vegetables.
4. Reduce the heat to low and cover with the lid. Let it cook for 3 minutes. Transfer the pan into your oven and bake for 10 minutes until fully settled.
5. Reduce the heat to low and cover with your lid. Let it cook for 3 minutes. Transfer the pan into your oven and then bake for another 10 minutes. Serve hot.

NUTRITION: Calories: 189 Fat: 13g Carbs: 6g Protein: 12g

58. Cheesy Olives Bread

Preparation Time: 1 hour and 40 minutes
Cooking Time: 30 minutes
Servings: 10

INGREDIENTS:

- 4 cups whole-wheat flour
- 3 tbsps. Oregano, chopped
- 2 tsps. Dry yeast
- ¼ cup olive oil
- 1 ½ cups black olives, pitted and sliced
- 1 cup of water
- ½ cup feta cheese, crumbled

DIRECTIONS:

1. In a bowl, mix the flour with the water, the yeast, and the oil. Stir and knead your dough very well. Put the dough in a bowl, cover with plastic wrap, and keep in a warm place for 1 hour.
2. Divide the dough into 2 bowls and stretch each ball well. Add the rest of the ingredients to each ball and tuck them inside. Knead the dough well again.
3. Flatten the balls a bit and leave them aside for 40 minutes more. Transfer the balls to a baking sheet lined with parchment paper, make a small slit in each, and bake at 425F for 30 minutes.
4. Serve the bread as a Mediterranean breakfast.

NUTRITION: Calories 251 Fat: 7.3g Carbs: 39.7g Protein: 6.7g

59. Sweet Potato Tart

Preparation Time: 10 minutes
Cooking Time: 1 hour and 10 minutes
Servings: 8

INGREDIENTS:

- 2 pounds' sweet potatoes, peeled and cubed
- ¼ cup olive oil + a drizzle
- 7 oz. Feta cheese, crumbled
- 1 yellow onion, chopped
- 2 eggs, whisked
- ¼ cup almond milk
- 1 tbsp. Herbs de Provence
- A pinch of salt and black pepper
- 6 phyllo sheets

DIRECTIONS:

1. In a bowl, combine the potatoes with half of the oil, salt, and pepper, toss, spread on a baking sheet lined with parchment paper, and roast at 400F for 25 minutes.
2. Meanwhile, heat a pan with half of the remaining oil over medium heat, add the onion, and sauté for 5 minutes.
3. In a bowl, combine the eggs with the milk, feta, herbs, salt, pepper, onion, sweet potatoes, and the rest of the oil and toss.
4. Arrange the phyllo sheets in a tart pan and brush them with a drizzle of oil. Add the sweet potato mix and spread it well into the pan.
5. Bake covered with tin foil at 350F for 20 minutes. Remove the tin foil, bake the tart for 20 minutes more, cool it down, slice, and serve for breakfast.

NUTRITION: Calories 476 Fat: 16.8g Carbs: 68.8g Protein: 13.9g

60. Stuffed Pita Breads

Preparation Time: 5 minutes
Cooking Time: 15 minutes
Servings: 4

INGREDIENTS:

- 1 ½ tbsp olive oil
- 1 tomato, cubed
- 1 garlic clove, minced
- 1 red onion, chopped
- ¼ cup parsley, chopped
- 15 oz. Canned fava beans, drained and rinsed
- ¼ cup lemon juice
- Salt and black pepper to the taste
- 4 whole-wheat pita bread pockets

DIRECTIONS:

1. Heat a pan with the oil over medium heat, add the onion, stir, and sauté for 5 minutes. Add the rest of the ingredients, stir, and cook for 10 minutes more
2. Stuff the pita pockets with this mix and serve for breakfast.

NUTRITION: Calories 382 Fat: 1.8g Carbs: 66g Protein: 28.5g

61. Blueberries Quinoa

Preparation Time: 5 minutes
Cooking Time: 0 minutes
Servings: 4

INGREDIENTS:

- 2 cups almond milk
- 2 cups quinoa, already cooked
- ½ tsp cinnamon powder
- 1 tbsp. Honey
- 1 cup blueberries
- ¼ cup walnuts, chopped

DIRECTIONS:

1. In a bowl, mix the quinoa with the milk and the rest of the ingredients, toss, divide into smaller bowls and serve for breakfast.

NUTRITION: Calories 284 Fat: 14.3g Carbs: 15.4g Protein: 4.4g

62. Endives, Fennel and Orange Salad

Preparation Time: 5 minutes
Cooking Time: 0 minutes
Servings: 4

INGREDIENTS:

- 1 tbsp. Balsamic vinegar
- 2 garlic cloves, minced
- 1 tsp. Dijon mustard
- 2 tbsps. Olive oil
- 1 tbsp. Lemon juice
- Sea salt and black pepper to taste
- ½ cup black olives, pitted and chopped
- 1 tbsp. Parsley, chopped
- 7 cups baby spinach
- 2 endives, shredded
- 3 medium navel oranges, peeled and cut into segments
- 2 bulbs fennel, shredded

DIRECTIONS:

1. In a salad bowl, combine the spinach with the endives, oranges, fennel, and the rest of the ingredients, toss and serve for breakfast.

NUTRITION: Calories 97 Fat: 9.1g Carbs: 3.7g Protein: 1.9g

63. Raspberries and Yogurt Smoothie

Preparation Time: 5 minutes
Cooking Time: 0 minutes
Servings: 2
INGREDIENTS:

- 2 cups raspberries
- ½ cup Greek yogurt
- ½ cup almond milk
- ½ tsp vanilla extract

DIRECTIONS:

1. In your blender, combine the raspberries with the milk, vanilla, and the yogurt, pulse well, divide into 2 glasses and serve for breakfast.

NUTRITION: Calories 245 Fat: 9.5g Carbs: 5.6g Protein: 1.6g

64. Homemade Muesli

Preparation Time: 15 minutes
Cooking Time: 20 minutes
Servings: 8
INGREDIENTS:

- 3 ½ cups rolled oats
- ½ cup wheat bran
- ½ tsp kosher salt
- ½ tsp ground cinnamon
- ½ cup sliced almonds
- ¼ cup raw pecans, coarsely chopped
- ¼ cup raw pepitas (shelled pumpkin seeds)
- ½ cup unsweetened coconut flakes
- ¼ cup dried apricots, coarsely chopped
- ¼ cup dried cherries

DIRECTIONS:

1. Take a medium bowl and combine the oats, wheat bran, salt, and cinnamon. Stir well. Place the mixture onto a baking sheet.
2. Next place the almonds, pecans, and pepitas onto another baking sheet and toss. Pop both trays into the oven and heat to 350°F. Bake for 10-12 minutes. Remove from the oven and pop to one side.
3. Leave the nuts to cool but take the one with the oats, sprinkle with the coconut, and pop back into the oven for 5 minutes more. Remove and leave to cool.
4. Find a large bowl and combine the contents of both trays then stir well to combine. Throw in the apricots and cherries and stir well. Pop into an airtight container until required.

NUTRITION: Calories 250 Fat: 10g Carbs: 36g Protein: 7g

65. Tangerine and Pomegranate Breakfast Fruit Salad

Preparation Time: 15 minutes
Cooking Time: 20 minutes
Servings: 5
INGREDIENTS:

- For the grains:
- 1 cup pearl or hulled barley
- 3 cups of water
- 3 tbsps. Olive oil, divided
- ½ tsp kosher salt
- For the fruit:
- ½ large pineapple, peeled and cut into 1 ½" chunks
- 6 tangerines
- 1 ¼ cups pomegranate seeds
- 1 small bunch of fresh mint
- For the dressing:
- 1/3 cup honey
- Juice and finely grated zest of 1 lemon
- Juice and finely grated zest of 2 limes
- ½ tsp kosher salt
- ¼ cup olive oil
- ¼ cup toasted hazelnut oil (olive oil is fine too)

DIRECTIONS:

1. Place the grain into a strainer and rinse well. Grab 2 baking sheets, line with paper, and add the grain. Spread well to cover then leave to dry.
2. Next, place the water into a saucepan and pop over medium heat. Place a skillet over medium heat, add 2 tbsps. Of the oil then add the barley. Toast for 2 minutes.
3. Add the water and salt and bring to a boil. Reduce to simmer and cook for 40 minutes until most of the liquid has been absorbed. Turn off the heat and leave to stand for 10 minutes to steam cook the rest.
4. Meanwhile, grab a medium bowl and add the honey, juices, zest, and salt, and stir well. Add the olive oil then nut oil and stir again. Pop until the fridge until needed.
5. Remove the lid from the barley then place it onto another prepared baking sheet and leave to cool. Drizzle with oil and leave to cool completely then pop into the fridge.
6. When ready to serve, divide the grains, pineapple, orange, pomegranate, and mint between the bowls. Drizzle with the dressing then serve and enjoy.

NUTRITION: Calories 400 Fat: 23g Carbs: 50g Protein: 3g

JUICE & SMOOTHIES

66. Mango Agua Fresca

Preparation time: 5 minutes.
Cooking time: 0 minutes.
Servings: 2
Ingredients:

- 2 fresh mangoes, diced
- 1(½) cups water
- 1 teaspoon fresh lime juice
- Maple syrup to taste
- 2 cups ice
- 2 slices fresh lime for garnish
- 2 fresh mint sprigs for garnish

Directions:

1. Put the mangoes, lime juice, maple syrup, and water to a blender. Process until creamy and smooth.
2. Divide the beverage into two glasses, then garnish each glass with ice, lime slice, and mint sprig before serving.

Nutrition: Calories: 230 Fat: 1.3g Carbs: 57.7g Fiber: 5.4g Protein: 2.8g

67. Light Ginger Tea

Preparation time: 5 minutes.
Cooking time: 10 to 15 minutes.
Servings: 2
Ingredients:

- 1 small ginger knob, sliced into four 1-inch chunks
- 4 cups water
- Juice of 1 large lemon
- Maple syrup to taste

Directions:

1. Add the ginger knob and water in a saucepan, then simmer over medium heat for 10 to 15 minutes.
2. Turn off the heat, then mix in the lemon juice. Strain the liquid to remove the ginger, then fold in the maple syrup and serve.

Nutrition: Calories: 32 Fat: 0.1g Carbs: 8.6g Fiber: 0.1g Protein: 0.1g

68. Classic Switchel

Preparation time: 5 minutes.
Cooking time: 0 minutes.
Servings: 4
Ingredients:

- 1-inch piece ginger, minced
- 2 tablespoons apple cider vinegar
- 2 tablespoons maple syrup
- 4 cups water
- ¼ teaspoon sea salt, optional

Directions:

1. Combine all the ingredients in a glass. Stir to mix well.
2. Serve immediately or chill in the refrigerator for an hour before serving.

Nutrition: Calories: 110 Fat: 0g Carbs: 28.0g Fiber: 0g Protein: 0g

69. Lime and Cucumber Electrolyte Drink

Preparation time: 5 minutes.
Cooking time: 0 minutes.
Servings: 4
Ingredients:

- ¼ cup chopped cucumber
- 1 tablespoon fresh lime juice
- 1 tablespoon apple cider vinegar
- 2 tablespoons maple syrup
- ¼ teaspoon sea salt, optional
- 4 cups water

Directions:

1. Combine all the ingredients in a glass. Stir to mix well. Refrigerate overnight before serving.

Nutrition: Calories: 114 Fat: 0.1g Carbs: 28.9g Fiber: 0.3g Protein: 0.3g

70. Easy and Fresh Mango Madness

Preparation time: 5 minutes.
Cooking time: 0 minutes.
Servings: 4
Ingredients:

- 1 cup chopped mango
- 1 cup chopped peach
- 1 banana
- 1 cup strawberries
- 1 carrot, peeled and chopped
- 1 cup water

Directions:

1. Put all the ingredients to a food processor, then blitz until glossy and smooth.
2. Serve immediately or chill in the refrigerator for an hour before serving.

Nutrition: Calories: 376 Fat: 22.0g Carbs: 19.0g Fiber: 14.0g Protein: 5.0g

71. Simple Date Shake

Preparation time: 10 minutes.
Cooking time: 0 minutes.
Servings: 2
Ingredients:

- 5 Medjool dates, pitted, soaked in boiling water for 5 minutes
- ¾ cup unsweetened coconut milk
- 1 teaspoon vanilla extract
- ½ teaspoon fresh lemon juice
- ¼ teaspoon sea salt, optional
- 1(½) cups ice

Directions:

1. Put all the ingredients to a food processor, then blitz until it has a milkshake and smooth texture. Serve immediately.

Nutrition: Calories: 380 Fat: 21.6g Carbs: 50.3g Fiber: 6.0g Protein: 3.2g

72. Beet and Clementine Protein Smoothie

Preparation time: 10 minutes.
Cooking time: 0 minutes.
Servings: 3
Ingredients:

- 1 small beet, peeled and chopped
- 1 clementine, peeled and broken into segments
- ½ ripe banana
- ½ cup raspberries
- 1 tablespoon chia seeds
- 2 tablespoons almond butter
- ¼ teaspoon vanilla extract
- 1 cup unsweetened almond milk
- 1/8 teaspoon fine sea salt, optional

Directions:

1. Combine all the ingredients to a food processor, then pulse on high for 2 minutes or until glossy and creamy. Refrigerate for an hour and serve chilled.

Nutrition: Calories: 526 Fat: 25.4g Carbs: 61.9g Fiber: 17.3g Protein: 20.6g

73. Matcha Limeade

Preparation time: 10 minutes.
Cooking time: 0 minutes.
Servings: 4
Ingredients:

- 2 tablespoons matcha powder
- ¼ cup raw agave syrup
- 3 cups water, divided
- 1 cup fresh lime juice
- 3 tablespoons chia seeds

Directions:

1. Lightly simmer the matcha, agave syrup, and 1 cup of water in a saucepan over medium heat. Keep stirring until no matcha lumps.
2. Pour the matcha mixture into a large glass, add the remaining ingredients, and mix well.
3. Refrigerate for at least an hour before serving.

Nutrition: Calories: 15 Fat: 4.5g Carbs: 26.8g Fiber: 5.3g Protein: 3.7g

74. Fruit Infused Water

Preparation time: 5 minutes.
Cooking time: 0 minutes.
Servings: 2
Ingredients:

- 3 strawberries, sliced
- 5 mint leaves
- ½ of orange, sliced
- 2 cups of water

Directions:

1. Divide fruits and mint between two glasses, pour in water, stir until just mixed, and refrigerate for 2 hours.
2. Serve straight away.

Nutrition: Calories: 5.4 Fat: 0.1g Carbs: 1.3g Protein: 0.1g Fiber: 0.4g

75. Hazelnut and Chocolate Milk

Preparation time: 5 minutes.
Cooking time: 0 minutes.
Servings: 2
Ingredients:

- 2 tablespoons cocoa powder
- 4 dates, pitted
- 1 cup hazelnuts
- 3 cups of water

Directions:

1. Place all the ingredients in the order to a food processor or blender and then pulse for 2 to 3 minutes at high speed until smooth.
2. Pour the smoothie into two glasses and then serve.

Nutrition: Calories: 120 Fat: 5g Carbs: 19g Protein: 2g Fiber: 1g

76. Banana Milk

Preparation time: 5 minutes.
Cooking time: 0 minutes.
Servings: 2
Ingredients:

- 2 dates
- 2 medium bananas, peeled
- 1 teaspoon vanilla extract, unsweetened
- 1/2 cup ice
- 2 cups of water

Directions:

1. Place all the ingredients in the order to a food processor or blender and then pulse for 2 to 3 minutes at high speed until smooth.
2. Pour the smoothie into two glasses and then serve.

Nutrition: Calories: 79 Fat: 0g Carbs: 19.8g Protein: 0.8g Fiber: 6g

77. Apple, Carrot, Celery, and Kale Juice

Preparation time: 5 minutes.
Cooking time: 0 minutes.
Servings: 2
Ingredients:

- 5 curly kale
- 2 green apples, cored, peeled, chopped
- 2 large stalks celery
- 4 large carrots, cored, peeled, chopped

Directions:

1. Process all the ingredients in the order in a juicer or blender and then strain it into two glasses.
2. Serve straight away.

Nutrition: Calories: 183 Fat: 2.5g Carbs: 46g Protein: 13g Fiber: 3g

78. Sweet and Sour Juice

Preparation time: 5 minutes.
Cooking time: 0 minutes.
Servings: 2
Ingredients:

- 2 medium apples, cored, peeled, chopped
- 2 large cucumbers, peeled
- 4 cups chopped grapefruit
- 1 cup mint

Directions:

1. Process all the ingredients in the order in a juicer or blender and then strain it into two glasses.
2. Serve straight away.

Nutrition: Calories: 90 Fat: 0g Carbs: 23g Protein: 0g Fiber: 9g

79. Green Lemonade

Preparation time: 5 minutes.
Cooking time: 0 minutes.
Servings: 2
Ingredients:

- 10 large stalks of celery, chopped
- 2 medium green apples, cored, peeled, chopped
- 2 medium cucumbers, peeled, chopped
- 2 inches' piece of ginger
- 10 stalks of kale, chopped
- 2 cups parsley

Directions:

1. Process all the ingredients in the order in a juicer or blender and then strain it into two glasses. Serve straight away.

Nutrition: Calories: 102.3 Fat: 1.1g Carbs: 26.2g Protein: 4.7g Fiber: 8.5g

80. Pineapple and Spinach Juice

Preparation time: 5 minutes.
Cooking time: 0 minutes.
Servings: 2
Ingredients:

- 2 medium red apples, cored, peeled, chopped
- 3 cups spinach
- ½ of a medium pineapple, peeled
- 2 lemons, peeled

Directions:

1. Process all the ingredients in the order in a juicer or blender and then strain it into two glasses.
2. Serve straight away.

Nutrition: Calories: 131 Fat: 0.5g Carbs: 34.5g Protein: 1.7g Fiber: 5g

81. Strawberry, Blueberry, and Banana Smoothie

Preparation time: 5 minutes.
Cooking time: 0 minutes.
Servings: 2
Ingredients:

- 1 tablespoon hulled hemp seeds
- ½ cup of frozen strawberries
- 1 small frozen banana
- ½ cup frozen blueberries
- 2 tablespoons cashew butter
- ¾ cup cashew milk, unsweetened

Directions:

1. Place all the ingredients in the order to a food processor or blender and then pulse for 2 to 3 minutes at high speed until smooth.
2. Pour the smoothie into two glasses and then serve.

Nutrition: Calories: 334 Fat: 17g Carbs: 46g Protein: 7g Fiber: 7g

82. Mango, Pineapple, and Banana Smoothie

Preparation time: 5 minutes.
Cooking time: 0 minutes.
Servings: 2
Ingredients:

- 2 cups pineapple chunks
- 2 frozen bananas
- 2 medium mangoes, destoned, cut into chunks
- 1 cup almond milk, unsweetened
- Chia seeds as needed for garnishing

Directions:

1. Place all the ingredients in the order to a food processor or blender and then pulse for 2 to 3 minutes at high speed until smooth.
2. Pour the smoothie into two glasses and then serve.

Nutrition: Calories: 287 Fat: 1.2g Carbs: 73.3g Protein: 3.5g Fiber: 8g

83. Blueberry and Banana Smoothie

Preparation time: 5 minutes.
Cooking time: 0 minutes.
Servings: 2
Ingredients:

- 2 frozen bananas
- 2 cups frozen blueberries
- 2 cups almond milk, unsweetened
- 1/2 teaspoon cinnamon
- Dash of vanilla extract

Directions:

1. Place all the ingredients in the order to a food processor or blender and then pulse for 2 to 3 minutes at high speed until smooth.
2. Pour the smoothie into two glasses and then serve.

Nutrition: Calories: 244 Fat: 3.8g Carbs: 51.5g Protein: 4g Fiber: 7.3g

84. Chard, Lettuce, and Ginger Smoothie

Preparation time: 5 minutes.
Cooking time: 0 minutes.
Servings: 2
Ingredients:

- 10 Chard leaves, chopped
- 1-inch piece of ginger, chopped
- 10 lettuce leaves, chopped
- ½ teaspoon black salt
- 2 pears, chopped
- 2 teaspoons coconut sugar
- ¼ teaspoon ground black pepper
- ¼ teaspoon salt
- 2 tablespoons lemon juice
- 2 cups of water

Directions:

1. Place all the ingredients in the order to a food processor or blender and then pulse for 2 to 3 minutes at high speed until smooth.
2. Pour the smoothie into two glasses and then serve.

Nutrition: Calories: 514 Fat: 0g Carbs: 15g Protein: 4g Fiber: 4g

85. Red Beet, Pear, and Apple Smoothie

Preparation time: 5 minutes.
Cooking time: 0 minutes.
Servings: 2
Ingredients:

- 1/2 of medium beet, peeled, chopped
- 1 tablespoon chopped cilantro
- 1 orange, juiced
- 1 medium pear, chopped
- 1 medium apple, cored, chopped
- 1/4 teaspoon ground black pepper
- 1/8 teaspoon rock salt
- 1 teaspoon coconut sugar
- 1/4 teaspoons salt
- 1 cup of water

Directions:

1. Place all the ingredients in the order to a food processor or blender and then pulse for 2 to 3 minutes at high speed until smooth.
2. Pour the smoothie into two glasses and then serve.

Nutrition: Calories: 132 Fat: 0g Carbs: 34g Protein: 1g Fiber: 5g

86.   Berry and Yogurt Smoothie

Preparation time: 5 minutes.
Cooking time: 0 minutes.
Servings: 2
Ingredients:

- 2 small bananas
- 3 cups frozen mixed berries
- 1(½) cup cashew yogurt
- 1/2 teaspoon vanilla extract, unsweetened
- 1/2 cup almond milk, unsweetened

Directions:

1. Place all the ingredients in the order to a food processor or blender and then pulse for 2 to 3 minutes at high speed until smooth.
2. Pour the smoothie into two glasses and then serve.

Nutrition: Calories: 326 Fat: 6.5g Carbs: 65.6g Protein: 8g Fiber: 8.4g

87.   Chocolate and Cherry Smoothie

Preparation time: 5 minutes.
Cooking time: 0 minutes.
Servings: 2
Ingredients:

- 4 cups frozen cherries
- 2 tablespoons cocoa powder
- 1 scoop of protein powder
- 1 teaspoon maple syrup
- 2 cups almond milk, unsweetened

Directions:

1. Place all the ingredients in the order to a food processor or blender and then pulse for 2 to 3 minutes at high speed until smooth.
2. Pour the smoothie into two glasses and then serve.

Nutrition: Calories: 324 Fat: 5g Carbs: 75.1g Protein: 7.2g Fiber: 11.3g

88.   Strawberry and Chocolate Milkshake

Preparation time: 5 minutes.
Cooking time: 0 minutes.
Servings: 2
Ingredients:

- 2 cups frozen strawberries
- 3 tablespoons cocoa powder
- 1 scoop protein powder
- 2 tablespoons maple syrup
- 1 teaspoon vanilla extract, unsweetened
- 2 cups almond milk, unsweetened

Directions:

1. Place all the ingredients in the order to a food processor or blender and then pulse for 2 to 3 minutes at high speed until smooth.
2. Pour the smoothie into two glasses and then serve.

Nutrition: Calories: 199 Fat: 4.1g Carbs: 40.5g Protein: 3.7g Fiber: 5.5g

89.   Trope-Kale Breeze

Preparation time: 5 minutes.
Cooking time: 0 minutes.
Servings: 3 to 4 cups.
Ingredients:

- 1 cup chopped pineapple (frozen or fresh)
- 1 cup chopped mango (frozen or fresh)
- ½ to 1 cup chopped kale
- ½ avocado
- ½ cup coconut milk
- 1 cup water, or coconut water
- 1 teaspoon matcha green tea powder (optional)

Directions:

1. Purée everything to a blender until smooth, adding more water (or coconut milk) if needed.

Nutrition: Calories: 566 Fat: 36g Carbs: 66g Fiber: 12g Protein: 8g

90.   Zobo Drink

Preparation time: 5 minutes.
Cooking time: 10 minutes.
Servings: 8
Ingredients:

- 2 cups dried hibiscus petals (zobo leaves), rinsed
- Pineapple rind from 1 pineapple
- 1 cup of granulated sugar
- 1 teaspoon fresh ginger, grated
- 10 cups of water

Directions:

1. Add water, ginger, and sugar into the pot and mix well.
2. Then add zobo leaves and pineapple rind.
3. Cover and cook on High for 10 minutes. Open and discard solids. Chill and serve.

Nutrition: Calories: 65 Carbs: 7g Fat: 2.6g Protein: 1.14g

91.   Basil Lime Green Tea

Preparation time: 5 minutes.
Cooking time: 4 minutes.
Servings: 8
Ingredients:

- 8 cups of filtered water
- 10 bags of green tea
- ¼ cup of honey
- A pinch of baking soda
- Lime slices to taste
- Lemon slices to taste
- Basil leaves to taste

Directions:

1. Add water, honey, and baking soda to the pot and mix. Add the tea bags and cover. Cook on High for 4 minutes. Open and serve with lime slices, lemon slices, and basil leaves.

Nutrition: Calories: 32 Carbs: 8g Fat: 0g Protein: 0g

92.   Berry Lemonade Tea

Preparation time: 5 minutes.
Cooking time: 12 minutes.
Servings: 4
Ingredients:

- 3 tea bags
- 2 cups of natural lemonade
- 1 cup of frozen mixed berries
- 2 cups of water
- 1 lemon, sliced

Directions:
1. Put everything in the Instant Pot and cover. Cook on High for 12 minutes. Open, strain, and serve.

Nutrition: Calories: 21 Carbs: 8g Fat: 0.2g Protein: 0.4g

93. Turmeric Coconut Milk

Preparation time: 5 minutes.
Cooking time: 15 minutes.
Servings: 8
Ingredients:
- 13.5 ounces' coconut milk
- 3 cups filtered water
- 2 teaspoons turmeric powder
- 3 whole cloves
- 2 cinnamon sticks
- ½ teaspoon ginger powder
- A pinch of pepper
- 2 tablespoons honey

Directions:
1. Place everything except the honey in the pot. Cover and cook on High for 15 minutes. Remove cloves and cinnamon sticks. Add honey, mix and serve.

Nutrition: Calories: 42 Carbs: 9g Fat: 0g Protein: 0g

94. Swedish Glögg

Preparation time: 5 minutes.
Cooking time: 15 minutes.
Servings: 1
Ingredients:
- ½ cup of orange juice
- ½ cup of water
- 1 piece of ginger cut into ½ pieces
- 1 whole clove
- 1 opened cardamom pods
- 2 tablespoons orange zest
- 1 cinnamon stick
- 1 whole allspice
- 1 vanilla bean

Directions:
1. Add everything in the pot. Cover and cook on High for 15 minutes. Open and serve.

Nutrition: Calories: 194 Carbs: 41g Fat: 3g Protein: 1.7g

95. Kale Smoothie

Preparation time: 5 minutes.
Cooking time: 0 minutes.
Servings: 2
Ingredients:
- 2 cups chopped kale leaves
- 1 banana, peeled
- 1 cup frozen strawberries
- 1 cup unsweetened almond milk
- 4 Medjool dates, pitted and chopped

Directions:
1. Put all the ingredients to a food processor, then blitz until glossy and smooth.
2. Serve immediately or chill in the refrigerator for an hour before serving.

Nutrition: Calories: 663 Fat: 10.0g Carbs: 142.5g Fiber: 19.0g Protein: 17.4g

96. Hot Tropical Smoothie

Preparation time: 5 minutes.
Cooking time: 0 minutes.
Servings: 4
Ingredients:
- 1 cup frozen mango chunks
- 1 cup frozen pineapple chunks
- 1 small tangerine, peeled and pitted
- 2 cups spinach leaves
- 1 cup coconut water
- ¼ teaspoon cayenne pepper, optional

Directions:
1. Add all the ingredients to a food processor, then blitz until the mixture is smooth and combine well.
2. Serve immediately or chill in the refrigerator for an hour before serving.

Nutrition: Calories: 283 Fat: 1.9g Carbs: 67.9g Fiber: 10.4g Protein: 6.4g

97. Cranberry and Banana Smoothie

Preparation time: 5 minutes.
Cooking time: 0 minutes.
Servings: 4
- 1 cup frozen cranberries
- 1 large banana, peeled
- 4 Medjool dates, pitted and chopped
- 1(½) cups unsweetened almond milk

Directions:
1. Add all the ingredients to a food processor, then process until the mixture is glossy and well mixed.
2. Serve immediately or chill in the refrigerator for an hour before serving.

Nutrition: Calories: 616 Fat: 8.0g Carbs: 132.8g Fiber: 14.6g Protein: 15.7g

98. Super Smoothie

Preparation time: 5 minutes.
Cooking time: 0 minutes.
Servings: 4
Ingredients:
- 1 banana, peeled
- 1 cup chopped mango
- 1 cup raspberries
- ¼ cup rolled oats
- 1 carrot, peeled
- 1 cup chopped fresh kale
- 2 tablespoons chopped fresh parsley
- 1 tablespoon flaxseeds
- 1 tablespoon grated fresh ginger
- ½ cup unsweetened soy milk
- 1 cup water

Directions:
1. Put all the ingredients to a food processor, then blitz until glossy and smooth.
2. Serve immediately or chill in the refrigerator for an hour before serving.

Nutrition: Calories: 550 Fat: 39.0g Carbs: 31.0g Fiber: 15.0g Protein: 13.0g

99. Kiwi and Strawberry Smoothie

Preparation time: 5 minutes.
Cooking time: 0 minutes.
Servings: 3
Ingredients:

- 1 kiwi, peeled
- 5 medium strawberries
- ½ frozen banana
- 1 cup unsweetened almond milk
- 2 tablespoons hemp seeds
- 1 to 2 teaspoons maple syrup
- ½ cup spinach leaves
- Handful broccoli sprouts

Directions:

1. Put all the ingredients to a food processor, then blitz until creamy and smooth.
2. Serve immediately or chill in the refrigerator for an hour before serving.

Nutrition: Calories: 562 Fat: 28.6g Carbs: 63.6g Fiber: 15.1g Protein: 23.3g

100. Banana and Chai Chia Smoothie

Preparation time: 5 minutes.
Cooking time: 0 minutes.
Servings: 3
Ingredients:

- 1 banana
- 1 cup alfalfa sprouts
- 1 tablespoon chia seeds
- ½ cup unsweetened coconut milk
- 1 to 2 soft Medjool dates, pitted
- ¼ teaspoon ground cinnamon
- 1 tablespoon grated fresh ginger
- 1 cup water
- Pinch ground cardamom

Directions:

1. Add all the ingredients to a blender, then process until the mixture is smooth and creamy. Add water or coconut milk if necessary. Serve immediately.

Nutrition: Calories:477 Fat: 41.0g Carbs: 31.0g Fiber: 14.0g Protein: 8.0g

101. Summer Smoothie

Preparation Time: 5 Minutes
Cooking Time: 5 minutes
Servings 1
Ingredients:

- 1/2 cup Greek yogurt
- 2 cups raspberries
- 1 nectarine
- 1 cup ice

Directions

1. In a blender merge all ingredients and blend until smooth
2. Pour smoothie in a glass and serve

Nutrition: Calories: 140 Carbs: 7g Fat: 13g Fiber: 3g Protein: 1g

102. Green Smoothie

Preparation Time: 5 Minutes
Cooking Time: 5 minutes
Servings 1
Ingredients:

- 1 cup almond milk
- 1 tablespoon honey
- 1 banana
- 2 cups spinach
- 1/4 cucumber

Directions

1. In a blender merge all ingredients and blend until smooth
2. Pour smoothie in a glass and serve

Nutrition Calories: 238 Fat: 12g Protein: 1g Sodium 4mg Fiber: 5g Carbs: 35g Sugar: 27g

103. Tropical Smoothie

Preparation Time: 5 Minutes
Cooking Time: 5 minutes
Servings 1
Ingredients:

- 1 banana
- 1 pineapple
- 1 cup mango
- 1 cup almond milk

Directions

1. In a blender merge all ingredients and blend until smooth
2. Pour smoothie in a glass and serve

Nutrition: Calories: 191 Fat: 14g Protein: 5g Sodium 3mg Fiber: 7g Carbs: 13g Sugar: 2g

104. Berry Smoothie

Preparation Time: 5 Minutes
Cooking Time: 5 minutes
Servings 1
Ingredients:

- 1 banana
- 4 cups pineapple juice
- 1 cup ice
- 4 oz. blueberries
- 4 oz. blackberries
- 1 tablespoon honey

Directions

1. In a blender merge all ingredients and blend until smooth
2. Pour smoothie in a glass and serve

Nutrition: Calories: 193 Fat: 14g Protein: 1g Sodium: 15mg Fiber: 3g Carbs: 18g

105. Citrus Smoothie

Preparation Time: 5 Minutes
Cooking Time: 5 minutes
Servings 1
Ingredients:

- 1 cup carrot juice
- 1 banana
- 1 cup pineapple juice
- 1 cup ice

Directions

1. In a blender merge all ingredients and blend until smooth
2. Pour smoothie in a glass and serve

Nutrition; Calories: 101 Fat: 0g Protein: 1g Sodium: 2mg Fiber: 5g Carbs: 27g

106. Pomegranate Smoothie

Preparation Time: 5 Minutes
Cooking Time: 5 minutes
Servings 1
Ingredients:

- 1 cup pomegranate juice
- 1 cup yogurt
- 1 cup berries
- 1 cup ice
- 1 cinnamon

Directions

1. In a blender merge all ingredients and blend until smooth
2. Pour smoothie in a glass and serve

Nutrition Calories: 97 Fat: 0g Protein: 3g Sodium: 36mg Fiber: 6g Carbs: 23g Sugar: 10g

107. Mango Smoothie

Preparation Time: 5 Minutes
Cooking Time: 5 minutes
Servings 1
Ingredients:

- 1 cup orange juice
- 1/4 cup vanilla yogurt
- 1 cup mango
- 1 carrot
- 1 cup Ice

DIRECTIONS

1. In a blender merge all ingredients and blend until smooth
2. Pour smoothie in a glass and serve

Nutrition: Calories: 367 Fat: 24.9g Saturated Fat: 15.1g Protein: 26.6g Carbs: 13.7g Fiber: 3.6g Sugar: 7g

108. Green Citrus Smoothie

Preparation Time: 10 Minutes
Cooking Time: 0 Minutes
Servings: 2
Ingredients:

- 1 cup chopped watercress
- 1 large grapefruit, peeled
- 2 medium oranges, peeled
- 1 medium banana, peeled
- 1 cup water, divided

Directions:

1. Place watercress, grapefruit, oranges, banana, and 1/2 cup water in a blender and blend until thoroughly combined.
2. Add remaining water while blending until desired texture is achieved.

Nutrition: Calories 162 Fat 1g Protein 3g Sodium 7mg Fiber 7g Carbs 41g Sugar 27g

109. Cherry Pear Smoothie

Preparation Time: 10 Minutes
Cooking Time: 0 Minutes
Servings: 2
Ingredients:

- 1 cup chopped iceberg lettuce
- 2 medium pears, cored
- 1 medium banana, peeled
- 1/2 cup pitted cherries
- 1/2 teaspoon vanilla bean pulp
- 2 cups unsweetened vanilla almond milk, divided

Directions:

1. Place lettuce, pears, banana, cherries, vanilla bean pulp, and 1 cup almond milk in a blender and blend until thoroughly combined.
2. Add remaining almond milk while blending until desired texture is achieved.

Nutrition: Calories 216 Fat 3g Protein 3g Sodium 175mg Fiber 8g Carbs 48g Sugar 30g

110. Apple Peach Smoothie

Preparation Time: 10 Minutes
Cooking Time: 0 Minutes
Servings: 2
Ingredients:

- 2 tablespoons rolled oats
- 1 cup chopped watercress
- 2 medium peaches, pitted
- 2 medium apples, cored and peeled
- 2 cups unsweetened vanilla almond milk, divided

Directions:

1. Place oats, watercress, peaches, apples, and 1 cup almond milk in a blender and blend until thoroughly combined.
2. Add remaining almond milk while blending until desired texture is achieved.

Nutrition: Calories 198 Fat 4g Protein 4g Sodium 172mg Fiber 7g Carbs 43g Sugar 31g

111. Zucchini Apple Smoothie

Preparation Time: 10 Minutes
Cooking Time: 0 Minutes
Servings: 2
Ingredients:

- 1 cup spinach
- 1 medium zucchini, chopped
- 3 medium carrots, peeled and chopped
- 2 medium apples, cored and peeled
- 2 cups water, divided

Directions:

1. Place spinach, zucchini, carrots, apples, and 1 cup water in a blender and blend until thoroughly combined.
2. Add remaining water while blending until desired texture is achieved.

Nutrition: Calories 163 Fat 1g Protein 4g Sodium 90mg Fiber 9g Carbs 40g Sugar 28g

112. Farmers' Market Smoothie

Preparation Time: 10 Minutes
Cooking Time: 0 Minutes
Servings: 2
Ingredients:

- 1 cup chopped romaine lettuce
- 2 medium tomatoes
- 1 medium zucchini, chopped
- 2 medium stalks celery, chopped
- 1 medium cucumber, chopped
- 1/2 cup chopped green onions
- 2 cloves garlic, peeled
- 2 cups water, divided

Directions:

1. Place romaine, tomatoes, zucchini, celery, cucumber, green onions, garlic, and 1 cup water in a blender and blend until thoroughly combined.
2. Add remaining 1 cup water, if needed, while blending until desired texture is achieved.

Nutrition: Calories 86 Fat 1g Protein 5g Sodium 59mg Fiber 6g Carbs 17g Sugar 11g

113. Sweet Asparagus Smoothie

Preparation Time: 10 Minutes
Cooking Time: 0 Minutes
Servings: 2
Ingredients:

- 1 cup chopped watercress
- 1 cup chopped asparagus
- 1 small lemon, peeled
- 1 large orange, peeled
- 1 cup water, divided

Directions:

1. Place watercress, asparagus, lemon, orange, and 1/2 cup water in a blender and blend until thoroughly combined.
2. Add remaining water while blending until desired texture is achieved.

Nutrition: Calories 65 Fat 0g Protein 3g Sodium 9mg Fiber 4g Carbs 16g Sugar 10g

114. Orange Broccoli Smoothie

Preparation Time: 10 Minutes
Cooking Time: 0 Minutes
Servings: 2
Ingredients:

- 1 cup chopped romaine lettuce
- 1 cup chopped broccoli
- 1 medium zucchini, chopped
- 2 medium carrots, peeled and chopped
- 2 cups water, divided

Directions:

1. Place romaine, broccoli, zucchini, carrots, and 1 cup water in a blender and blend until thoroughly combined.
2. Add remaining water while blending until desired texture is achieved.

Nutrition: Calories 71 Fat 1g Protein 4g Sodium 72mg Fiber 5g Carbs 15g Sugar 8g

115. Sweet Citrus Smoothie

Preparation Time: 10 Minutes
Cooking Time: 0 Minutes
Servings: 2
Ingredients:

- 1 cup chopped watercress
- 1 large grapefruit, peeled
- 2 medium oranges, peeled
- 1 (1/2) piece gingerroot, peeled
- 1/2 medium lemon, peeled
- 1 cup water, divided

Directions:

1. Place watercress, grapefruit, oranges, gingerroot, lemon, and 1/2 cup water in a blender and blend until thoroughly combined.
2. Add remaining water while blending until desired texture is achieved.

Nutrition: Calories 136 Fat 0g Protein 3g Sodium 7mg Fiber 7g Carbs 35g Sugar 24g

116. The Green Go-Getter Smoothie

Preparation Time: 10 Minutes
Cooking Time: 0 Minutes
Servings: 1
Ingredients:

- 1 cup spinach
- 2 medium green apples, peeled and cored
- 1/2 medium banana, peeled
- 1 cup water, divided

Directions:

1. Place spinach, apples, banana, and 1/2 cup water in a blender and blend until thoroughly combined.
2. Continue adding remaining water while blending until desired texture is achieved.

Nutrition: Calories 241 Fat 1g Protein 2g Sodium 29mg Fiber 11g Carbs 63g Sugar 44g

117. Clementine Smoothie

Preparation Time: 5 Minutes
Cooking Time: 5 minutes
Servings 1
Ingredients:

- 4 oz. clementine juice
- 2 oz. oats
- 2 oz. blueberries
- 2 pears
- 1 tablespoon honey
- 1 tsp. mixed spice

Directions

1. In a blender merge all ingredients and blend until smooth
2. Pour smoothie in a glass and serve

Nutrition: Calories 86 Fat 1g Protein 5g Sodium 59mg Fiber 6g Carbs 17g

118. Avocado Smoothie

Preparation Time: 5 Minutes
Cooking Time: 5 minutes
Servings 1
Ingredients:

- 1 banana
- 2 tablespoons cacao powder
- 1 tsp. coconut oil
- 1 avocado
- 1 tsp. vanilla extract
- 2 tablespoons honey
- 1 cup ice

Directions

1. In a blender merge all ingredients and blend until smooth
2. Pour smoothie in a glass and serve

Nutrition: Calories: 185 Fat: 7g Protein: 3g Sodium: 309mg Fiber: 15g Carbs: 29g

119. Pear Smoothie

Preparation Time: 5 Minutes
Cooking Time: 5 minutes
Servings 1
Ingredients:

- 2 pears
- 1 banana
- 1 cup almond milk
- 1/2 cup vanilla yoghurt
- 1 tsp. cinnamon

Directions

1. In a blender merge all ingredients and blend until smooth
2. Pour smoothie in a glass and serve

Nutrition: Calories: 32 Carbs: 2g Fat: 0.1g Fiber: 1g Protein: 1g

120. Breakfast Smoothie

Preparation Time: 5 Minutes
Cooking Time: 5 minutes
Servings 1
Ingredients:

- 1 banana
- 1 tsp. coffee
- 1 tsp. cinnamon
- 1 tsp. honey
- 1 cup milk

Directions

1. In a blender merge all ingredients and blend until smooth
2. Pour smoothie in a glass and serve

Nutrition: Calories: 140 Carbs: 7g Fat: 13g Fiber: 3g Protein: 1g

121. Banana Smoothie

Preparation Time: 5 Minutes
Cooking Time: 5 minutes
Servings 1
Ingredients:

- 2 tablespoons cocoa powder
- 1 cup ice
- 1 banana
- 1 cup skimmed milk

Directions

1. In a blender merge all ingredients and blend until smooth
2. Pour smoothie in a glass and serve

Nutrition: Calories: 193 Fat: 14g Protein: 1g Sodium: 15mg Fiber: 3g Carbs: 18g Sugar: 13g

122. Green Juice Smoothie

Preparation Time: 5 Minutes
Cooking Time: 5 minutes
Servings 1
Ingredients:

- 2 apples
- 2 celery sticks
- 1 cucumber
- 1/2 cup kale leaves
- 1/4 lemon

Directions

1. In a blender merge all ingredients and blend until smooth
2. Pour smoothie in a glass and serve

Nutrition: Calories 86 Fat 1g Protein 5g Sodium 59mg Fiber 6g Carbs 17g

123. Spicy Smoothie

Preparation Time: 5 Minutes
Cooking Time: 5 minutes
Servings 1
Ingredients:

- 1 banana
- 2 oz. baby spinach
- 1 cup mango
- 1/4 tsp. jalapeno pepper
- 1 cup water

Directions

1. In a blender merge all ingredients and blend until smooth
2. Pour smoothie in a glass and serve

Nutrition: Calories 528 Fat: 39g Carbs: 25g Fiber: 9g Sugar: 10g

124. Coconut Smoothie

Preparation Time: 5 Minutes
Cooking Time: 5 minutes
Servings 1

Ingredients:

- 1 mango
- 1 banana
- 1 cup coconut milk
- 1 cup pineapple chunks
- 2 tablespoons coconut flakes

Directions

1. In a blender merge all ingredients and blend until smooth
2. Pour smoothie in a glass and serve

Nutrition: Calories: 140 Carbs: 7g Fat: 13g Fiber: 3g Protein: 1g

125. Simple Smoothie Super food

Preparation Time: 5 Minutes
Cooking Time: 5 minutes
Servings 2

Ingredients:

- 2 tsps. Chia seeds
- 1 tbsp. Matcha green tea powder
- 1 cup of fresh spinach for the baby
- 1 cup of frozen banana chopped
- 1/2 c. of chilled unpleasantly chopped almond milk
- 1 c. of fresh and fresh kale chopped
- 1/2 c. of frozen bananas chunks

Directions:

1. Pulse all ingredients smoothly in a high-speed blender.
2. Serve immediately with 2 big glasses of portion.

Nutrition: Calories 65 Fat 0g Protein 3g Sodium 9mg Fiber 4g Carbs 16g Sugar 10g

126. Classic Lentil Soup with Swiss Chard

Preparation time: 10 minutes
Cooking Time: 25 minutes
Servings: 5
Ingredients:

- 2 tablespoons olive oil
- 1 white onion, chopped
- 1 teaspoon garlic, minced
- 2 large carrots, chopped
- 1 parsnip, chopped
- 2 stalks celery, chopped
- 2 bay leaves
- 1/2 teaspoon dried thyme
- 1/4 teaspoon ground cumin
- 5 cups roasted vegetable broth
- 1 ¼ cups brown lentils, soaked overnight and rinsed
- 2 cups Swiss chard, torn into pieces

Directions:
1. In a heavy-bottomed pot, heat the olive oil over a moderate heat. Now, sauté the vegetables along with the spices for about 3 minutes until they are just tender.
2. Add in the vegetable broth and lentils, bringing it to a boil. Immediately turn the heat to a simmer and add in the bay leaves. Let it cook for about 15 minutes or until lentils are tender.
3. Add in the Swiss chard, cover and let it simmer for 5 minutes more or until the chard wilts.
4. Serve in individual bowls and enjoy!

Nutrition: Calories: 148; Fat: 7.2g; Carbs: 14.6g; Protein: 7.7g

127. Spicy Winter Farro Soup

Preparation time: 10 minutes
Cooking Time: 30 minutes
Servings: 4
Ingredients:

- 2 tablespoons olive oil
- 1 medium-sized leek, chopped
- 1 medium-sized turnip, sliced
- 2 Italian peppers, seeded and chopped
- 1 jalapeno pepper, minced
- 2 potatoes, peeled and diced
- 4 cups vegetable broth
- 1 cup farro, rinsed
- 1/2 teaspoon granulated garlic
- 1/2 teaspoon turmeric powder
- 1 bay laurel
- 2 cups spinach, turn into pieces

Directions:
1. In a heavy-bottomed pot, heat the olive oil over a moderate heat. Now, sauté the leek, turnip, peppers and potatoes for about 5 minutes until they are crisp-tender.
2. Add in the vegetable broth, farro, granulated garlic, turmeric and bay laurel; bring it to a boil.
3. Immediately turn the heat to a simmer. Let it cook for about 25 minutes or until farro and potatoes have softened.
4. Add in the spinach and remove the pot from the heat; let the spinach sit in the residual heat until it wilts. Bon appétit!

Nutrition: Calories: 298; Fat: 8.9g; Carbs: 44.6g; Protein: 11.7g

128. Rainbow Chickpea Salad

Preparation time: 15 minutes
Cooking Time: 0 minutes
Servings: 4
Ingredients:

- 16 ounces canned chickpeas, drained
- 1 medium avocado, sliced
- 1 bell pepper, seeded and sliced
- 1 large tomato, sliced
- 2 cucumbers, diced
- 1 red onion, sliced
- 1/2 teaspoon garlic, minced
- 1/4 cup fresh parsley, chopped
- 1/4 cup olive oil
- 2 tablespoons apple cider vinegar
- 1/2 lime, freshly squeezed
- Sea salt and ground black pepper, to taste

Directions:
1. Toss all the Ingredients in a salad bowl.
2. Place the salad in your refrigerator for about 1 hour before serving.
3. Bonappétit!

Nutrition: Calories: 378; Fat: 24g; Carbs: 34.2g; Protein: 10.1g

129. Roasted Asparagus and Avocado Salad

Preparation time: 10 minutes
Cooking Time: 15 minutes
Servings: 4
Ingredients:

- 1-pound asparagus, trimmed, cut into bite-sized pieces
- 1 white onion, chopped
- 2 garlic cloves, minced
- 1 Roma tomato, sliced
- 1/4 cup olive oil
- 1/4 cup balsamic vinegar
- 1 tablespoon stone-ground mustard
- 2 tablespoons fresh parsley, chopped
- 1 tablespoon fresh cilantro, chopped
- 1 tablespoon fresh basil, chopped
- Sea salt and ground black pepper, to taste
- 1 small avocado, pitted and diced
- 1/2 cup pine nuts, roughly chopped

Directions:
1. Begin by preheating your oven to 420 degrees F.
2. Toss the asparagus with 1 tablespoon of the olive oil and arrange them on a parchment-lined roasting pan.
3. Bake for about 15 minutes, rotating the pan once or twice to promote even cooking. Let it cool completely and place in your salad bowl.
4. Toss the asparagus with the vegetables, olive oil, vinegar, mustard and herbs. Salt and pepper to taste.
5. Toss to combine and top with avocado and pine nuts. Bon appétit!

Nutrition: Calories: 378; Fat: 33.2g; Carbs: 18.6g; Protein: 7.8g

130. Creamed Pinto Bean Salad with Pine Nuts

Preparation time: 10 minutes
Cooking Time: 5 minutes
Servings: 5

Ingredients:

- 1 ½ pounds pinto beans, trimmed
- 2 medium tomatoes, diced
- 2 bell peppers, seeded and diced
- 4 tablespoons shallots, chopped
- 1/2 cup pine nuts, roughly chopped
- 1/2 cup vegan mayonnaise
- 1 tablespoon deli mustard
- 2 tablespoons fresh basil, chopped
- 2 tablespoons fresh parsley, chopped
- 1/2 teaspoon red pepper flakes, crushed
- Sea salt and freshly ground black pepper, to taste

Directions:

1. Boil the pinto beans in a large saucepan of salted water until they are just tender or about 2 minutes.
2. Drain and let the beans cool completely; then, transfer them to a salad bowl. Toss the beans with the remaining ingredients.
3. Taste and adjust the seasonings. Bon appétit!

Nutrition: Calories: 308; Fat: 26.2g; Carbs: 16.6g; Protein: 5.8g

131. Cannellini Bean Soup with Kale

Preparation time: 10 minutes
Cooking Time: 25 minutes
Servings: 5

Ingredients:

- 1 tablespoon olive oil
- 1/2 teaspoon ginger, minced
- 1/2 teaspoon cumin seeds
- 1 red onion, chopped
- 1 carrot, trimmed and chopped
- 1 parsnip, trimmed and chopped
- 2 garlic cloves, minced
- 5 cups vegetable broth
- 12 ounces Cannellini beans, drained
- 2 cups kale, torn into pieces
- Sea salt and ground black pepper, to taste

Directions:

1. In a heavy-bottomed pot, heat the olive over medium-high heat. Now, sauté the ginger and cumin for 1 minute or so.
2. Now, add in the onion, carrot and parsnip; continue sautéing an additional 3 minutes or until the vegetables are just tender.
3. Add in the garlic and continue to sauté for 1 minute or until aromatic.
4. Then, pour in the vegetable broth and bring to a boil. Immediately reduce the heat to a simmer and let it cook for 10 minutes.
5. Fold in the Cannellini beans and kale; continue to simmer until the kale wilts and everything is thoroughly heated. Season with salt and pepper to taste.
6. Ladle into individual bowls and serve hot. Bon appétit!

Nutrition: Calories: 188; Fat: 4.7g; Carbs: 24.5g; Protein: 11.1g

132. Hearty Cream of Mushroom Soup

Preparation time: 10 minutes
Cooking Time: 15 minutes
Servings: 5

Ingredients:

- 2 tablespoons soy butter
- 1 large shallot, chopped
- 20 ounces Cremini mushrooms, sliced
- 2 cloves garlic, minced
- 4 tablespoons flaxseed meal
- 5 cups vegetable broth
- 1 1/3 cups full-fat coconut milk
- 1 bay leaf
- Sea salt and ground black pepper, to taste

Directions:

1. In a stockpot, melt the vegan butter over medium-high heat. Once hot, cook the shallot for about 3 minutes until tender and fragrant.
2. Add in the mushrooms and garlic and continue cooking until the mushrooms have softened. Add in the flaxseed meal and continue to cook for 1 minute or so.
3. Add in the remaining ingredients. Let it simmer, covered and continue to cook for 5 to 6 minutes more until your soup has thickened slightly.
4. Bon appétit!

Nutrition: Calories: 308; Fat: 25.5g; Carbs: 11.8g; Protein: 11.6g

133. Authentic Italian Panzanella Salad

Preparation time: 10 minutes
Cooking Time: 35 minutes
Servings: 3

Ingredients:

- 3 cups artisan bread, broken into 1-inch cubes
- 3/4-pound asparagus, trimmed and cut into bite-sized pieces
- 4 tablespoons extra-virgin olive oil
- 1 red onion, chopped
- 2 tablespoons fresh lime juice
- 1 teaspoon deli mustard
- 2 medium heirloom tomatoes, diced
- 2 cups arugula
- 2 cups baby spinach
- 2 Italian peppers, seeded and sliced
- Sea salt and ground black pepper, to taste

Directions:

1. Arrange the bread cubes on a parchment-lined baking sheet. Bake in the preheated oven at 310 degrees F for about 20 minutes, rotating the baking sheet twice during the baking time; reserve.
2. Turn the oven to 420 degrees F and toss the asparagus with 1 tablespoon of olive oil. Roast the asparagus for about 15 minutes or until crisp-tender.
3. Toss the remaining Ingredients in a salad bowl; top with the roasted asparagus and toasted bread.
4. Bon!

Nutrition: Calories: 334; Fat: 20.4g; Carbs: 33.3g; Protein: 8.3g

134. Quinoa and Black Bean Salad

Preparation time: 10 minutes
Cooking Time: 15 minutes + chilling time
Servings: 4
Ingredients:

- 2 cups water
- 1 cup quinoa, rinsed
- 16 ounces canned black beans, drained
- 2 Roma tomatoes, sliced
- 1 red onion, thinly sliced
- 1 cucumber, seeded and chopped
- 2 cloves garlic, pressed or minced
- 2 Italian peppers, seeded and sliced
- 2 tablespoons fresh parsley, chopped
- 2 tablespoons fresh cilantro, chopped
- 1/4 cup olive oil
- 1 lemon, freshly squeezed
- 1 tablespoon apple cider vinegar
- 1/2 teaspoon dried dill weed
- 1/2 teaspoon dried oregano
- Sea salt and ground black pepper, to taste

Directions:

1. Place the water and quinoa in a saucepan and bring it to a rolling boil. Immediately turn the heat to a simmer.
2. Let it simmer for about 13 minutes until the quinoa has absorbed all of the water; fluff the quinoa with a fork and let it cool completely. Then, transfer the quinoa to a salad bowl.
3. Add the remaining Ingredients to the salad bowl and toss to combine well. Bon appétit!

Nutrition: Calories: 433; Fat: 17.3g; Carbs: 57g; Protein: 15.1g

135. Rich Bulgur Salad with Herbs

Preparation time: 10 minutes
Cooking Time: 20 minutes + chilling time
Servings: 4
Ingredients:

- 2 cups water
- 1 cup bulgur
- 12 ounces canned chickpeas, drained
- 1 Persian cucumber, thinly sliced
- 2 bell peppers, seeded and thinly sliced
- 1 jalapeno pepper, seeded and thinly sliced
- 2 Roma tomatoes, sliced
- 1 onion, thinly sliced
- 2 tablespoons fresh basil, chopped
- 2 tablespoons fresh parsley, chopped
- 2 tablespoons fresh mint, chopped
- 2 tablespoons fresh chives, chopped
- 4 tablespoons olive oil
- 1 tablespoon balsamic vinegar
- 1 tablespoon lemon juice
- 1 teaspoon fresh garlic, pressed
- Sea salt and freshly ground black pepper, to taste
- 2 tablespoons nutritional yeast
- 1/2 cup Kalamata olives, sliced

Directions:

1. In a saucepan, bring the water and bulgur to a boil. Immediately turn the heat to a simmer and let it cook for about 20 minutes or until the bulgur is tender and water is almost absorbed. Fluff with a fork and spread on a large tray to let cool.
2. Place the bulgur in a salad bowl followed by the chickpeas, cucumber, peppers, tomatoes, onion, basil, parsley, mint and chives.

3. In a small mixing dish, whisk the olive oil, balsamic vinegar, lemon juice, garlic, salt and black pepper. Dress the salad and toss to combine.
4. Sprinkle nutritional yeast over the top, garnish with olives and serve at room temperature. Bon appétit!

Nutrition: Calories: 408; Fat: 18.3g; Carbs: 51.8g; Protein: 13.1g

136. Classic Roasted Pepper Salad

Preparation time: 10 minutes
Cooking Time: 15 minutes + chilling time
Servings: 3
Ingredients:

- 6 bell peppers
- 3 tablespoons extra-virgin olive oil
- 3 teaspoons red wine vinegar
- 3 garlic cloves, finely chopped
- 2 tablespoons fresh parsley, chopped
- Sea salt and freshly cracked black pepper, to taste
- 1/2 teaspoon red pepper flakes
- 6 tablespoons pine nuts, roughly chopped

Directions:

1. Broil the peppers on a parchment-lined baking sheet for about 10 minutes, rotating the pan halfway through the cooking time, until they are charred on all sides.
2. Then, cover the peppers with a plastic wrap to steam. Discard the skin, seeds and cores.
3. Slice the peppers into strips and toss them with the remaining ingredients. Place in your refrigerator until ready to serve. Bon appétit!

Nutrition: Calories: 178; Fat: 14.4g; Carbs: 11.8g; Protein: 2.4g

137. Hearty Winter Quinoa Soup

Preparation time: 10 minutes
Cooking Time: 25 minutes
Servings: 4
Ingredients:

- 2 tablespoons olive oil
- 1 onion, chopped
- 2 carrots, peeled and chopped
- 1 parsnip, chopped
- 1 celery stalk, chopped
- 1 cup yellow squash, chopped
- 4 garlic cloves, pressed or minced
- 4 cups roasted vegetable broth
- 2 medium tomatoes, crushed
- 1 cup quinoa
- Sea salt and ground black pepper, to taste
- 1 bay laurel
- 2 cup Swiss chard, tough ribs removed and torn into pieces
- 2 tablespoons Italian parsley, chopped

Directions:

1. In a heavy-bottomed pot, heat the olive over medium-high heat. Now, sauté the onion, carrot, parsnip, celery and yellow squash for about 3 minutes or until the vegetables are just tender.
2. Add in the garlic and continue to sauté for 1 minute or until aromatic.
3. Then, stir in the vegetable broth, tomatoes, quinoa, salt, pepper and bay laurel; bring to a boil. Immediately reduce the heat to a simmer and let it cook for 13 minutes.
4. Fold in the Swiss chard; continue to simmer until the chard wilts.
5. Ladle into individual bowls and serve garnished with the fresh parsley. Bon appétit!

Nutrition: Calories: 328; Fat: 11.1g; Carbs: 44.1g; Protein: 13.3g

138. Almond and Tomato Salad

Preparation time: 15 minutes
Cooking time: 10 minutes
Servings: 4
Ingredients:

- 1 cup arugula/ rocket
- 7 oz fresh tomatoes, sliced or chopped
- 2 teaspoons olive oil
- 2 cups kale
- 1/2 cup almonds

Directions:

1. Put oil into your pan and heat it on a medium heat. Add tomatoes into the pan and fry for about 10 minutes. Once cooked, allow it to cool. Combine all salad ingredients in a bowl and serve.

Nutrition: Calories 355 Fat 19.1 g Carbs 8.3 g Protein 33 g

139. Strawberry Spinach Salad

Preparation time: 15 minutes
Cooking time: 0 minutes
Servings: 4
Ingredients:

- 5 cups baby spinach
- 2 cups strawberries, sliced
- 2 tablespoons lemon juice
- 1/2 teaspoon Dijon mustard
- 1/4 cup olive oil
- 3/4 cup toasted almonds, chopped
- 1/4 red onion, sliced
- Salt, pepper, to taste

Directions:

1. Take a large bowl and mix Dijon mustard with lemon juice in it, and slowly add olive oil and combine. Season the mixture with black pepper and salt.
2. Now, mix strawberries, half cup of almonds, and sliced onion in a bowl. Pour the dressing on top and toss to combine. Serve the salad topped with almonds and vegan cheese.

Nutrition: Calories 116 Fat 3 g Carbs 13 g Protein 6 g

140. Apple Spinach Salad

Preparation time: 15 minutes
Cooking time: 0 minutes
Servings: 4
Ingredients:

- 5 ounces fresh spinach
- 1/4 red onion, sliced
- 1 apple, sliced
- 1/4 cup sliced toasted almonds

For the Dressing:

- 3 tablespoons red wine vinegar
- 1/3 cup olive oil
- 1 minced garlic clove
- 2 teaspoons Dijon mustard
- Salt, pepper, to taste

Directions:

1. Combine red wine vinegar, olive oil, garlic, and Dijon mustard in a bowl. Season with black pepper and salt.
2. In a separate bowl mix fresh spinach, apple, onion, toasted almonds. Pour the dressing on top and toss to combine. Serve

Nutrition: Calories 232 Fat 20.8 g Carbs 10 g Protein 3 g

141. Kale Power Salad

Preparation time: 15 minutes
Cooking time: 40 minutes
Servings: 2
Ingredients:

- 1 bunch kale, ribs removed and chopped
- 1/2 cup quinoa
- 1 tablespoon olive oil
- 1/2 lime, juiced
- ½ teaspoon salt
- 1 tablespoon olive oil
- 1 red rose potato, cut into small cubes
- 1 teaspoon ground cumin
- 3/4 teaspoons salt
- 1/2 teaspoon smoked paprika
- 1 lime, juiced
- 1 avocado, sliced into long strips
- 1 tablespoon olive oil
- 1 tablespoon cilantro leaves
- 1 jalapeno, deseeded, membranes removed and chopped
- salt
- ¼ cup pepitas

Directions:

1. Rinse quinoa in a running water for 2 minutes. Mix 2 cups water and rinsed quinoa in a pot, reduce heat to simmer and cook for 15 minutes.
2. Remove quinoa from heat and let rest, covered, for 5 minutes. Uncover pot, drain excess water and fluff quinoa with a fork. Let cool.
3. Warm-up olive oil in a pan over medium heat. Add chopped red rose potatoes and toss. Add smoked paprika, cumin and salt. Mix to combine.
4. Add ¼ cup water once pan is sizzling. Cover the pan then adjust heat to low. Cook for 10 minutes, stirring occasionally. Uncover pan, raise heat to medium and cook for 7 minutes. Set aside to cool.
5. Transfer kale to a bowl and add salt to it and massage with hands. Scrunch handfuls of kale in your hands. Repeat until kale is darker in color.
6. Mix 2 tablespoons olive oil, ½ teaspoon salt and 1 lime juice in a bowl. Add over the kale and toss to coat.
7. Add 2 avocados, 2 lime juices, 2 tablespoons olive oil, jalapeno, cilantro leaves and salt in a blender. Blend well and season the avocado sauce.
8. Toast pepitas in a skillet over medium low heat for 5 minutes, stirring frequently. Add quinoa to the kale bowl and toss to combine well.
9. Divide kale and quinoa mixture into 4 bowls. Top with red rose potatoes, avocado sauce, and pepitas. Enjoy!

Nutrition: Calories 250 Fat 11 g Carbs 25 g Protein 9 g

142. Falafel Kale Salad with Tahini Dressing

Preparation time: 15 minutes
Cooking time: 0 minutes
Servings: 4
Ingredients:

- 12 balls Vegan Falafels
- 6 cups kale, chopped
- 1/2 red onion, thinly sliced
- 2 slices pita bread, cut in squares
- 1 jalapeño, chopped
- Tahini Dressing
- 1-2 lemons, juiced

Directions:
1. In a mixing bowl, combine kale and lemon juice and toss well to mix. Place into the refrigerator. Divide kale among four bowls.
2. Top with three Falafel balls, red onion, jalapeño and pita slices. Top with tahini dressing and serve.

Nutrition: Calories 178 Fat 2.8 g Carbs 16 g Protein 4 g

143. Fig and Kale Salad

Preparation time: 15 minutes
Cooking time: 0 minutes
Servings: 2

Ingredients:
- 1 ripe avocado
- 2 tablespoons lemon juice
- 3 ½ oz kale, packed, stems removed and cut into large sized bits
- 1 carrot, shredded
- 1 yellow zucchini, diced
- 4 fresh figs
- ¼ cup ground flaxseed
- 1 cup mixed green leaves
- 1 teaspoon sea salt

Directions:
1. Add kale to a bowl with avocado, lemon juice and sea salt. Massage together until kale wilts. Add in zucchini, carrot and 2 cups mixed green leaves. Fold in figs and remaining ingredients. Toss and serve.

Nutrition: Calories 255 Fat 12.5 g Carbs 35 g Protein 6 g

144. Cucumber Avocado Toast

Preparation time: 15 minutes
Cooking time: 0 minutes
Servings: 2

Ingredients:
- 1 cucumber, sliced
- 2 sprouted (essene) bread slices, toasted
- ¼ handful basil leaves, chopped
- 4 tablespoons avocado, mashed
- Salt and pepper, to taste
- 1 teaspoon lemon juice

Directions:
1. Combine lemon juice together with the mashed avocado, and then spread the mixture on two bread slices.
2. Top with cucumber slices along with the finely chopped basil leaves. Generously sprinkle with salt and pepper and enjoy!

Nutrition: Calories 232 Fat 14 g Carbs 24 g Protein 5 g

145. Kale and Cucumber Salad

Preparation time: 15 minutes
Cooking time: 50 minutes
Servings: 2

Ingredients:
- 1 garlic clove
- 3 ½ oz fresh ginger
- 1/2 green Thai chili
- 1 ½ tablespoons sugar
- 1 ½ tablespoons fish sauce
- 1 ½ tablespoons vegetable oil
- 1 English cucumber, thinly sliced
- 1 bunch red Russian kale, ribs and stems removed; leaves torn into small pieces
- 1 Persian cucumber, thinly sliced

- 2 tablespoons fresh lime juice
- 1 small red onion, sliced
- 1 teaspoon sugar
- 2 tablespoons cilantro, chopped
- Salt, to taste

Directions:
1. Heat the broiler and broil ginger, with skin for 50 minutes, turning once. Let cool and slice. Blend chili, ginger, garlic, sugar, fish sauce, oil and 2 tablespoon water in a blender until paste forms.
2. Toss ¼ cup dressing and kale in a bowl and coat well. Massage with hands until kale softens.
3. Toss Persian and English cucumbers, lime juice, onion and sugar in a bowl and season with salt. Let it sit for 10 minutes.
4. Add the cucumber mixture to the bowl with kale and toss to combine. Top with cilantro and serve.

Nutrition: Calories 160 Fat 8 g Carbs 22 g Protein 3 g

146. Mexican Quinoa

Preparation time: 15 minutes
Cooking time: 8 minutes
Servings: 4

Ingredients:
- 1 cup quinoa, uncooked and rinsed
- 1 ½ cup vegetable broth
- 3 cups diced tomatoes
- 2 cups frozen corn
- 1 cup fresh parsley, chopped
- 1 onion, chopped
- 3 cloves of garlic, minced
- 2 bell peppers, chopped
- 1 tablespoon paprika powder
- ½ tablespoon cumin
- 2 tablespoons olive oil
- 2 tablespoons lime juice
- 2 green onions, chopped
- salt and pepper

Directions:
1. Place a large pot over medium heat. Add olive oil. Cook onions for 3 minutes. Add garlic, bell peppers and cook for 5 minutes.
2. Add the remaining ingredients except for lime juice, green onions and parsley. Cover and cook for about 20 minutes, keep checking to make sure the quinoa doesn't stick and burn.
3. Add lime juice, green onions and parsley. Season the dish with salt and pepper before serving.

Nutrition: Calories 231 Fat 17.8 g Carbs 19 g Protein 2 g

147. Mediterranean Parsley Salad

Preparation time: 15 minutes
Cooking time: 0 minutes
Servings: 2

Ingredients:
- ½ red onion, thinly sliced
- 1 cups parsley, chopped
- 1 Roma tomato, seeded and diced
- 6 mints, chopped
- 3 tablespoons currants, died
- 1 green chili, minced
- 1 tablespoon lemon
- 2 tablespoons olive oil
- 1/8 teaspoon sumac
- 1/8 teaspoon pepper, cracked
- ¼ teaspoon salt

Directions:
1. Mix lemon juice, olive oil, sumac, salt and pepper in a bowl and whisk to combine well. Toss parsley with the remaining ingredients in a separate bowl. Add the olive oil mixture to it and toss well and serve.

Nutrition: Calories 110 Fat 8 g Carbs 7 g Protein 1 g

148. Tomatoes Parsley Salad

Preparation time: 15 minutes
Cooking time: 0 minutes
Servings: 2
Ingredients:
- 2 cups curly parsley leaves, packed
- 1 teaspoon garlic, minced
- 3/4 cup oil-packed sundried tomatoes, drained and julienned
- 2 tablespoons olive oil
- ½ cup basil leaves
- 2 tablespoons rice vinegar
- 1 shallot, minced
- 1 garlic clove, minced
- Salt and black pepper, to taste

Directions:
1. Wash parsley, dry and add to a bowl. Add garlic and tomatoes. Toss well. Wash basil and dry it. Add it to a blender and add vinegar, oil, salt and pepper to it. Blend until smooth.
2. Add garlic and shallots to the dressing. Add the dressing over salad and toss well. Divide among 6 salad plates and serve.

Nutrition: Calories 245 Fat 19.8 g Carbs 12 g Protein 7 g

149. Lemon Parsley Quinoa Salad

Preparation time: 15 minutes
Cooking time: 0 minutes
Servings: 2
Ingredients:
- 1 tablespoon lemon juice
- 3 cups quinoa, cooked
- ¼ cup olive oil
- 1 ½ teaspoons lemon zest
- 1 cup Italian flat-leaf parsley, tightly packed
- ½ bell pepper, diced
- Salt and black pepper, to taste

Directions:
1. Cook quinoa according to package instructions. Put a splash of water and heat in a microwave. Mix lemon juice and lemon zest in a bowl and whisk in olive oil.
2. Add salt and pepper. Add parsley, rice and diced pepper. Mix well and season with salt and pepper. Enjoy!

Nutrition: Calories 207 Fat 9 g Carbs 28 g Protein 2.6 g

150. Green Lentil Salad

Preparation time: 10 minutes
Cooking Time: 20 minutes + chilling time
Servings: 5
Ingredients:
- 1 ½ cups green lentils, rinsed
- 2 cups arugula
- 2 cups Romaine lettuce, torn into pieces
- 1 cup baby spinach
- 1/4 cup fresh basil, chopped
- 1/2 cup shallots, chopped
- 2 garlic cloves, finely chopped
- 1/4 cup oil-packed sun-dried tomatoes, rinsed and chopped
- 5 tablespoons extra-virgin olive oil

- 3 tablespoons fresh lemon juice
- Sea salt and ground black pepper, to taste

Directions:
1. In a large-sized saucepan, bring 4 ½ cups of the water and red lentils to a boil.
2. Immediately turn the heat to a simmer and continue to cook your lentils for a further 15 to 17 minutes or until they've softened but not mushy. Drain and let it cool completely.
3. Transfer the lentils to a salad bowl; toss the lentils with the remaining Ingredients until well combined.
4. Serve chilled or at room temperature. Bon appétit!

Nutrition: Calories: 349; Fat: 15.1g; Carbs: 40.9g; Protein: 15.4g

151. Rainbow Fruit Salad

Preparation time: 10 minutes
Cooking time: 0 minute
Servings: 4
Ingredients:
For the Fruit Salad:
- 1 pound strawberries, hulled, sliced
- 1 cup kiwis, halved, cubed
- 1 1/4 cups blueberries
- 1 1/3 cups blackberries
- 1 cup pineapple chunks

For the Maple Lime Dressing:
- 2 teaspoons lime zest
- 1/4 cup maple syrup
- 1 tablespoon lime juice

Directions:
1. Prepare the salad, and for this, take a bowl, place all its ingredients and toss until mixed. Set the dressing, and for this, take a small bowl, place all its ingredients and whisk well. Drizzle the dressing over salad, toss until coated and serve.

Nutrition: Calories: 180 Fat: 10 g Protein: 2 g Carbs: 19 g Fiber: 2 g

152. Turkish Tuna with Bulgur and Chickpea Salad

Preparation time: 10 minutes
Cooking time: 30 minutes
Servings: 4
Ingredients:
- 16 oz. tuna, 4 steaks
- 1/2 cup bulgur
- 12 oz. chickpeas
- 4 teaspoons lemon zest, grated
- 1/4 cup Italian parsley, chopped
- 1/4 cup extra-virgin olive oil
- 1/4 teaspoon ground pepper
- 1/2 teaspoon salt

Directions:
1. Boil water and keep the bulgur in your bowl.
2. Add 2 inches of the water.
3. Mix your bulgur with 1 tablespoon of oil, pepper, salt, and the lemon zest.
4. Add the chickpeas and parsley.
5. Stir well to combine.
6. Now heat the remaining oil in your skillet over medium heat.
7. Add the tuna. Sear both sides until they become brown.

8. The tuna should flake easily with your fork. Transfer to a plate.
9. In the meantime, bring together 1/4 teaspoon salt and the remaining lemon zest in a bowl.
10. Transfer your tuna fish to a serving platter.
11. Sprinkle lemon zest and serve with the bulgur.

Nutrition: Calories 459 Carbs 43g Fiber 8g, Sugar 0.2g, Cholesterol 44mgFat 16g Protein 36g

153. Watermelon and Arugula Salad

Preparation time: 10 Minutes
Cooking time: 40 minutes
Servings: 6
Ingredients:

- 4 cups watermelon, cut in 1-inch cubes
- 3 cup arugula
- 1 lemon, zested
- 1/2 cup feta cheese, crumbled
- 1/4 cup fresh mint, chopped
- 1 tbsp. fresh lemon juice
- 3 tbsp. olive oil
- Fresh ground black pepper
- Salt to taste

Directions:
1. Combine oil, zest, juice and mint in a large bowl. Stir together.
2. Add watermelon and gently toss to coat. Add remaining Ingredients and toss to combine. Taste and adjust seasoning as desired.
3. Seal and chill at least 1 hour before serving.

Nutrition: Calories 148 Carbs 10g Protein 4g Fat 11g Sugar 7g Fiber 1g

154. Beet and Orange Salad

Preparation time: 10 Minutes
Cooking time: 0 minutes
Servings: 3
Ingredients:

- 2 oranges, peeled, seeded and sectioned
- 2 beets, trimmed, peeled and sliced
- 4 cups fresh arugula
- 3 tablespoons olive oil
- 2 tablespoon balsamic vinegar
- Salt, as required

Directions:
1. In a large bowl, merge all ingredients and gently, toss to coat.
2. Serve immediately.

Nutrition: Calories: 216 Fat: 14.5g Saturated Fat: 2.1g Protein: 3g Carbs: 22.1g Fiber: 4.7g Sugar: 17.4g

155. Broccoli and Carrot Salad

Preparation time: 10 Minutes
Cooking time: 0 minutes
Servings: 2
Ingredients:

- 1 small head broccoli with stem
- 2 medium carrots, peeled and spiralized with Blade C
- 1/4 cup red onion, chopped
- 3 hard-boiled organic eggs, chopped
- 1/4 cup fresh basil, chopped

- 1 garlic clove, minced
- 1/2 teaspoon lime zest, grated freshly
- 2 tablespoons extra-virgin olive oil
- 1 tablespoon fresh lime juice
- Water, as required
- Salt and ground black pepper, as required
- 2 tablespoons pumpkin seeds, roasted

Directions:
1. Cut the broccoli florets into bite-sized pieces.
2. Spiralized the stem with Blade C.
3. Transfer the chopped broccoli florets and spiralized stem into a large serving bowl.
4. Add the carrot, onion and egg into the bowl with broccoli and mix.
5. In a food processor, attach remaining ingredients except pumpkin seeds and pulse until well combined.
6. Pour mixture over vegetables and gently, toss to coat.
7. Garnish with pumpkin seeds and serve.

Nutrition: Calories: 329 Fat: 24.9g Saturated Fat: 8.6g Protein: 14.1g Carbs: 16.7g Fiber: 4.9g Sugar: 6g

156. Zoodles and Radish Salad

Preparation time: 10 Minutes
Cooking time: 0 minutes
Servings: 4
Ingredients:

- 2 tablespoons fresh lemon juice
- 2 teaspoons fresh lemon zest, grated
- 1/2 teaspoon Dijon mustard
- 1/2 teaspoon garlic powder
- Salt and ground black pepper, as required
- 1/3 cup olive oil
- 3 medium zucchinis, spiralized with Blade C
- 1 bunch radishes, thinly sliced

Directions:
1. For dressing: in a small bowl, attach the lemon juice, lemon zest, Dijon mustard, garlic powder, salt and black pepper and merge until well combined.
2. Slowly, add the oil, beating continuously until well combined.
3. In a large bowl, add the zucchini noodles, radishes and dressing and toss to coat well.
4. Serve immediately.

Nutrition: Calories: 178 Fat: 17.2g Saturated Fat: 2.5g Protein: 2.2g Carbs: 6.9g Fiber: 2.4g Sugar: 3.6g

157. Greens Salad

Preparation time: 10 Minutes
Cooking time: 20 minutes
Servings: 6
Ingredients:

- 11/2 teaspoons fresh ginger, grated finely
- 2 tablespoons apple cider vinegar
- 3 tablespoons olive oil
- 1 teaspoon sesame oil, toasted
- 3 teaspoons raw honey, divided
- 1/2 teaspoon red pepper flakes, divided
- Salt, as required

- 1 tablespoon water
- 2 tablespoons raw sunflower seeds
- 1 tablespoon raw pumpkin seeds, shelled
- 1 tablespoon raw sesame seeds
- 10 ounces mixed salad greens

Directions:

1. For dressing in a bowl, add the ginger, vinegar, both oils, 1 teaspoon of honey, 1/4 teaspoon of the red pepper flakes and salt and beat until well combined.
2. Set aside.
3. In another bowl, add the remaining honey, remaining red pepper flakes and water and mix until well combined.
4. Warmth a medium nonstick skillet over medium heat and cook all the seeds for about 3 minutes, stirring continuously.
5. Stir in the honey mixture and cook for about 3 minutes, stirring continuously.
6. Transfer the seeds mixture onto a parchment paper and set aside to cool completely.
7. Break the seeds mixture into small pieces.
8. In a large bowl, add the greens, 2 teaspoons of the dressing and a little salt and toss to coat well.
9. With your hands, rub the greens for about 30 seconds.
10. Add the remaining dressing and seeds pieces and toss to coat well.
11. Serve immediately.

Nutrition: Calories: 153 Fat: 14.6g Saturated Fat: 2.1g Protein: 2.2g Carbs: 8.4g Fiber: 0.6g Sugar: 4.4g

158. Quinoa and Mango Salad

Preparation time: 10 Minutes
Cooking time: 15 minutes
Servings: 2
Ingredients:

- 1 large cucumber, spiralized with Blade C
- 1/2 cup mango, peeled, pitted and cubed
- 1/2 cup cooked quinoa
- 1/4 cup dried cranberries
- 3 tablespoons raw pumpkin seeds, shelled
- 1/2 teaspoon fresh ginger, grated
- 1-2 fresh basil leaves, chopped
- Salt and ground black pepper, as required
- 3 teaspoons balsamic vinegar
- 3 teaspoons extra-virgin olive oil

Directions

1. In a large serving bowl, attach all the ingredients and toss to coat well.
2. Serve immediately.

Nutrition: Calories: 345 Fat: 15.9g Saturated Fat: 2.5g Protein: 10.6g Carbs: 42.9g Fiber: 5.5g Sugar: 8.8g

159. Beef and Plum Salad

Preparation time: 15 Minutes
Cooking time: 10 minutes
Servings: 4
Ingredients:

- 4 teaspoons fresh lemon juice, divided
- 1 1/2 tablespoons extra-virgin olive oil, divided
- Salt and ground black pepper, as required
- 1 pound grass-fed flank steak, trimmed
- Cooking spray, as required
- 1 teaspoon raw honey
- 8 cups fresh baby arugula
- 3 plums, pitted and sliced thinly

Directions

1. In a large bowl, place 1 teaspoon of lemon juice, 1 1/2 teaspoons of oil, salt and black pepper and mix well.
2. Add the steak and coat with mixture generously.
3. Grease a nonstick skillet with a little cooking spray and heat over medium-high heat.
4. Add the beef steak and cook for about 5-6 minutes per side.
5. Set the steak onto a cutting board and set aside for about 10 minutes before slicing.
6. With a sharp knife, cut the beef steak diagonally across grain in desired size slices.
7. In a large bowl, add the remaining lemon juice, oil, honey, sea salt and black pepper and beat well.
8. Add the arugula and toss well.
9. Divide arugula onto 4 serving plates.
10. Top with beef slices and plum slices evenly and serve.

Nutrition: Calories: 304 Fat: 15.1g Saturated Fat: 4.7g Protein: 33g Fiber: 1.3g Sugar: 7.6g

160. Salmon and Veggie Salad

Preparation time: 10 Minutes
Cooking time: 15 minutes
Servings: 2
Ingredients:

- 6 ounces grilled wild salmon, cut into bite-sized pieces
- 1 medium zucchini, spiralized with Blade C
- 1 medium cucumber, peeled and spiralized with Blade C
- 1/2 cup celery stalk, chopped
- 1/2 cup unsweetened coconut milk
- 1 small garlic clove, minced
- Salt and ground black pepper, as required
- 2 organic hard-boiled large eggs, peeled and chopped

Directions:

1. In a large serving bowl, mix together salmon, zucchini, cucumber and celery.
2. In another bowl, add the coconut milk, garlic and seasoning and mix until well combined.
3. Pour the coconut milk mixture over vegetables and gently, toss to coat.
4. Top with chopped eggs and serve.

Nutrition: Calories: 367 Fat: 24.9g Saturated Fat: 15.1g Protein: 26.6g Carbs: 13.7g Fiber: 3.6g Sugar: 7g

161. Carrot Apple Salad with Orange Dressing and Walnuts

Preparation time: 10 Minutes
Cooking time: 0 minutes
Servings: 6
Ingredients:

- 500 g carrots
- 1 large red apple
- 4 tbsp. walnuts

For the dressing:

- 5 tbsp. oil
- 3 tbsp. vinegar
- 1 orange
- 1 cm fresh ginger
- some salt and pepper

Directions

1. For the dressing, squeeze the orange in a large bowl. Grate the ginger and add it.
2. Add oil, vinegar, salt and pepper and stir everything well.
3. Peel the carrots
4. Wash, peel and core the apple.
5. Grate the carrots and apple directly into a bowl. Mix everything together and let it steep in the refrigerator for 30 minutes.
6. Roughly chop walnuts and sprinkle over the salad when serving.

Nutrition: Calories: 121 Fat: 8.3g Carbs: 11.2g Protein: 2.8g

162. Bruschetta

Preparation time: 10 Minutes
Cooking time: 5 minutes
Servings: 6
Ingredients:

- 4 spring onions or spring onions
- 2 cloves of garlic
- 1 pot of fresh oregano
- 1 pot of fresh basil
- 3 teaspoons of vegetable oil
- 8 tomatoes
- 1 stick of baguette

Directions:

1. Cut into the tomatoes and put them in boiling water for a short time, then remove the skin.
2. After you have peeled off the skin, the tomatoes are pitted and cut into small pieces.
3. Pluck the leaves from the basil and oregano bushes and chop them into small pieces.
4. Chop the spring onions and the garlic into small pieces.
5. Put everything in a bowl and add the oil.
6. Season to taste with salt.
7. Cut the baguette into slices and fry in a pan with oil until crispy.
8. Cover it with the salad immediately afterwards. Serve immediately.

Nutrition: Calories: 165 Fat: 9 g Carbs: 3 g Protein: 9 g

163. Rocket, carrot and mango salad

Preparation time: 10 Minutes
Cooking time: 5 minutes
Servings: 6
Ingredients:

- 125 g rocket
- 2 carrots
- 3/4 ripe mangoes
- possibly pine nuts
- 3 tbsp. olive oil
- 3 tbsp. light balsamic vinegar
- some nutmeg
- salt and pepper
- Salad herbs, freeze-dried or fresh

Directions

1. Carefully wash the rocket in cold water and spin dry with a salad spinner.
2. Grate the carrots as finely as possible.
3. Dice the mango meat
4. Put the rocket, carrots and mango in a bowl.
5. Mix a dressing from the oil, vinegar, the spices and herbs, pour over the colorful salad and mix well. If desired, lightly toast the pine nuts in a pan and pour over the salad before serving. Caution: after a certain moment, they burn up very quickly. Always watch and stir the pine nuts.

Nutrition: Calories: 323 Fat: 11 g Carbs: 6 g Protein: 14.3 g

164. Tabbouleh

Preparation time: 10 Minutes
Cooking time: 5 minutes
Servings: 6
Ingredients:

- 200 g fine-grain bulgur
- 6 tomatoes
- 1 cucumber
- 4 spring onions
- 1 handful of freshly chopped parsley
- 1 handful of freshly chopped peppermint
- 1 lemons
- 2 tbsp. olive oil
- salt and pepper

Directions:

1. Set boiling water over the tomatoes, peels them and cut into small cubes.
2. Peel and core the cucumber and cut into small cubes.
3. Cut the spring onion into thin slices.
4. Mix the tomatoes, cucumber and spring onions with the parsley and mint.
5. Add lemon juice and olive oil.
6. Merge everything and season with salt and pepper.
7. Mix in the bulgur.
8. Chill for four hours and let it steep. Stir well 2-3 times in between.

Nutrition: Calories 148 Carbs 10g Protein 4g Fat 11g Sugar 7g Fiber 1g

165. Savory pickled sun-dried tomatoes

Preparation time: 10 Minutes
Cooking time: 5 minutes
Servings: 6
Ingredients:

- 400 g of dried tomato without oil
- 1 bunch of basil
- 1 bunch of parsley
- 2 tbsp. capers in brine
- 1 tbsp. sweet paprika powder
- 1 teaspoon hot chili powder
- 1 teaspoon turmeric
- 2 cloves of garlic
- 1 dash of vinegar
- 200 ml of olive oil
- Screw jars or canning jars

Directions:

1. Try the tomatoes first. If they are already very salty, soak the tomatoes in water for 20-30 minutes at room temperature and then rinse them well.
2. Set the tomatoes in a saucepan, cover them with just a little water and add a dash of vinegar. Set to a boil and cook for two minutes. Pour into a sieve and drain well.
3. Set the basil leaves from the stems and finely chop the parsley.
4. Drain the capers and roughly chop them.
5. Peel the garlic cloves and cut into wafer-thin slices.
6. Put tomatoes, herbs, capers and garlic in a bowl and mix well together with the paprika, chili and turmeric powder.
7. Place the tomatoes flat in glasses and squeeze them lightly. Set up with olive oil so that the tomatoes are covered. Screw on glasses.
8. Let it steep for about a week. Finished!

Nutrition: Calories: 323 Fat: 11 g Carbs: 6 g Protein: 14.3 g

166. Pea salad with avocado and mint

Preparation time: 10 Minutes
Cooking time: 5 minutes
Servings: 4
Ingredients:

- 500 g fresh peas
- 1 avocado
- 5 fresh mint leaves
- 1 splash of fresh lemon juice
- salt and pepper
- olive oil

Directions:

1. Steam or stew the peas until they are firm to the bite. Then let it cool down.
2. Peel the avocado and cut into cubes
3. Put the peas and avocado in a bowl.
4. Add pepper, salt, olive oil, lemon juice and finely chopped mint and mix carefully.

Nutrition: Calories: 195 Fat: 14.1g Carbs: 13.2g Protein: 3.9g

167. Avocado - salsa with jacket potatoes

Preparation time: 10 Minutes
Cooking time: 5 minutes
Servings: 4
Ingredients:

- 8 waxy potatoes
- 2 ripe avocados
- 1 lemon juice
- 1 shallot
- 1/2 green chili pepper or some cayenne pepper
- 1 ripe tomato
- 2 sprigs of coriander green
- flat leaf parsley
- some chives
- salt and pepper
- Salt water

Directions:

1. Boil the potatoes in salted water. Depending on your taste, the peel may or may not stay on the potatoes.
2. Skin the avocados and then mash them with a fork.
3. Cut the shallot and the tomato into small cubes. Also cut the chili and herbs into small pieces.
4. Mix everything together and season with salt, pepper and the juice of one lemon. Serve as a dip with the potatoes.

Nutrition: Calories 282 Fat 17g Total Carbs 5 gTotal Sugars 0.5g Protein 11.9g

168. Mediterranean zucchini

Preparation time: 10 Minutes
Cooking time: 5 minutes
Servings: 2
Ingredients:

- 1 medium zucchini
- 2 cloves of garlic
- 1 lemon
- salt and pepper
- Paprika powder, noble sweet
- olive oil
- possibly frozen herbs (8 herbs)

Directions:

1. Cut the zucchini into thick slices and place them in a bowl.
2. Squeeze the lemon and pour over the zucchini. Peel and press the garlic cloves or cut into small cubes and mix with a little olive oil. Season with salt, pepper and paprika.
3. Add herbs as desired. Mix well and let steep for about 1 hour.
4. Fry the zucchini slices on the grill or in a pan.

Nutrition: Calories: 121 Fat: 8.3g Carbs: 11.2g Protein: 2.8g

169. Acorn Squash, Chickpea and Couscous Soup

Preparation time: 10 minutes
Cooking Time: 20 minutes
Servings: 4

Ingredients:

- 2 tablespoons olive oil
- 1 shallot, chopped
- 1 carrot, trimmed and chopped
- 2 cups acorn squash, chopped
- 1 stalk celery, chopped
- 1 teaspoon garlic, finely chopped
- 1 teaspoon dried rosemary, chopped
- 1 teaspoon dried thyme, chopped
- 2 cups cream of onion soup
- 2 cups water
- 1 cup dry couscous
- Sea salt and ground black pepper, to taste
- 1/2 teaspoon red pepper flakes
- 6 ounces canned chickpeas, drained
- 2 tablespoons fresh lemon juice

Directions:

1. In a heavy-bottomed pot, heat the olive over medium-high heat. Now, sauté the shallot, carrot, acorn squash and celery for about 3 minutes or until the vegetables are just tender.
2. Add in the garlic, rosemary and thyme and continue to sauté for 1 minute or until aromatic.
3. Then, stir in the soup, water, couscous, salt, black pepper and red pepper flakes; bring to a boil. Immediately reduce the heat to a simmer and let it cook for 12 minutes.
4. Fold in the canned chickpeas; continue to simmer until heated through or about 5 minutes more.
5. Ladle into individual bowls and drizzle with the lemon juice over the top. Bon appétit!

Nutrition: Calories: 378; Fat: 11g; Carbs: 60.1g; Protein: 10.9g

170. Cabbage Soup with Garlic Crostini

Preparation time: 10 minutes
Cooking Time: 1 hour
Servings: 4

Ingredients:
Soup:

- 2 tablespoons olive oil
- 1 medium leek, chopped
- 1 cup turnip, chopped
- 1 parsnip, chopped
- 1 carrot, chopped
- 2 cups cabbage, shredded
- 2 garlic cloves, finely chopped
- 4 cups vegetable broth
- 2 bay leaves
- Sea salt and ground black pepper, to taste
- 1/4 teaspoon cumin seeds
- 1/2 teaspoon mustard seeds
- 1 teaspoon dried basil
- 2 tomatoes, pureed

Crostini:

- 8 slices of baguette
- 2 heads garlic
- 4 tablespoons extra-virgin olive oil

Directions:

1. In a soup pot, heat 2 tablespoons of the olive over medium-high heat. Now, sauté the leek, turnip, parsnip and carrot for about 4 minutes or until the vegetables are crisp-tender.
2. Add in the garlic and cabbage and continue to sauté for 1 minute or until aromatic.
3. Then, stir in the vegetable broth, bay leaves, salt, black pepper, cumin seeds, mustard seeds, dried basil and pureed tomatoes; bring to a boil. Immediately reduce the heat to a simmer and let it cook for about 20 minutes.
4. Meanwhile, preheat your oven to 375 degrees F. Now, roast the garlic and baguette slices for about 15 minutes. Remove the crostini from the oven.
5. Continue baking the garlic for 45 minutes more or until very tender. Allow the garlic to cool.
6. Now, cut each head of the garlic using a sharp serrated knife in order to separate all the cloves.
7. Squeeze the roasted garlic cloves out of their skins. Mash the garlic pulp with 4 tablespoons of the extra-virgin olive oil.
8. Spread the roasted garlic mixture evenly on the tops of the crostini. Serve with the warm soup. Bon appétit!

Nutrition: Calories: 408; Fat: 23.1g; Carbs: 37.6g; Protein: 11.8g

171. Cream of Pinto Bean Soup

Preparation time: 10 minutes
Cooking Time: 35 minutes
Servings: 4

Ingredients:

- 1 tablespoon sesame oil
- 1 onion, chopped
- 1 green pepper, seeded and chopped
- 2 russet potatoes, peeled and diced
- 2 garlic cloves, chopped
- 4 cups vegetable broth
- 1-pound pinto beans, trimmed
- Sea salt and ground black pepper, to season
- 1 cup full-fat coconut milk

Directions:

1. In a heavy-bottomed pot, heat the sesame over medium-high heat. Now, sauté the onion, peppers and potatoes for about 5 minutes, stirring periodically.
2. Add in the garlic and continue sautéing for 1 minute or until fragrant.
3. Then, stir in the vegetable broth, pinto beans, salt and black pepper; bring to a boil. Immediately reduce the heat to a simmer and let it cook for 20 minutes.
4. Puree the pinto beans mixture using an immersion blender until creamy and uniform.
5. Return the pureed mixture to the pot. Fold in the coconut milk and continue to simmer until heated through or about 5 minutes longer.
6. Ladle into individual bowls and serve hot. Bon appétit!

Nutrition: Calories: 410; Fat: 19.6g; Carbs: 50.6g; Protein: 13.3g

172. Traditional French Onion Soup

Preparation time: 10 minutes
Cooking Time: 1 hour 30 minutes
Servings: 4

Ingredients:

- 2 tablespoons olive oil
- 2 large yellow onions, thinly sliced
- 2 thyme sprigs, chopped
- 2 rosemary sprigs, chopped
- 2 teaspoons balsamic vinegar
- 4 cups vegetable stock

- Sea salt and ground black pepper, to taste

Directions:

1. In pan or Dutch oven, heat the olive oil over a moderate heat. Now, cook the onions with thyme, rosemary and 1 teaspoon of the sea salt for about 2 minutes.
2. Now, turn the heat to medium-low and continue cooking until the onions caramelize or about 50 minutes.
3. Add in the balsamic vinegar and continue to cook for a further 15 more. Add in the stock, salt and black pepper and continue simmering for 20 to 25 minutes.
4. Serve with toasted bread and enjoy!

Nutrition: Calories: 129; Fat: 8.6g; Carbs: 7.4g; Protein: 6.3g

173. Roasted Carrot Soup

Preparation time: 10 minutes
Cooking Time: 50 minutes
Servings: 4

Ingredients:

- 1 ½ pounds carrots
- 4 tablespoons olive oil
- 1 yellow onion, chopped
- 2 cloves garlic, minced
- 1/3 teaspoon ground cumin
- Sea salt and white pepper, to taste
- 1/2 teaspoon turmeric powder
- 4 cups vegetable stock
- 2 teaspoons lemon juice
- 2 tablespoons fresh cilantro, roughly chopped

Directions:

1. Start by preheating your oven to 400 degrees F. Place the carrots on a large parchment-lined baking sheet; toss the carrots with 2 tablespoons of the olive oil.
2. Roast the carrots for about 35 minutes or until they've softened.
3. In a heavy-bottomed pot, heat the remaining 2 tablespoons of the olive oil. Now, sauté the onion and garlic for about 3 minutes or until aromatic.
4. Add in the cumin, salt, pepper, turmeric, vegetable stock and roasted carrots. Continue to simmer for 12 minutes more.
5. Puree your soup with an immersion blender. Drizzle lemon juice over your soup and serve garnished with fresh cilantro leaves. Bon appétit!

Nutrition: Calories: 264; Fat: 18.6g; Carbs: 20.1g; Protein: 7.4g

174. Arugula with Fruits and Nuts

Preparation Time: 10 Minutes
Cooking Time: 5 Minutes
Servings: 1

Ingredients:

- ½ cup arugula
- ½ peach
- ½ red onion
- ¼ cup blueberries
- 5 walnuts, chopped
- 1 tbsp. extra-virgin olive oil
- 2 tbsp. red wine vinegar
- 1 spring of fresh basil

Directions:

1. Halve the peach and remove the seed. Heat a grill pan and grill it briefly on both sides. Cut the red onion into thin half-rings. Roughly chop the pecans.
2. Heat a pan and roast the pecans in it until they are fragrant.
3. Place the arugula on a plate and spread peaches, red onions, blueberries, and roasted pecans over it.

4. Put all the ingredients for the dressing in a food processor and mix to an even dressing. Drizzle the dressing over the salad.

Nutrition: Calories: 160 Fat: 7g Carbs: 25g Protein: 3g

175. Broccoli Salad

Preparation Time: 25 Minutes
Cooking Time: 10 Minutes
Servings: 2

Ingredients:

- 1 head of broccoli
- 1/2 red onion
- 2 carrots, grated
- ¼ cup red grapes
- 2 1/2 tbsp. Coconut yogurt
- 1 tbsp. Water
- 1 tsp. mustard
- 1 pinch salt

Directions:

1. Cut the broccoli into florets and cook for 8 minutes. Cut the red onion into thin half-rings. Halve the grapes. Mix coconut yogurt, water, and mustard with a pinch of salt to make the dressing.
2. Drain the broccoli and rinse with ice-cold water to stop the cooking process.
3. Mix the broccoli with the carrot, onion, and red grapes in a bowl. Serve the dressing separately on the side.

Nutrition: Calories: 230 Fat: 18g Carbs: 35g Protein: 10g

176. Brunoise Salad

Preparation Time: 10 Minutes
Cooking Time: 0 Minutes
Servings: 2

Ingredients:

- 1 tomato
- 1 zucchini
- ½ red bell pepper
- ½ yellow bell pepper
- ½ red onion
- 3 springs fresh parsley
- ½ lemon
- 2 tbsp. olive oil

Directions:

1. Finely dice tomatoes, zucchini, peppers, and red onions to get a brunoise. Mix all the cubes in a bowl. Chop parsley and mix in the salad. Squeeze the lemon over the salad and add the olive oil.
2. Season with salt and pepper.

Nutrition: Calories: 84 Carbs: 3g Fat: 4g Protein: 0g

177. Brussels Sprouts and Ricotta Salad

Preparation Time: 15 Minutes
Cooking Time: 0 Minutes
Servings: 2

Ingredients:

- 1 ½ cups Brussels sprouts, thinly sliced
- 1 green apple cut "à la julienne."
- ½ red onion
- 8 walnuts, chopped
- 1 tsp. extra-virgin olive oil
- 1 tbsp. lemon juice
- 1 tbsp. orange juice
- 4 oz. ricotta cheese

Directions:

1. Put the red onion in a cup and cover it with boiling water. Let it rest 10 minutes, then drain and pat with kitchen paper. Slice Brussels sprouts as thin as you can, cut the apple à la julienne (sticks).
2. Mix Brussels sprouts, onion, and apple and season them with oil, salt, pepper, lemon juice, and orange juice and spread it on a serving plate.
3. Spread small spoonful of ricotta cheese over Brussels sprouts mixture and top with chopped walnuts.

Nutrition: Calories: 353, Fat: 4.8g, Carbs: 28.1g, Protein: 28.3g

178. Celery and Raisins Snack Salad

Preparation Time: 10 Minutes
Cooking Time: 0 Minutes
Servings: 4

Ingredients:

- ½ cup raisins
- 4 cups celery, sliced
- ¼ cup parsley, chopped
- ½ cup walnuts, chopped
- Juice of ½ lemon
- 2 tbsp. olive oil
- Salt and black pepper to taste

Directions:

1. In a salad bowl, mix celery with raisins, walnuts, parsley, lemon juice, oil, and black pepper, toss.
2. Divide into small cups and serve as a snack.

Nutrition: Calories 120 , Fat 1g, Carbs 6g, Protein 5g

179. Dijon Celery Salad

Preparation Time: 10 Minutes
Cooking Time: 0 Minutes
Servings: 4

Ingredients:

- ½ cup lemon juice
- 1/3 cup Dijon mustard
- 2/3 cup olive oil
- Black pepper to taste
- 2 apples, cored, peeled, and cubed
- 1 bunch celery roughly chopped
- ¾ cup walnuts, chopped

Directions:

1. In a salad bowl, mix celery and its leaves with apple pieces and walnuts.
2. Add black pepper, lemon juice, mustard, and olive oil, whisk well, add to your salad, toss, divide into small cups and serve.

Nutrition: Calories 125 , Fat 2g, Carbs 7g, Protein 7g

180. Fresh Endive Salad

Preparation Time: 10 Minutes
Cooking Time: 0 Minutes
Servings: 1

Ingredients:

- ½ red endive
- 1 orange
- 1 tomato
- 1/2 cucumber
- 1/2 red onion

Directions:

1. Cut off the hard stem of the endive and remove the leaves. Peel the orange and cut the pulp into wedges.
2. Cut the tomatoes and cucumbers into small pieces. Cut the red onion into thin half-rings.

3. Place the endive boats on a plate; spread the orange wedges, tomato, cucumber, and red onion over the boats. Drizzle some olive oil and fresh lemon juice and serve.

Nutrition: Calories: 112 Fat: 11g Carbs: 2g Protein: 0g

181. Green Creamy Soup

Preparation Time: 10 minutes
Cooking Time: 30 minutes
Servings: 2

INGREDIENTS

- 5 ounces fresh pinto beans, thinly sliced
- 8 ounces fresh Brussels sprouts, sliced
- 5 cups low-sodium, fat-free vegetable broth
- 1½ cups frozen peas, defrosted
- 4 tablespoons olive oil
- 1 white onion, chopped
- 1 tablespoon freshly squeezed lemon juice
- 4 cloves fresh garlic, minced
- 1 large leek, slice both white parts and sliced green parts thinly but keep them separate
- 1 teaspoon ground coriander
- 1 cup low-fat milk
- Salt and freshly ground pepper to taste
- Croutons for garnish

DIRECTIONS

1. Take out a large skillet and place it over low heat. Add the olive oil and allow the oil to heat up slightly.
2. Add onion and garlic. Cook them until they turn fragrant and soft. Make sure that you do not allow them to turn brown.
3. Add the green parts of the Brussels sprouts, leek, and pinto beans to the skillet. Add the broth and mix the ingredients well. Bring the broth to a boil. When it starts boiling, lower the heat and let simmer for about 12 minutes.
4. Add lemon juice, peas, and coriander. Let the broth continue to simmer for another 10 minutes, or until the vegetables become tender.
5. Remove the broth mixture from heat and allow it to cool slightly. Transfer the mixture to a blender and pulse until they turn smooth.
6. Take out a saucepan and add the white parts of leek. Add the blended mixture into the saucepan. Place the saucepan over medium high heat and allow the soup to boil. Reduce the heat to low and allow the soup to simmer for about 5 minutes
7. Take out another bowl and add flour and milk. Whisk them until they turn smooth.
8. Add salt and pepper to taste, if preferred.

NUTRITION: Calories: 163 Protein: 4 g Fat: 8 g Carbs: 15 g

182. Orzo and Lemon Chicken Soup

Preparation Time: 10 minutes
Cooking Time: 40 minutes
Servings: 2

INGREDIENTS

- 12 ounces skinless, boneless chicken breasts
- 1 tablespoon olive oil
- ½ cup chopped celery
- ½ cup chopped white onion
- 6 cups low-sodium, fat-free chicken broth

- ½ cup sliced carrot
- ½ cup orzo
- ¼ cup chopped fresh dill
- Salt and freshly ground pepper to taste
- Lemon halves

DIRECTIONS

1. Take out a large pot and place it over medium heat. Add olive oil to it and allow it to heat.
2. Add celery and onion. Cook them until the onions are fragrant and the celery is soft.
3. Add chicken, chicken broth, and carrot to the mixture. Add salt and pepper to taste, if preferred.
4. Increase the temperature to medium high heat and allow the broth to boil. When it starts boiling, reduce heat and allow the soup to simmer for about 20 minutes, or until the chicken is cooked.
5. Take out the chicken from the pot, transfer it to a bowl and allow it to cool. Cover the pot so that the ingredients inside are simmering. When the chicken is sufficiently cool, shred the chicken into small pieces.
6. Open the cover of the pot and add orzo. Increase the heat to medium high and allow the broth to boil for about 8 minutes. Make sure that the cover is back on the pot during the boiling process.
7. Remove pot from heat and add dill and the shredded chicken broth.
8. Squeeze lemon juice into the broth. Serve immediately.

NUTRITION: Calories: 248 Protein: 25 g Fat: 4 g Carbs: 23 g

183. Chilled Avocado Soup

Preparation Time: 50 minutes
Cooking Time: 0 minutes
Servings: 2

INGREDIENTS

- 3 medium ripe avocados, halved, seeded, peeled, and cut to chunks
- 2 cloves fresh garlic, minced
- 2 cups low-sodium, fat-free chicken broth, divided
- ½ cucumber, peeled and chopped
- ½ cup chopped white onion
- ¼ cup finely diced carrot
- Thin avocado slices for garnish
- Paprika to sprinkle
- Salt and freshly ground pepper to taste
- Hot red pepper sauce to taste

DIRECTIONS

1. Place 6 bowls into the freezer and allow them to chill for half an hour.
2. In the meantime, take out your blender and add garlic, cucumber, avocados, onion, carrot, and 1 cup broth. Blend all the ingredients together until they turn smooth.
3. Add the remaining broth. Add the salt and pepper and hot sauce to taste, if preferred.
4. Blend all the ingredients again until they are smooth.
5. Take out the chilled bowls and pour the blended ingredients into them.
6. This time, place the bowls in the refrigerator for another 1 hour.
7. When you are ready to serve, top the soup with paprika and slices of avocado.
8. Serve chilled.

NUTRITION: Calories: 255 Protein: 4 g Fat: 22 g Carbs: 15 g

184. Broccoli and Potato Soup

Preparation Time: 10 minutes
Cooking Time: 25 minutes
Servings: 2

INGREDIENTS

- 2 cups escarole leaves, rinsed and drained
- 3 tablespoons all-purpose flour
- 3 cups fresh broccoli florets
- 3 scallions, sliced
- 2 cups smoked Gouda cheese, shredded and more for garnish
- 2 cups low-sodium, fat-free chicken broth
- 1 cup almond milk
- 3 medium red-gold potatoes, chopped
- 2 cloves fresh garlic, minced
- Salt and freshly ground pepper to taste

DIRECTIONS

1. Take out a large pot and place it over medium high heat. Add potatoes, garlic, and chicken broth. Bring the mixture to a boil and reduce the heat to low. Allow the mixture to simmer for a while until you notice the potatoes begin to soften
2. Use a fork and mash the potatoes slightly.
3. Add broccoli, milk, and scallions. Continue to heat to a simmer until broccoli turns tender and crispy.
4. Bring down the heat to low and then add the Gouda cheese. Continue stirring until the sauce thickens and the cheese melts.
5. Add salt and pepper for seasoning, if preferred. Serve the soup in 4 equal portions.
6. Add additional cheese and escarole as toppings.

NUTRITION: Calories: 350 Protein: 17 g Fat: 14 g Carbs: 42 g

185. Tortellini and Vegetable Soup

Preparation Time: 10 minutes
Cooking Time: 30 minutes
Servings: 2

INGREDIENTS

- 32 ounces' low-sodium, fat-free chicken broth
- 3 cups fresh chicken-filled tortellini
- 1 large white onion, chopped
- 4 cloves fresh garlic, chopped
- 3 celery stalks, chopped
- 1 teaspoon minced chives
- 2 14.5-ounce cans diced tomatoes, undrained
- 2 tablespoons olive oil
- 1 teaspoon dried sweet basil
- 1 cup frozen corn
- 1 teaspoon dried thyme
- 1 cup chopped carrot
- 1 cup frozen cut pinto beans
- 1 cup diced raw potato

DIRECTIONS

1. Take out a large pot and place it over medium heat. Add garlic, onion, celery, and olive oil. Sauté until you notice the onion and garlic become fragrant and soft.
2. Add potato, basil, carrot, beans, broth, thyme, corn, and chives. Increase the heat to medium high and then bring the broth to a boil.
3. When it starts boiling, reduce the heat and cover the pot. Allow the mixture to simmer for about 15 minutes, or until the vegetables become tender.
4. Add tortellini and tomatoes. Remove the cover and allow the soup to simmer uncovered for about 5 minutes.
5. Serve hot.

NUTRITION: Calories: 213 Protein: 7 g Fat: 7 g Carbs: 26 g

186. *Traditional Oyster Soup*

Preparation Time: 10 minutes
Cooking Time: 15 minutes
Servings: 2
INGREDIENTS

- 2 pints (about 32 ounces) fresh shucked oysters, undrained
- 4 tablespoons olive oil
- 1 cup finely chopped celery
- 3 (12-ounce) cans low-fat evaporated milk
- 6 tablespoons minced shallots
- 2 pinches of cayenne pepper (add more if you like more spice)
- Toasted bread squares
- Salt and freshly ground pepper to taste

DIRECTIONS

1. Start with the oysters. Drain the liquid from them in a small bowl. Set the liquid aside since we are going to use it. Place the oysters separately.
2. Run the liquid through a strainer to remove any solid materials.
3. Take out a large pot and place it over medium heat. Add olive oil into it. Toss in oysters, celery, and shallots.
4. Allow the ingredients to simmer for about 5 minutes, or until you notice the edges of the oysters begin to curl.
5. Take a separate pot (or pan) and then heat the oyster liquid and milk. When the mixture is sufficiently warm, then pour it over the oysters. Stir all the ingredients together.
6. Add salt and pepper, and cayenne pepper to taste.
7. Serve soup warm with toasted bread squares as toppings or on the side.

NUTRITION: Calories: 311 Protein: 23 g Fat: 11 g Carbs: 22 g

187. *Eggplant Soup*

Preparation Time: 10 minutes
Cooking Time: 30 minutes
Servings: 2
INGREDIENTS

- 3 tablespoons olive oil
- 1 (14-ounce) can low-sodium tomato
- ½ cup chopped white onion
- 2 tablespoons Italian bread crumbs
- 2 cloves fresh garlic, minced
- 2 cups low sodium, fat-free chicken broth
- ½ cup shredded reduced-fat mozzarella cheese
- 1 small eggplant, halved and sliced thinly (about 2 cups)

DIRECTIONS

1. Preheat the oven to 500° F. We are aiming for a broiling temperature. An oven's broiling temperature is anywhere from 500° F to 550° F.
2. If you feel that you want to increase the temperature, feel free to do so when you place the dish in the oven.
3. Take out a nonstick pan and place it over medium heat. Add olive oil into the pan and allow it to heat. Add the eggplant and cook for about 5 minutes, stirring occasionally.
4. Add garlic and onion and continue cooking until you notice the eggplant turn into a golden-brown color.
5. Add broth and sauce. Increase the heat to medium high and then allow the mixture to boil.
6. When it starts boiling, lower the heat to a simmer. Continue to cook until the soup thickens.
7. Take out a baking tray and line it with tin foil. Use 2 oven-safe crock bowls and place them on the tray. Split the soup into equal portions and pour them into the bowls.
8. Top with bread crumbs, and mozzarella cheese.
9. Allow the dish to broil for about 2 to 3 minutes, or until cheese has melted and turned golden.
10. Serve hot.

NUTRITION: Calories: 274 Protein: 9 g Fat: 17 g Carbs: 23 g

188. *Cheesy Keto Zucchini Soup*

Preparation time: 15 minutes
Cooking time: 20 minutes
Servings: 2
INGREDIENTS:

- ½ medium onion, peeled and chopped
- 1 cup bone broth
- 1 tablespoon coconut oil
- 1½ zucchinis, cut into chunks
- ½ tablespoon nutrition al yeast
- Dash of black pepper
- ½ tablespoon parsley, chopped, for garnish
- ½ tablespoon coconut cream, for garnish

DIRECTIONS:

1. Melt the coconut oil in a large pan over medium heat and add onions. Sauté for about 3 minutes and add zucchinis and bone broth.
2. Reduce the heat to simmer for about 15 minutes and cover the pan. Add nutrition al yeast and transfer to an immersion blender.
3. Blend until smooth and season with black pepper. Top with coconut cream and parsley to serve.

NUTRITION: Calories: 154 Carbs: 8.9g Fats: 8.1g Proteins: 13.4g

189. *Spring Soup with Poached Egg*

Preparation time: 15 minutes
Cooking time: 10 minutes
Servings: 2
INGREDIENTS:

- 32 oz vegetable broth
- 2 eggs
- 1 head romaine lettuce, chopped
- Salt, to taste

DIRECTIONS:

1. Bring the vegetable broth to a boil and reduce the heat. Poach the eggs for 5 minutes in the broth and remove them into 2 bowls.
2. Stir in romaine lettuce into the broth and cook for 4 minutes. Dish out in a bowl and serve hot.

NUTRITION: Calories: 158 Carbs: 6.9g Fats: 7.3g Proteins: 15.4g

190. Mint Avocado Chilled Soup

Preparation time: 15 minutes
Cooking time: 0 minutes
Servings: 2

INGREDIENTS:

- 2 romaine lettuce leaves
- 1 Tablespoon lime juice
- 1 medium ripe avocado
- 1 cup coconut milk, chilled
- 20 fresh mint leaves
- Salt to taste

DIRECTIONS:

1. Put all the ingredients in a blender and blend until smooth. Refrigerate for about 10 minutes and serve chilled.

NUTRITION: Calories: 432 Carbs: 16.1g Fats: 42.2g Proteins: 5.2g

191. Easy Butternut Squash Soup

Preparation time: 15 minutes
Cooking time: 1 hour & 35 minutes
Servings: 4

INGREDIENTS:

- 1 small onion, chopped
- 4 cups chicken broth
- 1 butternut squash
- 3 tablespoons coconut oil
- Salt, to taste
- Nutmeg and pepper, to taste

DIRECTIONS:

1. Put oil and onions in a large pot and add onions. Sauté for about 3 minutes and add chicken broth and butternut squash.
2. Simmer for about 1 hour on medium heat and transfer into an immersion blender. Pulse until smooth and season with salt, pepper and nutmeg.
3. Return to the pot and cook for about 30 minutes. Dish out and serve hot.

NUTRITION: Calories: 149 Carbs: 6.6g Fats: 11.6g Proteins: 5.4g

192. Cauliflower, Leek & Bacon Soup

Preparation time: 15 minutes
Cooking time: 1 hour & 35 minutes
Servings: 4

INGREDIENTS:

- 4 cups chicken broth
- ½ cauliflower head, chopped
- 1 leek, chopped
- Salt and black pepper, to taste
- 5 bacon strips

DIRECTIONS:

1. Put the cauliflower, leek and chicken broth into the pot and cook for about 1 hour on medium heat. Transfer into an immersion blender and pulse until smooth.
2. Return the soup into the pot and microwave the bacon strips for 1 minute. Cut the bacon into small pieces and put into the soup.
3. Cook on for about 30 minutes on low heat. Season with salt and pepper and serve.

NUTRITION: Calories: 185 Carbs: 5.8g Fats: 12.7g Proteins: 10.8g

193. Swiss Chard Egg Drop Soup

Preparation time: 15 minutes
Cooking time: 10 minutes
Servings: 4

INGREDIENTS:

- 3 cups bone broth
- 2 eggs, whisked
- 1 teaspoon ground oregano
- 3 tablespoons butter
- 2 cups Swiss chard, chopped
- 2 tablespoons coconut aminos
- 1 teaspoon ginger, grated
- Salt and black pepper, to taste

DIRECTIONS:

1. Heat the bone broth in a saucepan and add whisked eggs while stirring slowly. Add the swiss chard, butter, coconut aminos, ginger, oregano and salt and black pepper. Cook for about 10 minutes and serve hot.

NUTRITION: Calories: 185 Carbs: 2.9g Fats: 11g Proteins: 18.3g

194. Mushroom Spinach Soup

Preparation time: 15 minutes
Cooking time: 10 minutes
Servings: 4

INGREDIENTS:

- 1 cup spinach, cleaned and chopped
- 100g mushrooms, chopped
- 1 onion
- 6 garlic cloves
- ½ teaspoon red chili powder
- Salt and black pepper, to taste
- 3 tablespoons buttermilk
- 1 teaspoon almond flour
- 2 cups chicken broth
- 3 tablespoons butter
- ¼ cup fresh cream for garnish

DIRECTIONS:

1. Heat butter in a pan and add onions and garlic. Sauté for about 3 minutes and add spinach, salt and red chili powder.
2. Sauté for about 4 minutes and add mushrooms. Transfer into a blender and blend to make a puree. Return to the pan and add buttermilk and almond flour for creamy texture.
3. Mix well and simmer for about 2 minutes. Garnish with fresh cream and serve hot.

NUTRITION: Calories: 160 Carbs: 7g Fats: 13.3g Proteins: 4.7g

195. Delicate Squash Soup

Preparation time: 15 minutes
Cooking time: 27 minutes
Servings: 5
INGREDIENTS:

- 1½ cups beef bone broth
- 1small onion, peeled and grated.
- ½ teaspoon sea salt
- ¼ teaspoon poultry seasoning
- 2small Delicata Squash, chopped
- 2 garlic cloves, minced
- 2tablespoons olive oil
- ¼ teaspoon black pepper
- 1 small lemon, juiced
- 5 tablespoons sour cream

DIRECTIONS:

1. Put Delicata Squash and water in a medium pan and bring to a boil. Reduce the heat and cook for about 20 minutes. Drain and set aside.
2. Put olive oil, onions, garlic and poultry seasoning in a small sauce pan. Cook for about 2 minutes and add broth. Allow it to simmer for 5 minutes and remove from heat.
3. Whisk in the lemon juice and transfer the mixture in a blender. Pulse until smooth and top with sour cream.

NUTRITION: Calories: 109 Carbs: 4.9g Fats: 8.5g Proteins: 3g

196. Broccoli Soup

Preparation time: 15 minutes
Cooking time: 37 minutes
Servings: 6
INGREDIENTS:

- 3 tablespoons ghee
- 5 garlic cloves
- 1 teaspoon sage
- ¼ teaspoon ginger
- 2 cups broccoli
- 1 small onion
- 1 teaspoon oregano
- ½ teaspoon parsley
- Salt and black pepper, to taste
- 6 cups vegetable broth
- 4 tablespoons butter

DIRECTIONS:

1. Put ghee, onions, spices and garlic in a pot and cook for 3 minutes. Add broccoli and cook for about 4 minutes. Add vegetable broth, cover and allow it to simmer for about 30 minutes.
2. Transfer into a blender and blend until smooth. Add the butter to give it a creamy delicious texture and flavor

NUTRITION: Calories: 183 Carbs: 5.2g Fats: 15.6g Proteins: 6.1g

197. Keto French Onion Soup

Preparation time: 15 minutes
Cooking time: 335 minutes
Servings: 6
INGREDIENTS:

- 5 tablespoons butter
- 500 g brown onion medium
- 4 drops liquid stevia
- 4 tablespoons olive oil
- 3 cups beef stock

DIRECTIONS:

1. Put the butter and olive oil in a large pot over medium low heat and add onions and salt. Cook for about 5 minutes and stir in stevia.
2. Cook for another 5 minutes and add beef stock. Reduce the heat to low and simmer for about 25 minutes. Dish out into soup bowls and serve hot.

NUTRITION: Calories: 198 Carbs: 6g Fats: 20.6g Proteins: 2.9g

198. Cauliflower and Thyme Soup

Preparation time: 15 minutes
Cooking time: 13 minutes
Servings: 6
INGREDIENTS:

- 2 teaspoons thyme powder
- 1 head cauliflower
- 3 cups vegetable stock
- ½ teaspoon matcha green tea powder
- 3 tablespoons olive oil
- Salt and black pepper, to taste
- 5 garlic cloves, chopped

DIRECTIONS:

1. Put the vegetable stock, thyme and matcha powder to a large pot over medium-high heat and bring to a boil. Add cauliflower and cook for about 10 minutes.
2. Meanwhile, put the olive oil and garlic in a small sauce pan and cook for about 1 minute. Add the garlic, salt and black pepper and cook for about 2 minutes.
3. Transfer into an immersion blender and blend until smooth. Dish out and serve immediately.

NUTRITION: Calories: 79 Carbs: 3.8g Fats: 7.1g Proteins: 1.3g

199. Homemade Thai Soup

Preparation time: 15 minutes
Cooking time: 8 hours
Servings: 12
INGREDIENTS:

- 1 lemongrass stalk, cut into large chunks
- 5 thick slices of fresh ginger
- 1 whole chicken
- 20 fresh basil leaves
- 1 lime, juiced
- 1 tablespoon salt

DIRECTIONS:

1. Place the chicken, 20 basil leaves, lemongrass, ginger, salt and water into the slow cooker. Cook for about 8 hours on low and

dish out into a bowl. Stir in fresh lime juice and basil leaves to serve.

NUTRITION: Calories: 182 Carbs: 8.9g Fats: 9.3g Proteins: 14.4g

200. Chicken Kale Soup

Preparation time: 15 minutes
Cooking time: 6 hours & 15 minutes
Servings: 6
INGREDIENTS:

- 2 pounds' chicken breast, skinless
- 1/3cup onion
- 1 tablespoon olive oil
- 14 ounces' chicken bone broth
- ½ cup olive oil
- 4 cups chicken stock
- ¼ cup lemon juice
- 5 ounces' baby kale leaves
- Salt, to taste

DIRECTIONS:

1. Season chicken with salt and black pepper. Heat olive oil over medium heat in a large skillet and add seasoned chicken.
2. Reduce the temperature and cook for about 15 minutes. Shred the chicken and place in the crock pot. Process the chicken broth and onions in a blender and blend until smooth.
3. Pour into crock pot and stir in the remaining ingredients. Cook on low for about 6 hours, stirring once while cooking.

NUTRITION: Calories: 266 Carbs: 33g Fats: 5.6g Proteins: 22g

201. Chicken Veggie Soup

Preparation time: 15 minutes
Cooking time: 1 hour & 30 minutes
Servings: 6
INGREDIENTS:

- 5 chicken thighs
- 12 cups water
- 1 tablespoon adobo seasoning
- 4 celery ribs
- 1 yellow onion
- 1½ teaspoons whole black peppercorns
- 6 sprigs fresh parsley
- 2 teaspoons coarse sea salt
- 2 carrots
- 6 mushrooms, sliced
- 2 garlic cloves
- 1 bay leaf
- 3 sprigs fresh thyme

DIRECTIONS:

1. Put water, chicken thighs, carrots, celery ribs, onion, garlic cloves and herbs in a large pot. Bring to a boil and reduce the heat to low.
2. Cover the pot and simmer for about 30 minutes. Dish out the chicken and shred it, removing the bones. Put the bones back into the pot and simmer for about 20 minutes.
3. Strain the broth, discarding the chunks and put the liquid back into the pot. Bring it to a boil and simmer for about 30 minutes.
4. Put the mushrooms in the broth and simmer for about 10 minutes. Dish out to serve hot.

NUTRITION: Calories: 250 Carbs: 6.4g Fats: 8.9g Proteins: 35.1g

202. Chicken Mulligatawny Soup

Preparation time: 15 minutes
Cooking time: 30 minutes
Servings: 10
INGREDIENTS:

- 1½ tablespoons curry powder
- 3 cups celery root, diced
- 2 tablespoons Swerve
- 10 cups chicken broth
- 5 cups chicken, chopped and cooked
- ¼ cup apple cider
- ½ cup sour cream
- ¼ cup fresh parsley, chopped
- 2 tablespoons butter
- Salt and black pepper, to taste

DIRECTIONS:

1. Combine the broth, butter, chicken, curry powder, celery root and apple cider in a large soup pot. Bring to a boil and simmer for about 30 minutes.
2. Stir in Swerve, sour cream, fresh parsley, salt and black pepper. Dish out and serve hot.

NUTRITION: Calories: 215 Carbs: 7.1g Fats: 8.5g Proteins: 26.4g

203. Buffalo Ranch Soup

Preparation time: 15 minutes
Cooking time: 30 minutes
Servings: 4
INGREDIENTS:

- 2 tablespoons parsley
- 2 celery stalks, chopped
- 6 tablespoons butter
- 1 cup heavy whipping cream
- 4 cups chicken, cooked and shredded
- 4 tablespoons ranch dressing
- ¼ cup yellow onions, chopped
- 8 oz cream cheese
- 8 cups chicken broth
- 7 hearty bacon slices, crumbled

DIRECTIONS:

1. Heat butter in a pan and add chicken. Cook for about 5 minutes and add 1½ cups water. Cover and cook for about 10 minutes.
2. Put the chicken and rest of the ingredients into the saucepan except parsley and cook for about 10 minutes. Top with parsley and serve hot.

NUTRITION: Calories: 478 Carbs: 7.5g Fats: 23.6g Proteins: 56.6g

204. Traditional Chicken Soup

Preparation time: 15 minutes
Cooking time: 1 hour & 30 minutes
Servings: 6

INGREDIENTS:

- 3 pounds' chicken
- 4 quarts' water
- 4 stalks celery
- 1/3 large red onion
- 1 large carrot
- 3 garlic cloves
- 2 thyme sprigs
- 2 rosemary sprigs
- Salt and black pepper, to taste

DIRECTIONS:

1. Put water and chicken in the stock pot on medium high heat. Bring to a boil and allow it to simmer for about 10 minutes.
2. Add onion, garlic, celery, salt and pepper and simmer on medium low heat for 30 minutes. Add thyme and carrots and simmer on low for another 30 minutes.
3. Dish out the chicken and shred the pieces, removing the bones. Return the chicken pieces to the pot and add rosemary sprigs. Simmer for about 20 minutes at low heat and dish out to serve.

NUTRITION: Calories: 314 Carbs: 3.3g Fats: 7g Proteins: 66.2g

205. Noodle Soup

Preparation time: 15 minutes
Cooking time: 20 minutes
Servings: 6

INGREDIENTS:

- 1 onion, minced
- 1 rib celery, sliced
- 3 cups chicken, shredded
- 3 eggs, lightly beaten
- 1 green onion, for garnish
- 2 tablespoons coconut oil
- 1 carrot, peeled and thinly sliced
- 2 teaspoons dried thyme
- 2½ quarts homemade bone broth
- ¼ cup fresh parsley, minced
- Salt and black pepper, to taste

DIRECTIONS:

1. Heat coconut oil over medium-high heat in a large pot and add onions, carrots, and celery. Cook for about 4 minutes and stir in the bone broth, thyme and chicken.
2. Simmer for about 15 minutes and stir in parsley. Pour beaten eggs into the soup in a slow steady stream.
3. Remove soup from heat and let it stand for about 2 minutes. Season with salt and black pepper and dish out to serve.

NUTRITION: Calories: 226 Carbs: 3.5g Fats: 8.9g Proteins: 31.8g

206. Chicken Cabbage Soup

Preparation time: 15 minutes
Cooking time: 26 minutes
Servings: 8

INGREDIENTS:

- 2 celery stalks
- 2 garlic cloves, minced
- 4 oz. Butter
- 6 oz. Mushrooms, sliced
- 2 tablespoons onions, dried and minced
- 1 teaspoon salt
- 8 cups chicken broth
- 1 medium carrot
- 2 cups green cabbage, sliced into strips
- 2 teaspoons dried parsley
- ¼ teaspoon black pepper
- 1½ rotisserie chickens, shredded

DIRECTIONS:

1. Melt butter in a large pot and add celery, mushrooms, onions and garlic into the pot. Cook for about 4 minutes and add broth, parsley, carrot, salt and black pepper.
2. Simmer for about 10 minutes and add cooked chicken and cabbage. Simmer for an additional 12 minutes until the cabbage is tender. Dish out and serve hot.

NUTRITION: Calories: 184 Carbs: 4.2g Fats: 13.1g Proteins: 12.6g

207. Carrot and Red Lentil Soup

Preparation Time: 5 minutes
Cooking Time: 20-30 minutes
Servings: 2

INGREDIENTS:

- 2 onions, minced
- 2 tablespoons dried parsley flakes
- 2 teaspoons ground allspice
- 2 teaspoons ground cumin
- 2 teaspoons ground turmeric
- 1-½ teaspoon salt
- 1 teaspoon garlic powder
- 1 teaspoon ground cardamom
- 1 teaspoon ground cinnamon
- 1 teaspoon pepper
- 0.6 lb. Dried red lentils
- 1 medium carrot, finely chopped
- 1 celery rib, finely chopped
- 1 tablespoon olive oil
- 4 quarts of vegetable broth

DIRECTIONS:

1. In a saucepan add olive oil, onion, carrots, and salt; cook for a few seconds.
2. Add red lentils, pepper, cardamom, garlic, cinnamon, celery, turmeric, cumin, all spices, parsley, and pepper; mix well.
3. Add vegetable broth and cover with a lid. Let it cook on low flame for 20-25 minutes or until lentil is tender.
4. Serve and enjoy.

NUTRITION: Calories – 318, Fat – 97 g, Carbs – 60 g, Protein – 1.7 g

208. White Bean Soup

Preparation Time: 5 minutes
Cooking Time: 35 minutes
Servings: 2

INGREDIENTS:

- 1 tablespoon virgin olive oil
- 1 red onion (chopped)
- 1 garlic clove (minced)
- 1 celery stalk (chopped)
- 1 cup spinach (fresh, finely chopped)
- 1 tablespoon lemon juice (fresh squeezed)
- 2x 16-ounce cans white kidney beans (drained, rinsed)
- 2 cups chicken broth (or a 14-ounce can of low-sodium chicken broth)
- ¼ teaspoon thyme (dried)
- ½ teaspoon black pepper
- 1 ½ cups water

DIRECTIONS:

1. Place a large saucepan on your stove. Add the virgin olive oil to your pan and turn the heat to medium-high. Add the celery, chopped onions, and minced garlic to the pan and allow them to cook for 5 minutes.
2. Add the white kidney beans, chicken broth, water, thyme, and black pepper to the saucepan.
3. Allow the liquid to come to a boil, then reduce heat to medium-low and let the soup simmer for 15 minutes.
4. Transfer two cups of the bean and vegetables from the saucepan to a bowl. Use a slotted spoon to get as little of the liquid as possible. Set the bowl to the side.
5. Use an emulsion blender to blend the remaining soup mixture in the saucepan. You want to get a nice smooth consistency.
6. If you do not have an emulsion blender you can use a regular stand-alone blender. Just work in batches to blend everything. Once everything has been thoroughly blended, return back to your saucepan.
7. Add the 2 cups of beans and vegetable mixture that you removed earlier back into the soup. Bring the soup back up to a boil, stirring occasionally.
8. Add in the spinach to the soup; after 2 minutes it should begin to wilt.
9. Turn the heat all the way off, and then stirs in the lemon juice just before serving.

NUTRITION: Calories – 185, Carbs - 23.8 g, Protein - 10 g, Fat - 5.2 g

209. Peas Soup

Preparation Time: 10 minutes
Cooking Time: 25 minutes
Servings: 2

INGREDIENTS:

- ¼ cup long-grain rice
- 4 cups chicken stock
- ¼ teaspoon ground black pepper
- ½ teaspoon Italian seasonings

DIRECTIONS:

1. Heat a saucepan with the stock.
2. Add all ingredients and bring the soup to boil.
3. Cook the soup for 5 minutes over the low heat.

NUTRITION: 95 calories 5.4g protein 6.1g Carbs

210. Red Lentil Soup

Preparation Time: 5 minutes
Cooking Time: 35 minutes
Servings: 5

INGREDIENTS:

- 8 cups chicken broth
- Cup red lentils
- 1 bell pepper, onion
- 1 tablespoon tomato paste
- 1 teaspoon chili powder

DIRECTIONS:

1. Melt 1 tsp. Olive oil in the saucepan and add onion and bell pepper.
2. Roast the vegetables for 5 minutes.
3. After this, add red lentils, tomato paste, chili powder, and chicken broth. Stir the soup well.
4. Cook the soup for 30 minutes over the medium heat.

NUTRITION: 225 calories 18.4g protein 29.3g Carbs

211. White Mushrooms Soup

Preparation Time: 10 minutes
Cooking Time: 25 minutes
Servings: 2

INGREDIENTS:

- 4 oz. White mushrooms, chopped
- ½ cup white onion, diced
- 1 teaspoon cayenne pepper
- 2 cups of water

DIRECTIONS:

1. Melt the 1 tbsp. Olive oil in the pan and add onion and mushrooms.
2. Cook the vegetables for 5 minutes over the medium heat.
3. Then add cayenne pepper and water.
4. Simmer the soup for 10 minutes.
5. Remove the soup from the heat.

NUTRITION: 142 calories 5.7g protein 5.2g Carbs

212. Lamb Soup

Preparation Time: 10 minutes
Cooking Time: 35 minutes
Servings: 2

INGREDIENTS:

- 9 oz. Lamb sirloin, sliced
- 5 cups of water
- 1 cup cauliflower, chopped
- 1 teaspoon dried dill
- 2 tablespoons tomato paste

DIRECTIONS:

1. Preheat the pan well and add lamb sirloin.
2. Roast it for 1 minute per side.
3. Then add water, ½ tsp. Ground black pepper, and dried dill.
4. Cook the meat for 20 minutes, covered.
5. Then add tomato paste and cauliflower. Stir the soup.
6. Cook the soup for 10 minutes.

NUTRITION: 144 calories 19g protein 3.2g Carbs

213. Lemon Zest Soup

Preparation Time: 10 minutes
Cooking Time: 15 minutes
Servings: 2

INGREDIENTS:

- 2 tablespoons lemon juice
- ½ teaspoon lemon zest, grated
- ¼ cup long-grain rice
- 4 cups chicken stock
- 1 celery stalk, chopped

DIRECTIONS:

1. Boil chicken stock then add rice, cook for 10 minutes.
2. Then add lemon zest and celery stalk. Cook the soup for 3 minutes more.
3. After this, add lemon juice and boil it for 2 minutes.

NUTRITION: 109 calories 3.2g protein 20.6g Carbs

214. Cucumber Avocado Watermelon Salad

Preparation Time: 15 Minutes
Cooking Time: 0 Minutes
Servings: 2

INGREDIENTS:

- 1 cucumber, sliced thin
- 1 lime's juice
- 1 avocado, small scooped into balls
- 2 tablespoons of basil, fresh
- 2 1/2 cups of watermelon, cubed
- 3 tablespoons of oil
- Salt & pepper, to taste

DIRECTIONS:

1. In a bowl, add all ingredients, toss gently and serve.

NUTRITION: Calories 113 Total Fat: 3 g Total carbs: 7 g Fiber: 17g Sugar: 3 g Protein: 10g Sodium: 128 mg

215. Cream of Cauliflower Broccoli Soup

Preparation Time: 15 Minutes
Cooking Time: 20 Minutes
Servings: 4

INGREDIENTS:

- Half chopped onion
- 1 chopped garlic clove
- 2 teaspoon of Sesame oil
- Broccoli & Cauliflower &: 5 oz., each, cut into florets
- 2 cups of vegetable stock
- 15 soaked Almonds
- Salt & pepper, to taste
- A pinch of nutmeg

DIRECTIONS:

1. In a pot, sauté broccoli, cauliflower, onion and garlic in hot sesame oil.
2. Add stock and let it come to a boil. Season with salt and pepper, cook for 10 minutes.
3. Take the puree out in a blender, pulse and add peeled almonds.
4. Pour in the stock, mix and add spices, adjust seasoning and serve.

NUTRITION: Calories 267 Total Fat: 7 g Total carbs: 7.9 g Fiber: 14.2 g Sugar: 5 g Protein: 9.8 g Sodium: 201 mg

216. Quinoa Pegan Salad Bowl

Preparation Time: 15 Minutes
Cooking Time: 0 Minutes
Servings: 4

INGREDIENTS:

- Half cucumber
- 1 cup of cooked quinoa
- Half cup of canned black bean, rinsed
- 1/4 cup of diced onion
- 1 cup of baby spinach leaves
- Half cup of shredded purple Cabbage

Dressing

- 3 teaspoon of Lemon juice
- black pepper, to taste
- 1 teaspoon of miso gluten-free paste

DIRECTIONS:

1. In a bowl, add all vegetables and toss.
2. In a separate bowl, add the dressing ingredients and whisk well.
3. Pour the dressing over salad, toss and serve.

NUTRITION: Calories 269 Total Fat: 7 g Total carbs: 50 g Fiber: 14.2 g Sugar: 5 g Protein: 11 g Sodium: 180 mg

217. Slaw Salad

Preparation Time: 15 Minutes
Cooking Time: 0 Minutes
Servings: 4

INGREDIENTS:

- 1 cup of arugula
- Half cup of shredded carrots
- Half can of roasted green peppers
- 1 cup of shredded green cabbage
- 1/4 cup of chopped green onion
- half sliced red onion
- half cup of shredded red cabbage
- 1/8 cup of chopped cilantro
- 2 tablespoons of salad dressing
- 1 tablespoon of chopped mint

DIRECTIONS:

1. In a bowl, add all ingredients, toss and serve.

NUTRITION: Calories 189 Total Fat: 2 g Total carbs: 5 g Fiber: 11 g Sugar: 3 g Protein: 12 g Sodium: 150 mg

218. Bacon, Brussels Sprout & Spinach Salad

Preparation Time: 15 Minutes
Cooking Time: 10 Minutes
Servings: 4
INGREDIENTS:

- 2 cups of Brussels sprouts, thinly sliced
- 3 tablespoons of wine vinegar
- 1/4 teaspoon of sugar
- 3 tablespoons of extra-virgin olive oil
- 1 1/2 teaspoon of caraway seed
- 8 slices of bacon
- Half-pound of chopped spinach

DIRECTIONS:

1. In a skillet, cook bacon until crispy, take it out on paper towels and crumble.
2. Add Brussels sprouts to the pan with seeds, cook for 1-2 minutes.
3. Add the rest of the ingredients to the pan, except for spinach. Cook for 1 minute.
4. Add spinach and cook for 1-2 minutes.
5. Before serving, add crispy bacon on top. Serve.

NUTRITION: Calories 293 Total Fat: 19g Total carbs: 12g Fiber: 17g Sugar: 1g Protein: 10g Sodium: 367mg

219. Golden Beet & Potato Soup

Preparation Time: 15 Minutes
Cooking Time: 45 Minutes
Servings: 5-6
INGREDIENTS:

- 2 tablespoons of cooking oil
- 4 cups of water
- 1 lb. of peeled Russet potatoes, cubed
- 2 lbs. peeled golden beets & chopped
- 1 teaspoon of salt
- 2 sweet chopped onions
- 1 tablespoon of lemon juice
- 4 peeled garlic cloves
- black pepper, to taste

DIRECTIONS:

1. Let the oven preheat to 400 F.
2. Toss the beets on a baking sheet with oil (half) and roast for 10 minutes.
3. On a different baking sheet, spread onion, peeled garlic and potatoes, toss with rest of the oil and roast for 30 minutes.
4. In a pan, add all roasted vegetables with water, salt and pepper.
5. Puree with a stick blender.
6. Add lemon juice and serve.

NUTRITION: Calories 265 Total fat: 12 g Total carbs: 13 g Fiber: 14 g Sugar: 5 g Protein: 14 g Sodium: 217mg

220. Thai Mango Avocado Salad

Preparation Time: 15 Minutes
Cooking Time: 10 Minutes
Servings: 5-6
INGREDIENTS:

- 1 tablespoon of Coconut Oil
- 1 cubed Avocado
- 1/4 cup of chopped Fresh Cilantro
- 1 cup of Mango
- Sea Salt, to taste
- 1/4 cup of sliced Fresh Mint
- 1 peeled Sweet Potato & sliced into ¼" thick
- 2/3 cup of diced Cucumber

For Sauce

- 2 teaspoons of paleo Fish Sauce
- 4 teaspoons of Lime Juice

DIRECTIONS:

1. Let the grill preheat to high.
2. Toss the potatoes in oil and grill for 3 to 4 minutes on one side, and let them cool.
3. Dice the potatoes and transfer them to a bowl.
4. Add the rest of the ingredients. Toss and serve.

NUTRITION: Calories 170 Total fat: 8.2 g Total carbs: 24.5 g Fiber: 17g Sugar: 1g Protein: 2.1 g Sodium: 305 mg

221. Warm Breakfast Salad

Preparation Time: 10 Minutes
Cooking Time: 10 Minutes
Servings: 4
INGREDIENTS:

- 1/3 cup of diced shallot
- 1 tablespoon of water
- 1 1/2 tablespoon of olive oil
- 1/4 teaspoon of sea salt & pepper, each
- 1/3 cup of blueberries
- 1 1/3 cup of peeled butternut squash, chopped
- 12 oz. of Coleslaw mix
- 1 tablespoon of balsamic vinegar
- 1 sliced avocado
- 1/4 teaspoon of minced garlic
- 4 eggs

DIRECTIONS:

1. In a bowl, add squash with one tablespoon of water and microwave for 2 or 2.5 minutes, covered with plastic wrap.
2. Drain and mash it well.
3. In a skillet, sauté onion in hot oil for 2 minutes. Add the rest of the ingredients except for avocado, blueberries, eggs and squash.
4. Cook for 1-2 minutes, with one tablespoon of water.
5. Take it out in a bowl, add blueberries.
6. Cook eggs sunny side up to desired consistency.
7. Serve slaw with eggs, avocado and mashed squash on the side.

NUTRITION: Calories 235 Total fat: 1.5 g Total carbs: 18 g Fiber: 7g Sugar: 6.5 g Protein: 9.2 g Sodium: 213 mg

222. Grilled Chicken Taco Salad

Preparation Time: 30 Minutes
Cooking Time: 20 Minutes
Servings: 4

INGREDIENTS:

- ¾ cup of salsa
- 1 cup of chopped cilantro, fresh
- 1 teaspoon of ground cumin
- 1 tablespoon of lime juice
- 1 can of (15 oz.) black beans, rinsed
- 2 tablespoons of chili powder
- 1 teaspoon of brown sugar
- 1 pound of chicken breast halved, skinless & boneless
- 1 teaspoon of ground coriander
- ¼ teaspoon of cayenne pepper
- 4 cups of shredded lettuce
- 1 tablespoon of olive oil
- 4 corn tortillas of 7"

DIRECTIONS:

1. Let the grill preheat to medium-high and oil spray the grates.
2. In a bowl, toss beans, cilantro (half), lime juice and salsa.
3. In a bowl, add the spices, oil and sugar, mix and rub all over chicken breasts.
4. Grill the chicken for 10-12 minutes, until the internal temperature reaches 165 F.
5. Grill the tortillas for 3-5 minutes.
6. Cut the chicken into strips and serve in tortillas with bean mixture and cilantro on top.

NUTRITION: Calories 470 Total fat: 18.7 g Total carbs: 44.4 g Fiber: 7g Sugar: 6.5 g Protein: 35.2 g Sodium: 831 mg

223. Butternut Squash Soup

Preparation Time: 10 Minutes
Cooking Time: 45 Minutes
Servings: 6

INGREDIENTS:

- 1 sweet chopped onion
- 3 lbs. of peeled butternut squash, chopped
- 1 diced carrot
- 1 sprig of fresh thyme
- 1 diced celery rib
- 1 tablespoon of olive oil
- 1 sprig of fresh rosemary
- 1/4 teaspoon of black pepper
- 3 cups of vegetable broth
- 1 peeled, chopped apple
- 3 minced garlic cloves

- 1/4 teaspoon of ground cinnamon
- 1 teaspoon of kosher salt

DIRECTIONS:

1. Sauté garlic, celery, carrots and onion for 3-5 minutes.
2. Add the rest of the ingredients and cook until squash is tender for 20-30 minutes; add more broth if it gets dry.
3. With a stick blender, puree the soup and adjust seasoning.
4. Serve.

NUTRITION: Calories 159 Total fat: 3 g Total carbs: 36 g Fiber: 6 g Sugar: 10 g Protein: 3 g Sodium: 876 mg

224. Tuscan Black Cabbage Soup

Preparation Time: 10 minutes
Cooking Time: 15 minutes
Servings: 2

INGREDIENTS:

- Pound Tuscan black cabbage
- Tablespoons further virgin olive oil
- Large onion, thinly sliced
- Celery stalk, thinly sliced
- Carrot, diced
- Medium potato, bare-assed and diced
- 5 cups vegetable broth or water
- Salt
- Freshly ground black pepper
- Slices wheaten bread
- Garlic cloves, peeled, and cut in half

DIRECTIONS

1. Wash the cabbage and take away the stalks. Withdraw skinny strips and heat the vegetable oil
2. In an exceedingly massive pot and cook the onion, celery, carrot, and potato for three minutes.
3. Add the cabbage and broth and bring to a boil cowl and simmer for one hour and you should After that you should Season it with salt & black pepper.
4. Meanwhile place the slices of bread on a baking receptacle and toast
5. In an exceedingly preheated 375 ·p kitchen appliance till they're golden.
6. Take away from the kitchen appliance and rub every slice with garlic.
7. Place the slices of bread into individual soup bowls and pour the new soup over them.
8. Serve at once.

NUTRITION: Calories: 456, Fats: 19g, Carbss: 27g, Protein: 8g

225. Potato Leek Soup

Preparation Time: 10 minutes
Cooking Time: 20 minutes
Servings: 5

INGREDIENTS:

- 4 tablespoons of olive oil
- 3 leeks
- 3 cups of onions, diced
- 1 lb. Of potatoes, diced
- 4 garlic cloves, chopped
- 1 tablespoon of thyme
- 6 cups of veggie stock
- ½ teaspoon of pepper
- 1 teaspoon of salt
- ½ cup of plant-based sour cream
- 2 tablespoons of chives, for garnishing

DIRECTIONS

1. Cut the leeks in half-length. Slice them into ¼-inch rounds.
2. Heat oil over medium heat in a pot or oven.
3. Add the leeks and sauté for 8 minutes.
4. Add the garlic. Sauté for 3 minutes more.
5. Add the thyme, potatoes, and stock. Boil. Turn the heat to a simmer for 20 minutes. Your potatoes should be tender.
6. Add the pepper and salt.
7. Blend in batches to make it very silky and smooth.
8. Return your soup to the pot. Simmer over low heat.
9. Stir the sour cream in. Serve with the chives.

NUTRITION: Calories 224 Carbss 31g Cholesterol 10mg Fat 13g Protein 4g Sugar 4g Fiber 4g Sodium 337mg

VEGAN RECIPES

226. Chipotle, Pinto, and Black Bean and Corn Succotash

Preparation Time: 5 Minutes
Cooking Time: 10 Minutes
Servings: 2
Ingredients:
- 2 tablespoons extra-virgin olive oil
- 1 1/2 cups fresh or frozen corn
- 1 cup black beans, chopped
- 2 green onions, white and green parts, sliced
- 1/2 tablespoon minced garlic
- 1 medium tomato, chopped
- 1 teaspoon chili powder
- 1/2 teaspoon chipotle powder
- 1/2 teaspoon ground cumin
- 1 (14-ounce) can pinto beans, drained and rinsed
- 1 teaspoon sea salt, or to taste

Directions:
1. Heat the olive oil in a large skillet over medium heat. Add the corn, black beans, green onions, and garlic and stir for 5 minutes.
2. Add the tomato, chili powder, chipotle powder, and cumin and stir for 3 minutes, until the tomato starts to soften.
3. In a bowl, mash some of the pinto beans with a fork. Add all of the beans to the skillet and stir for 2 minutes, until the beans are heated through.
4. Remove from the heat and stir in the salt. Serve hot or warm.

Nutrition: Calories: 391Fat: 16gCarbs: 53g Fiber: 15gSugar: 4g Protein: 15g Sodium: 253mg

227. Mixed Vegetable Medley

Preparation Time: 5 Minutes
Cooking Time: 20 Minutes
Servings: 2
Ingredients:
- 1 stick (1/2 cup) unsalted butter, divided
- 1 large potato, cut into 1/2-inch dice
- 1 onion, chopped
- 1/2 tablespoon minced garlic
- 1 cup pinto beans, chopped
- 2 ears fresh sweet corn, kernels removed
- 1 red bell pepper, seeded and cut into strips
- 2 cups sliced white mushrooms
- Salt
- Freshly ground black pepper

Directions:
1. Heat half of the butter in a large nonstick skillet over medium-high heat. When the butter is frothy, add the potato and cook, stirring frequently, for 15 minutes, until golden.
2. Turn the heat down slightly if the butter begins to burn.
3. Add the remaining butter, turn down the heat to medium, and add the onion, garlic, pinto beans, and corn. Cook, stirring frequently, for 5 minutes.
4. Add the red bell pepper and mushrooms. Stir for another 5 minutes, until the vegetables are tender and the mushrooms have browned but are still plump. Add more butter, if necessary.
5. Remove from heat and season with salt and pepper. Serve hot.

Nutrition: Calories: 688 Fat: 48g Carbs: 63g Fiber: 11g Sugar: 11g Protein: 11g Sodium: 360mg

228. Spicy Lentils with Spinach

Preparation Time: 5 Minutes
Cooking Time: 25 Minutes
Servings: 4
Ingredients:
- 1 cup dried red lentils, well-rinsed
- 2 1/2 cups water
- 1 tablespoon extra-virgin olive oil
- 1 tablespoon minced garlic
- 1 teaspoon ground cumin
- 1/2 teaspoon ground coriander
- 1/2 teaspoon turmeric
- 1/4 teaspoon cayenne pepper
- 1 medium tomato, chopped
- 1 (16-ounce) package spinach
- 1 teaspoon salt
- Freshly ground black pepper

Directions:
1. In a medium saucepan, bring the lentils and water to a boil.
2. Partially cover the pot, reduce the heat to medium, and simmer, stirring occasionally, until the lentils are tender, about 15 minutes.
3. Drain the lentils and set aside.
4. In a large nonstick skillet, heat the olive oil over medium heat. When hot, add the garlic, cumin, coriander, turmeric, and cayenne. Sauté for 2 minutes.
5. Stir in the tomato and cook for another 3 to 5 minutes, until the tomato begins to break apart and the mixture thickens somewhat.
6. Add handfuls of the spinach at a time, stirring until wilted.
7. Stir in the drained lentils and cook for another few minutes.
8. Season with salt and freshly ground black pepper and serve hot.

Nutrition: Calories: 237 Fat: 5g Carbs: 35g Fiber: 18g Sugar: 2g Protein: 16g Sodium: 677mg

229. Pinto and Black Bean Fry with Couscous

Preparation Time: 5 Minutes
Cooking Time: 20 Minutes
Servings: 4
Ingredients:
- 1/2 cup water
- 1/3 cup couscous (semolina or whole-wheat)
- 2 tablespoons extra-virgin olive oil
- 1 small onion, chopped
- 1/2 tablespoon minced garlic
- 1 cup black beans, cut into 1-inch pieces
- 1 cup fresh or frozen corn
- 1 1/2 teaspoons chili powder
- 1/2 teaspoon ground cumin
- 1 large tomato, finely chopped
- 1 (14-ounce) can pinto beans, drained and rinsed
- 1 teaspoon salt

Directions:

1. Bring the water to a boil in a small saucepan. Remove from the heat and stir in the couscous. Cover the pan and let sit for 10 minutes.
2. Gently fluff the couscous with a fork.
3. While the couscous is cooking, heat the olive oil in a large skillet over medium heat. Add the onion and garlic and stir for 1 minute.
4. Add the black beans and stir for 4 minutes, until they begin to soften.
5. Add the corn, stir for another 2 minutes, then add the chili powder and cumin, and stir to coat the vegetables.
6. Add the tomato and simmer for 3 or 4 minutes. Stir in the pinto beans and couscous and cook for 3 to 4 minutes, until everything is heated throughout. Stir often.
7. Stir in the salt and serve hot or warm.

Nutrition: Calories: 267 Fat: 8g Carbs: 41g Fiber: 10g Sugar: 4g Protein: 10g Sodium: 601mg

230. Indonesian-Style Spicy Fried Tempeh Strips

Preparation Time: 5 Minutes
Cooking Time: 20 Minutes
Servings: 4
Ingredients:

- 1 cup sesame oil, or as needed
- 1 (12-ounce) package tempeh, cut into narrow 2-inch strips
- 2 medium onions, sliced
- 1 1/2 tablespoons tomato paste
- 3 teaspoons tamari or soy sauce
- 1 teaspoon dried red chili flakes
- 1/2 teaspoon brown sugar
- 2 tablespoons lime juice

Directions:

1. Heat the sesame oil in a large wok or saucepan over medium-high heat. Add more sesame oil as needed to raise the level to at least 1 inch.
2. As soon as the oil is hot but not smoking, add the tempeh slices and cook, stirring frequently, for 10 minutes, until a light golden color on all sides.
3. Add the onions and stir for another 10 minutes, until the tempeh and onions are brown and crispy.
4. Remove with a slotted spoon and add to a large bowl lined with several sheets of paper towel.
5. While the tempeh and onions are cooking, whisk together the tomato paste, tamari or soy sauce, red chili flakes, brown sugar, and lime juice in a small bowl.
6. Remove the paper towel from the large bowl and pour the sauce over the tempeh strips. Mix well to coat.

Nutrition: Calories: 317 Fat: 23g Carbs: 15g Sugar: 4g Protein: 17g Sodium: 266mg

231. Vegetable Rice

Preparation Time: 5 Minutes
Cooking Time: 25 Minutes
Servings: 4
Ingredients:

- 3/4 cup uncooked short- or long-grain white rice
- 1 1/2 cups water
- 2 tablespoons sesame oil, divided
- 2 carrots, diced
- 1 tablespoon minced garlic
- 6 green onions, white and green parts, sliced and divided
- 2 tablespoons tamari or soy sauce
- 1/2 cup frozen green peas, defrosted

Directions:

1. Rinse the rice and add to a small saucepan. Add the water and bring to a boil.
2. Reduce the heat to low, cover, and simmer for 15 minutes, until the water is absorbed. Fluff with a fork and set aside.
3. While the rice is cooking, heat 1/2 tablespoon of the sesame oil in a large saucepan or wok over medium heat.
4. Cook without stirring for 5 minutes. Remove to a plate and cut into small strips. Set aside.
5. Return the saucepan or wok to the heat. Heat the remaining 2 1/2 tablespoons of sesame oil. Add the carrots and stir for 2 minutes.
6. Add the mushrooms, garlic, and the white parts of the green onions. Stir for 3 more minutes.
7. Add the cooked rice and tamari or soy sauce. Cook, stirring frequently, for 10 minutes, until the rice is sticky.
8. Toss in the green parts of the green onions, and peas and stir to mix. Remove from the heat and serve hot with extra tamari or soy sauce, if desired.

Nutrition: Calories: 271 Fat: 10g Carbs: 37g Fiber: 3g Sugar: 4g Protein: 9g Sodium: 567mg

232. Spanish-Style Saffron Rice with Black Beans

Preparation Time: 5 Minutes
Cooking Time: 25 Minutes
Servings: 4
Ingredients:

- 2 cups vegetable stock
- 1/4 teaspoon saffron threads (optional)
- 1 1/2 tablespoons extra-virgin olive oil
- 1 small red or yellow onion, halved and thinly sliced
- 1 tablespoon minced garlic
- 1 teaspoon turmeric
- 2 teaspoons paprika
- 1 cup long-grain white rice, well-rinsed
- 1 (14-ounce) can black beans, drained and rinsed
- 1/2 cup pinto beans, halved or quartered
- 1 small red bell pepper, chopped
- 1 teaspoon salt

Directions:

1. In a small pot, heat the vegetable stock until boiling. Add the saffron, if using, and remove from the heat.
2. Meanwhile, heat the olive oil in a large nonstick skillet over medium heat.
3. Add the onion, garlic, turmeric, paprika, and rice and stir to coat.
4. Pour in the stock, and mix in the black beans, pinto beans, and red bell pepper.
5. Bring to a boil, reduce the heat to medium-low, cover, and simmer until the rice is tender and most of the liquid has been absorbed, about 20 minutes.
6. Stir in the salt and serve hot.

Nutrition: Calories: 332 Fat: 5g Carbs: 63g Fiber: 9g Sugar: 2g Protein: 11g Sodium: 658mg

233. Simple Lemon Dal

Preparation Time: 5 Minutes
Cooking Time: 25 Minutes
Servings: 4
Ingredients:
For the lentils

- 1 cup dried red lentils, well-rinsed
- 2 1/2 cups water
- 1/2 teaspoon turmeric

- 1/2 teaspoon ground cumin
- 2 tablespoons lemon juice
- 1/3cup fresh parsley, chopped
- 1 teaspoon salt

For finishing
- 1 tablespoon extra-virgin olive oil
- 2 teaspoons minced garlic
- 1/2 teaspoon dried red chili flakes or ¼ teaspoon cayenne pepper

Directions:
1. Add the lentils to a medium saucepan and pour in the water. Stir in the turmeric and cumin and bring to a boil.
2. Reduce the heat to medium-low, cover, and simmer, stirring occasionally, for 20 minutes, until the lentils are soft and the mixture has thickened.
3. Stir in the lemon juice, parsley, and salt, and remove the pan from the heat.
4. In a small saucepan, heat the oil over medium-high heat. When hot, add the garlic and red chili flakes or cayenne, and stir for 1 minute.
5. Quickly pour the oil into the cooked lentils, cover, and let sit for 5 minutes.
6. Stir the lentils and serve immediately.

Nutrition: Calories: 207 Fat: 4g Carbs: 30g Fiber: 15g Sugar: 1g Protein: 13g Sodium: 589mg

234. Cauliflower Latke

Preparation Time: 15 minutes
Cooking Time: 30 minutes
Servings: 4
Ingredients:
- 12 oz. cauliflower rice, cooked
- 1 egg, beaten
- 1/3 cup cornstarch
- Salt and pepper to taste
- ¼ cup vegetable oil, divided
- Chopped onion chives

Directions:
1. Squeeze excess water from the cauliflower rice using paper towels.
2. Place the cauliflower rice in a bowl.
3. Stir in the egg and cornstarch.
4. Season with salt and pepper.
5. Fill 2 tablespoons of oil into a pan over medium heat.
6. Add 2 to 3 tablespoons of the cauliflower mixture into the pan.
7. Cook for 3 minutes each side.
8. Repeat until you've used up the rest of the batter.
9. Garnish with chopped chives.

Nutrition: 209 Calories 1.9g Fiber 3.4g Protein

235. Brussels sprouts Hash

Preparation Time: 30 minutes
Cooking Time: 20 minutes
Servings: 4
Ingredients:
- 1 lb. Brussels sprouts, sliced in half
- 1 tablespoon olive oil
- Salt and pepper to taste
- 2 teaspoons balsamic vinegar
- ¼ cup goat cheese, crumbled

Directions:
1. Preheat your oven to 400 degrees F.
2. Coat the Brussels sprouts with oil.
3. Sprinkle with salt and pepper.
4. Transfer to a baking pan.

5. Roast in the oven for 20 minutes.
6. Drizzle with the vinegar.
7. Sprinkle with the seeds and cheese before serving.

Nutrition: 117 Calories 4.8g Fiber 5.8g Protein

236. Brussels sprouts Chips

Preparation Time: 10 minutes
Cooking Time: 0 minute
Servings: 6
Ingredients:
- 3 tablespoons lemon juice
- ¼ cup olive oil
- Salt and pepper to taste
- 1 lb. Brussels sprouts, sliced thinly
- ½ cup pecans, toasted and chopped

Directions:
1. Mix the lemon juice, olive oil, salt and pepper in a bowl.
2. Toss the Brussels sprouts, and pecans in this mixture.

Nutrition: 245 Calories 6.4g Protein 5g Fiber

237. Vegan Potato Pancakes

Preparation Time: 5 minutes
Cooking Time: 10 minutes
Servings: 10
Ingredients:
- ½ yellow onion (grated)
- ¼ teaspoons baking powder
- Salt and pepper to taste
- 3 russet potato (grated)
- ½ cup all-purpose flour
- vegetable oil for frying
- 2 green onion (chopped)

Directions:
1. In a large bowl, mix everything together.
2. Heat about 1 tablespoon of oil in a frying pan over medium-high heat. Once hot, form a loose patty out of the potato mixture.
3. When the oil is hot, drop the patty directly into the frying pan.
4. After frying the bottom for a few minutes, flip over and fry the other side.
5. Repeat with remaining potato mixture until all of it is consumed. If necessary, add more oil to the pan.

Nutrition: 70 Calories 10g Carbs 2.1g Protein 1g Fat

238. Broccoli with Lemon

Preparation Time: 15 minutes
Cooking Time: 15 minutes
Servings: 8
Ingredients:
- 2 lemons, sliced in half
- 1 lb. broccoli
- 2 tablespoons sesame oil, toasted
- Salt and pepper to taste
- 1 tablespoon sesame seeds, toasted

Directions:
1. Fill oil into a pan over medium heat.
2. Add the lemons and cook until caramelized.
3. Transfer to a plate.
4. Put the broccoli in the pan and cook for 8 minutes.
5. Squeeze the lemons to release juice in a bowl.
6. Stir in the oil, salt and pepper.
7. Coat the broccoli rabe with the mixture.
8. Sprinkle seeds on top.

Nutrition: 59 Calories 4.1g Carbs 2.2g Protein

239. Vegan Green Spaghetti

Preparation Time: 2 to 3 hours
Cooking Time: 15 to 20 minutes
Servings: 8
INGREDIENTS:

- 4 roasted poblano chiles, chopped
- 2 chopped garlic cloves
- 1 cup of almond milk, unsweetened
- 2 tablespoon of olive oil
- 1 cup of soaked cashews
- 3 tablespoon of lemon juice
- Half chopped white onion
- Black Pepper, to taste
- 3 tablespoon of cilantro
- ¾ teaspoon of salt

Pasta

- Half cup of water
- Spaghetti: 26 oz.

DIRECTIONS:

1. Soak the cashews in boiling water for 2 to 3 hours.
2. Sauté onion in hot oil for 3 to 4 minutes, add garlic and cook for 1 to 2 minutes.
3. Add rest of the ingredients and blend with a stick blender, taste and adjust seasoning.
4. Cook pasta as per the pack's instructions, drain all bit half cup of water.
5. Add sauce to the pasta, toss well and serve.

NUTRITION: Calories 496 Total fat: 13 g Total carbs: 79 g Fiber: 0 g Sugar: 5.3 g Protein: 16 g Sodium: 269 mg

240. Grilled Fajitas with Jalapeño Sauce

Preparation Time: 1 hour & 10 minutes
Cooking Time: 25 minutes
Servings: 4
Ingredients:

- Marinade
- ¼ cup olive oil
- ¼ cup lime juice
- 2 garlic cloves, minced
- 1 teaspoon chili powder
- 1 teaspoon ground cumin
- 1 teaspoon dried oregano
- ½ teaspoon salt
- ½ teaspoon black pepper
- Jalapeño Sauce
- 6 jalapeno peppers stemmed, halved, and seeded
- 1–2 teaspoons olive oil
- 1 cup raw cashews, soaked and drained
- ½ cup almond milk
- ¼ cup water
- ¼ cup lime juice
- 2 teaspoons agaves
- ½ cup fresh cilantro
- Salt, to taste
- Grilled Vegetables
- ½ lb. asparagus spears, trimmed
- 2 large portobello mushrooms, sliced

- 1 large zucchini, sliced
- 1 red bell pepper, sliced
- 1 red onion, sliced

Directions:

1. Dump all the ingredients for the marinade in a large bowl.
2. Toss in all the veggies and mix well to marinate for 1 hour.
3. Meanwhile, prepare the sauce and brush the jalapenos with oil.
4. Grill the jalapenos for 5 minutes per side until slightly charred.
5. Blend the grilled jalapenos with other ingredients for the sauce in a blender.
6. Transfer this sauce to a separate bowl and keep it aside.
7. Now grill the marinated veggies in the grill until soft and slightly charred on all sides.
8. Pour the prepared sauce over the grilled veggies.
9. Serve.

Nutrition: Calories: 663 Fat: 68g Carbs: 20g Fiber: 2g Protein: 4g

241. Grilled Ratatouille Kebabs

Preparation Time: 1 hour & 15 minutes
Cooking Time: 10 minutes
Servings: 6
Ingredients:

- 3 tablespoons soy sauce
- 3 tablespoons balsamic vinegar
- 1 teaspoon dried thyme leaves
- 2 tablespoons extra virgin olive oil
- Veggies
- 1 zucchini, diced
- ½ red onion, diced
- ½ red capsicum, diced
- 2 tomatoes, diced
- 1 small eggplant, diced
- 8 button mushrooms, diced

Directions:

1. Toss the veggies with soy sauce, olive oil, thyme, and balsamic vinegar in a large bowl.
2. Thread the veggies alternately on the wooden skewers and reserve the remaining marinade.
3. Marinate these skewers for 1 hour in the refrigerator.
4. Preheat the grill over medium heat.
5. Grill the marinated skewers for 5 minutes per side while basting with the reserved marinade.
6. Serve fresh.

Nutrition: Calories: 166 Fat: 17g Carbs: 5g Fiber: 1g Protein: 1g

242. Tofu Hoagie Rolls

Preparation Time: 20 minutes
Cooking Time: 20 minutes
Servings: 6
Ingredients:

- ½ cup vegetable broth
- ¼ cup hot sauce
- 1 tablespoon vegan butter
- 1 (16 ounce) package tofu, pressed and diced
- 4 cups cabbage, shredded
- 2 medium apples, grated
- 1 medium shallot, grated
- 6 tablespoons vegan mayonnaise
- 1 tablespoon apple cider vinegar
- Salt and black pepper
- 4 6-inch hoagie rolls, toasted

Directions:

1. In a saucepan, combine broth with butter and hot sauce and bring to a boil.

2. Add tofu and reduce the heat to a simmer.
3. Cook for 10 minutes then remove from heat and let sit for 10 minutes to marinate.
4. Toss cabbage and rest of the ingredients in a salad bowl.
5. Prepare and set up a grill on medium heat.
6. Drain the tofu and grill for 5 minutes per side.
7. Lay out the toasted hoagie rolls and add grilled tofu to each hoagie
8. Add the cabbage mixture evenly between them then close it.
9. Serve.

Nutrition: Calories: 111 Fat: 11g Carbs: 5g Fiber: 0g Protein: 1g

243. Grilled Avocado with Tomatoes

Preparation Time: 10 minutes
Cooking Time: 15 minutes
Servings: 6
Ingredients:

- 3 avocados, halved and pitted
- 3 limes, wedged
- 1½ cup grape tomatoes
- 1 cup fresh corn
- 1 cup onion, chopped
- 3 serrano peppers
- 2 garlic cloves, peeled
- ¼ cup cilantro leaves, chopped
- 1 tablespoon olive oil
- Salt and black pepper to taste

Directions:

1. Prepare and set a grill over medium heat.
2. Brush the avocado with oil and grill it for 5 minutes per side.
3. Meanwhile, toss the garlic, onion, corn, tomatoes, and pepper in a baking sheet.
4. At 550 degrees F, roast the vegetables for 5 minutes.
5. Toss the veggie mix and stir in salt, cilantro, and black pepper.
6. Mix well then fill the grilled avocadoes with the mixture.
7. Garnish with lime.
8. Serve.

Nutrition: Calories: 56 Fat: 6g Carbs: 3g Fiber: 0g Protein: 1g

244. Grilled Tofu with Chimichurri Sauce

Preparation Time: 10 minutes
Cooking Time: 12 minutes
Servings: 4
Ingredients:

- 2 tablespoons plus 1 teaspoon olive oil
- 1 teaspoon dried oregano
- 1 cup parsley leaves
- ½ cup cilantro leaves
- 2 Fresno peppers, seeded and chopped
- 2 tablespoons white wine vinegar
- 2 tablespoons water
- 1 tablespoon fresh lime juice
- Salt and black pepper
- 1 cup couscous, cooked
- 1 teaspoon lime zest
- ¼ cup toasted pumpkin seeds
- 1 cup fresh spinach, chopped
- 1 (15.5 ounce) can kidney beans, rinsed and drained
- 1 (14 to 16 ounce) block tofu, diced
- 2 summer squashes, diced
- 3 spring onions, quartered

Directions:

1. In a saucepan, heat 2 tablespoons oil and add oregano over medium heat.
2. After 30 seconds add parsley, chili pepper, cilantro, lime juice, 2 tablespoons water, vinegar, salt and black pepper.
3. Mix well then blend in a blender.
4. Add the remaining oil, pumpkin seeds, beans and spinach and cook for 3 minutes.
5. Stir in couscous and adjust seasoning with salt and black pepper.
6. Prepare and set up a grill on medium heat.
7. Thread the tofu, squash, and onions on the skewer in an alternating pattern.
8. Grill these skewers for 4 minutes per side while basting with the green sauce.
9. Serve the skewers on top of the couscous with green sauce.
10. Enjoy.

Nutrition: Calories: 813 Fat: 83g Carbs: 25g Fiber: 1g Protein: 7g

245. Grilled Seitan with Creole Sauce

Preparation Time: 2 hours & 10 minutes
Cooking Time: 14 minutes
Servings: 4
Ingredients:
Grilled Seitan Kebabs:

- 4 cups seitan, diced
- 2 medium onions, diced into squares
- 8 bamboo skewers
- 1 can coconut milk
- 2½ tablespoons creole spice
- 2 tablespoons tomato paste
- 2 cloves of garlic

Creole Spice Mix:

- 2 tablespoons paprika
- 12 dried peri chili peppers
- 1 tablespoon salt
- 1 tablespoon freshly ground pepper
- 2 teaspoons dried thyme
- 2 teaspoons dried oregano

Directions:

1. Prepare the creole seasoning by blending all its ingredients and preserve in a sealable jar.
2. Thread seitan and onion on the bamboo skewers in an alternating pattern.
3. On a baking sheet, mix coconut milk with creole seasoning, tomato paste and garlic.
4. Soak the skewers in the milk marinade for 2 hours.
5. Prepare and set up a grill over medium heat.
6. Grill the skewers for 7 minutes per side.
7. Serve.

Nutrition: Calories: 407 Fat: 42g Carbs: 13g Fiber: 1g Protein: 4g

246. Pinto Beans Gremolata

Preparation Time: 15 minutes
Cooking Time: 10 minutes
Servings: 6
Ingredients:

- 1-pound fresh pinto beans
- 3 garlic cloves, minced
- Zest of 2 oranges
- 3 tablespoons minced fresh parsley
- 2 tablespoons pine nuts
- 3 tablespoons olive oil
- Sea salt
- Freshly ground black pepper

Directions:
1. Boil water over high heat. Cook pinto beans for 3 minutes. Drain r and rinse with cold water to stop the cooking.
2. Blend garlic, orange zest, and parsley.
3. In a huge sauté pan over medium-high heat, toast the pine nuts in the dry, hot pan for 3 minutes. Remove from the pan and set aside.
4. Cook olive oil in the same pan until it shimmers. Add the beans and cook, -stirring frequently, until heated through, about 2 minutes. Take pan away from the heat and add the parsley mixture and pine nuts. Season with salt and pepper. Serve immediately.

Nutrition: 98 Calories 2g Fiber 3g Protein

247. Minted Peas

Preparation Time: 5 minutes
Cooking Time: 5 minutes
Servings: 4
Ingredient:
- 1 tablespoon olive oil
- 4 cups peas, fresh or frozen (not canned)
- ½ teaspoon sea salt
- Freshly ground black pepper
- 3 tablespoons chopped fresh mint

Directions:
1. In a large sauté pan, cook olive oil over medium-high heat until hot. Add the peas and cook, about 5 minutes. Remove the pan from heat. Stir in the salt, season with pepper, and stir in the mint. Serve hot.

Nutrition: 90 Calories 5g Fiber 8g Protein

248. Sweet and Spicy Brussels Sprout Hash

Preparation Time: 10 minutes
Cooking Time: 15 minutes
Servings: 4
Ingredient:
- 3 tablespoons olive oil
- 2 shallots, thinly sliced
- 1½ pounds Brussel sprouts
- 3 tablespoons apple cider vinegar
- 1 tablespoon pure maple syrup
- ½ teaspoon sriracha sauce (or to taste)
- Sea salt
- Freshly ground black pepper

Directions:
1. In pan, cook olive oil over medium-high heat until it shimmers. Mix the shallots and Brussels sprouts and cook, stirring frequently, until the -vegetables soften and begin to turn golden brown, about 10 minutes. Stir in the vinegar, using a spoon to scrape any browned bits from the pan's bottom. Stir in the maple syrup and Sriracha.
1. Simmer, stirring frequently, until the liquid reduces, 3 to 5 minutes. Season and serve immediately.

Nutrition: 97 Calories 4g Fiber 7g Protein

249. Glazed Curried Carrots

Preparation Time: 5 minutes
Cooking Time: 15 minutes
Servings: 6
Ingredient:
- 1-pound carrots
- 2 tablespoons olive oil
- 2 tablespoons curry powder
- 2 tablespoons pure maple syrup
- Juice of ½ lemon

Directions:
1. Cook carrots with water over medium-high heat for 10 minutes. Drain and return them to the pan over medium-low heat.
2. Stir in the olive oil, curry powder, maple syrup, and lemon juice. Cook, stirring constantly, until the liquid reduces, about 5 minutes. Season well and serve immediately.

Nutrition: 91 Calories 5g Fiber 9g Protein

250. Pepper Medley

Preparation Time: 10 minutes
Cooking Time: 15 minutes
Servings: 4
Ingredient:
- 3 tablespoons olive oil
- 1 red bell pepper, sliced
- 1 orange bell pepper, sliced
- 1 yellow bell pepper, sliced
- 1 green bell pepper, sliced
- 2 garlic cloves, minced
- 3 tablespoons red wine vinegar
- 2 tablespoons chopped fresh basil

Directions:
1. Warm up olive oil over medium-high heat. Stir in the bell peppers and cook, stir, for 7 to 10 minutes. Cook garlic for 30 seconds. Add the vinegar, using a spoon to scrape any browned bits off the bottom of the pan.
2. Simmer until the vinegar reduces, 2 to 3 minutes. Season. Stir in the basil and serve immediately.

Nutrition: 96 Calories 3g Fiber 5g Protein

251. Garlicky Red Wine Mushrooms

Preparation Time: 10 minutes
Cooking Time: 15 minutes
Servings: 4
Ingredient:
- 3 tablespoons olive oil
- 2 cups sliced mushrooms
- 3 garlic cloves, minced
- ½ cup red wine
- 1 tablespoon dried thyme

Directions:
1. Cook olive oil over medium-high heat until it shimmers. Mix in the mushrooms and sit, untouched, until they release their liquid and begin to brown, about 5 minutes. Stir the mushrooms occasionally, cooking until softened and golden brown, about 5 minutes more. Cook garlic. Add the red wine and thyme, using a wooden spoon to scrape any browned bits off the pan's bottom.
2. Adjust heat to medium. Cook for 5 minutes. Season well and serve.

Nutrition: 98 Calories 4g Fiber 6g Protein

252. Sautéed Citrus Spinach

Preparation Time: 10 minutes
Cooking Time: 10 minutes
Servings: 4

Ingredient:

- 2 tablespoons olive oil
- 1 shallot, chopped
- 2 garlic cloves, minced
- 10 ounces' baby spinach
- Zest and juice of 1 orange

Directions:

1. Cook olive oil over medium-high heat. Cook the shallot for 3 minutes. Cook garlic for 30 seconds.
2. Add the spinach, orange juice, and orange zest. Cook for 2 minutes. Season with salt and pepper. Serve warm.

Nutrition: 91 Calories 4g Fiber 7g Protein

253. Lemon Broccoli Rabe

Preparation Time: 10 minutes
Cooking Time: 10 minutes
Servings: 4

Ingredient:

- 8 cups water
- Sea salt
- 2 bunches broccoli rabe, chopped
- 3 tablespoons olive oil
- 3 garlic cloves, minced
- Pinch of cayenne pepper
- Zest of 1 lemon

Directions:

1. Boil 8 cups of the water. Sprinkle a pinch of salt and the broccoli rabe. Cook until the broccoli rabe is slightly softened, about 2 minutes. Drain.
2. Heat olive oil over medium-high heat. Cook the garlic for 30 seconds. Stir in the broccoli rabe, cayenne, and lemon zest. Season with salt and black pepper. Serve immediately.

Nutrition: 99 Calories 7g Fiber 11g Protein

254. Spicy Swiss Chard

Preparation Time: 10 minutes
Cooking Time: 10 minutes
Servings: 4

Ingredient:

- 2 tablespoons olive oil
- 1 onion, chopped
- 2 bunches Swiss chard
- 3 garlic cloves, minced
- ½ teaspoon red pepper flakes (or to taste)
- Juice of ½ lemon

Directions:

1. In a big pot, cook olive oil over medium-high heat until it shimmers. Cook the onion and chard stems for 5 minutes.
2. Cook chard leaves for 1 minute. Stir in the garlic and pepper flakes. Cover and cook for 5 minutes. Stir in the lemon juice. Season with salt and serve immediately.

Nutrition: 94 Calories 5g Fiber 7g Protein

255. Red Peppers and Kale

Preparation Time: 5 minutes
Cooking Time: 15 minutes
Servings: 4

Ingredient:

- 2 bunches kale
- 3 tablespoons olive oil
- ½ onion, chopped
- 2 red bell peppers, cut into strips
- 3 garlic cloves, minced
- ¼ teaspoon red pepper flakes

Directions:

1. In steamer basket in a pan, steam the kale until it softens, 5 to 10 minutes. Remove from the heat and set aside.
2. Meanwhile, in a sauté pan, heat the olive oil over medium-high heat until it -shimmers. Cook onion and bell peppers for 5 minutes. Cook garlic for 30 seconds. Take out from heat and stir in the kale and red pepper flakes. Season and serve immediately.

Nutrition: 101 Calories 5g Fiber 10g Protein

256. Mashed Cauliflower with Roasted Garlic

Preparation Time: 5 minutes
Cooking Time: 10 minutes
Servings: 4

Ingredient:

- 2 heads cauliflower, cut into small florets
- 1 tablespoon olive oil
- 8 jarred roasted garlic cloves
- 2 teaspoons chopped fresh rosemary
- Sea salt
- Freshly ground black pepper
- 1 tablespoon chopped fresh chives

Directions:

1. Boil cauliflower florets for 9 minutes, then drain.
2. In a blender or food processor, combine the cauliflower, olive oil, garlic, and -rosemary and process until smooth. Season with salt and pepper. Stir in the chives and serve hot.

Nutrition: 88 Calories 1g Fiber 2g Protein

257. Steamed Broccoli with Walnut Pesto

Preparation Time: 5 minutes
Cooking Time: 10 minutes
Servings: 4

Ingredient:

- 1-pound broccoli florets
- 2 cups chopped fresh basil
- ¼ cup olive oil
- 4 garlic cloves
- ½ cup walnuts
- Pinch of cayenne pepper

Directions:

1. Put the broccoli in a large pot and cover with water. Bring to a simmer over medium-high heat and cook until the broccoli is tender, about 5 minutes.
2. Process basil, olive oil, garlic, walnuts, and cayenne for ten 1-second pulses, scraping down the bowl halfway through processing.
3. Drain and put again to the pan. Toss with the pesto. Serve immediately.

Nutrition: 101 Calories 3g Fiber 5g Protein

258. Roasted Asparagus with Balsamic Reduction

Preparation Time: 10 minutes
Cooking Time: 30 minutes
Servings: 4

Ingredient:

- 1½ pounds asparagus, trimmed
- 2 tablespoons olive oil
- ½ teaspoon sea salt
- ¼ teaspoon freshly ground black pepper
- 1/3 cup balsamic vinegar
- Juice and zest of 1 Meyer lemon

Directions:

1. Preheat the oven to 375°F. On a large rimmed baking sheet, throw the asparagus with the olive oil, salt, and pepper and then spread the asparagus out into a single layer. Roast for 23 minutes.
2. While roasting, put the vinegar in a small saucepan and bring it to a boil over medium-high heat. Decrease heat to low and simmer for 8 minutes.
3. When the asparagus is roasted, remove the baking sheet from the oven. Stir lemon juice and zest to coat. Drizzle the balsamic reduction over the top. Serve immediately.

Nutrition: 104 Calories 4g Fiber 8g Protein

259. Sweet and Sour Tempeh

Preparation Time: 10 minutes
Cooking Time: 8 minutes
Servings: 4

Ingredient:

- 1 cup pineapple juice
- 1 tablespoon unseasoned rice vinegar
- 1 tablespoon soy sauce
- 1 tablespoon cornstarch
- 2 tablespoons coconut oil
- 1-pound tempeh, cut into thin strips
- 6 green onions
- 1 green bell pepper, diced
- 4 garlic cloves, minced
- 2 cups prepared brown or white rice

Directions:

1. Blend pineapple juice, rice vinegar, soy sauce, and cornstarch and set aside.
2. In a wok or large sauté pan, heat the coconut oil over medium-high heat until it shimmers. Add the tempeh, green onions, and bell pepper and cook until vegetables soften, about 5 minutes.
3. Cook garlic. Stir in sauce and cook until it thickens. Serve over rice.

Nutrition: 95 Calories 2g Fiber 5g Protein

260. Fried Seitan Fingers

Preparation Time: 15 minutes
Cooking Time: 10 minutes
Servings: 4

INGREDIENT:

- 1 cup all-purpose flour
- 1 teaspoon garlic powder
- 1 teaspoon onion powder
- Pinch of cayenne pepper
- 1 teaspoon dried thyme
- ½ teaspoon sea salt
- ½ teaspoon freshly ground black pepper
- 1 cup soy milk
- 1 tablespoon lemon juice
- 2 tablespoons baking powder
- 2 tablespoons olive oil
- 8 ounces Seitan

DIRECTIONS:

1. In a shallow dish, incorporate flour, garlic powder, onion powder, cayenne, thyme, salt, and black pepper, whisking to mix thoroughly. In another shallow dish, whisk together the soy milk, lemon juice, and baking powder.
2. In sauté pan, cook the olive oil over medium-high heat. Dip each piece of seitan in the flour mixture, tapping off any excess flour. Next, dip the seitan in the soy milk mixture and then back in the flour mixture.
3. Fry for 4 minutes per side. Blot on paper towels before serving.

NUTRITION: 100 Calories 4g Fiber 8g Protein

261. Crusty Grilled Corn

Preparation Time: 10 minutes
Cooking Time: 15 minutes
Servings: 4

INGREDIENTS:

- 2 corn cobs
- 1/3 cup Vegenaise
- 1 small handful cilantro
- ½ cup breadcrumbs
- 1 teaspoon lemon juice

DIRECTIONS:

1. Preheat the gas grill on high heat.
2. Add corn grill to the grill and continue grilling until it turns golden-brown on all sides.
3. Mix the Vegenaise, cilantro, breadcrumbs, and lemon juice in a bowl.
4. Add grilled corn cobs to the crumbs mixture.
5. Toss well then serve.

NUTRITION: Calories: 253 Fat: 13g Protein: 31g Carbs: 3g Fiber: 0g

262. Grilled Carrots with Chickpea Salad

Preparation Time: 10 minutes
Cooking Time: 10 minutes
Servings: 8

INGREDIENTS:

- Carrots
- 8 large carrots
- 1 tablespoon oil
- 1 ½ teaspoon salt
- 1 teaspoon dried oregano
- 1 teaspoon dried thyme
- 2 teaspoons paprika powder
- 1 ½ tablespoon soy sauce
- ½ cup of water
- Chickpea Salad
- 14 oz. canned chickpeas
- 3 medium pickles
- 1 small onion
- A big handful of lettuce
- 1 teaspoon apple cider vinegar
- ½ teaspoon dried oregano
- ½ teaspoon salt
- Ground black pepper, to taste
- ½ cup vegan cream

DIRECTIONS:
1. Toss the carrots with all of its ingredients in a bowl.
2. Thread one carrot on a stick and place it on a plate.
3. Preheat the grill over high heat.
4. Grill the carrots for 2 minutes per side on the grill.
5. Toss the ingredients for the salad in a large salad bowl.
6. Slice grilled carrots and add them on top of the salad.
7. Serve fresh.

NUTRITION: Calories: 661 Fat: 68g Carbs: 17g Fiber: 2g Protein: 4g

263. Grilled Avocado Guacamole

Preparation Time: 10 minutes
Cooking Time: 25 minutes
Servings: 4
INGREDIENTS:
- ½ teaspoon olive oil
- 1 lime, halved
- ½ onion, halved
- 1 serrano chile, halved, stemmed, and seeded
- 3 Haas avocados, skin on
- 2–3 tablespoons fresh cilantro, chopped
- ½ teaspoon smoked salt

DIRECTIONS:
1. Preheat the grill over medium heat.
2. Brush the grilling grates with olive oil and place chile, onion, and lime on it.
3. Grill the onion for 10 minutes, chile for 5 minutes, and lime for 2 minutes.
4. Transfer the veggies to a large bowl.
5. Now cut the avocados in half and grill them for 5 minutes.
6. Mash the flesh of the grilled avocado in a bowl.
7. Chop the other grilled veggies and add them to the avocado mash.
8. Stir in remaining ingredients and mix well.
9. Serve.

NUTRITION: Calories: 165 Fat: 17g Carbs: 4g Fiber: 1g Protein: 1g

264. Lemon Artichoke Salad

Preparation time: 10 minutes
Cooking time: 0 minutes
Servings: 4
INGREDIENTS:
- 28 oz can artichoke hearts, drained and quartered
- 2 tbsp olive oil
- ¼ cup fresh parsley, chopped
- 2 garlic cloves, minced
- 1 lemon, chopped
- 10 oz can mushroom, drained and sliced
- Pepper
- Salt

DIRECTIONS:
1. Add all ingredients into the mixing bowl and toss well. Serve immediately and enjoy.

NUTRITION: Calories: 141 Fat: 7g Protein: 5.2g Carbs: 14.1g

265. Zucchini with mixed herbs

Preparation time: 10 minutes
Cooking time: 15 minutes
Servings: 4
INGREDIENTS:
- 1 lb. Zucchini, sliced
- 1 tsp dried mix herbs
- 1 garlic clove, minced
- 2 tbsp olive oil

DIRECTIONS:
1. Preheat the oven to 450 F/ 232 C. Add all ingredients into the large bowl and toss well.
2. Transfer the zucchini mixture to the baking dish and cook in preheated oven for 10 minutes. Return to the oven and cook for 5 minutes more. Serve and enjoy.

NUTRITION: Calories: 102 Fat: 8.7g Protein: 3.7g Carbs: 4.3g

266. Spaghetti Squash with Tomato Basil Cream

Preparation Time: 15 Minutes
Cooking Time: 45 Minutes
Servings: 2-3
Ingredients:

Spaghetti Squash

- 1 spaghetti squash, medium
- Salt & pepper to taste
- 2 teaspoon of olive oil

Tomato sauce

- 2 tablespoons of water
- Half teaspoon of salt
- 1 can of (15 oz.) diced roasted tomatoes
- ¼ cup of chopped fresh basil
- Half cup of soaked cashews

DIRECTIONS:
1. Let the oven preheat to 375 F.
2. Cut the squash in half, take the seeds and membrane out.
3. On the inside of the squash, rub some olive oil, and sprinkle with salt, garlic and pepper.
4. Bake for 35 minutes on a baking sheet, face down.
5. In a blender, add all ingredients of the sauce, pulse until smooth.
6. Shred the baked spaghetti into spaghetti.
7. In a pan, add oil on medium flame. Add spaghetti squash and sauce, toss and cook for 2-3 minutes.
8. Serve.

NUTRITION: Calories 257 Total fat: 12.9 g Total carbs: 31 g Fiber: 11.2 g Sugar: 4 g Protein: 6 g Sodium: 121 mg

267. Vegan Shepherd's Pie

Preparation Time: 15 Minutes
Cooking Time: 1 hour & 35 Minutes
Servings: 6

INGREDIENTS:

- Sea salt & black pepper, to taste
- 3 to 4 Tablespoons of vegan butter
- 3 pounds of peeled Yukon potatoes
- Filling
- 1 chopped onion
- 1 1/2 cups of rinsed brown lentils
- 2 minced cloves garlic
- 1 tablespoon of olive oil
- 4 cups of vegetable stock
- 2 tablespoons of tomato paste
- 10 oz. of frozen mixed vegetables
- 2 pinches of sea salt & pepper, each
- 2 teaspoon of fresh thyme

DIRECTIONS:

1. In a pot, add water and a generous amount of salt, boil it.
2. Add potatoes and cook for 20 to 30 minutes, covered.
3. Drain add to a bowl. Mash with vegan butter, salt and pepper.
4. Let the oven preheat to 425 F. Oil spray a 2 qt. baking dish.
5. In a pan, sauté garlic, onion for 5 minutes in hot oil.
6. Add tomato paste, salt and pepper, cook for 1 minute.
7. Add the rest of the ingredients, stir. Let it come to a boil, turn the heat low and simmer for 25 to 30 minutes.
8. Add frozen vegetables, cook for ten minutes.
9. Adjust seasoning. Pour in the prepared dish, add mashed potatoes on top, spread with a fork, and sprinkle with salt and pepper.
10. Bake for 10 to 15 minutes. Serve.

NUTRITION: Calories 396 Total fat: 1.6 g Total carbs: 72 g Fiber: 11.2 g Sugar: 4 g Protein: 17.7 g Sodium: 109 mg

268. Creamy Carrot Soup

Preparation time: 10 minutes
Cooking time: 45 minutes
Servings: 6

INGREDIENTS:

- 2 lb. Carrots, peeled and sliced
- 4 garlic cloves, chopped
- 2 leeks, sliced
- 2 tbsp olive oil
- 4 cups vegetable stock
- 1/2 tsp ground cumin
- 1/4 tsp ground coriander
- Pepper
- Salt

DIRECTIONS:

1. Heat olive oil in a saucepan over medium heat. Add carrots, cumin, coriander, garlic, leek, pepper, and salt and cook for 15 minutes. Add stock and stir well. Bring to boil.
2. Turn heat to low and simmer for 30 minutes. Puree the soup using an immersion blender until smooth. Serve and enjoy.

NUTRITION: Calories: 125 Fat: 5.1g Protein: 1.9g Carbs: 20.2g

269. Zucchini Noodles with Avocado Sauce

Preparation Time: 15 Minutes
Cooking Time: 0 Minutes
Servings: 2

INGREDIENTS:

- 1 1/4 cup of basil
- 1 avocado
- 1/3 cup of water
- 1 zucchini, spiralized into noodles
- 4 tablespoons of pine nuts
- 12 cherry tomatoes, sliced
- 2 tablespoons of lemon juice

DIRECTIONS:

1. In a blender, add all ingredients except for noodles and cherry tomatoes.
2. In a bowl, add puree, noodles and tomatoes. Toss well and serve.

NUTRITION: Calories 313 Total fat: 26.8 g Total carbs: 18.7 g Fiber: 9.7 g Sugar: 6.5 g Protein: 6.8 g Sodium: 22 mg

270. Avocado Tomato Salad

Preparation time: 10 minutes
Cooking time: 0 minutes
Servings: 4

INGREDIENTS:

- 2 avocados, diced
- ½ onion, diced
- 1 tbsp olive oil
- ¼ cup fresh cilantro, chopped
- 1 fresh lime juice
- 4 cups cherry tomatoes, halved
- Pepper
- Salt

DIRECTIONS:

1. Add all ingredients into the mixing bowl and toss well. Serve and enjoy.

NUTRITION: Calories: 276 Fat: 23.5g Protein: 3.7g Carbs: 17.9g

271. Vegan Vegetarian Curry

Preparation Time: 15 Minutes
Cooking Time: 40 Minutes
Servings: 6

INGREDIENTS:

- 12 ounces of cauliflower florets
- 10 ounces of eggplants, cubed
- 1 diced bell pepper
- 1 teaspoon of coarse salt
- 10 ounces of broccoli florets
- black pepper, to taste
- 6 tablespoons of olive oil

Aromatics
- 2 chopped shallots
- 2 tablespoons of chopped garlic
- 1 tablespoon of chopped ginger

Spices & Other
- 1 to 1.5 tablespoons of tamarind concentrate
- 14 ounces of canned coconut milk
- 1 teaspoon of cumin, turmeric and coriander powder
- 1 tablespoon of almond butter

DIRECTIONS:
1. Let the oven preheat to 420 F.
2. Spread vegetables on a baking sheet. Toss with salt, oil and pepper.
3. Bake for 25 to 30 minutes on the center rack.
4. In a skillet, add aromatics and saute in oil on medium heat for 2 minutes.
5. Add the spices, cook for 30 seconds.
6. Add the rest of the ingredients. Cook for 2 to 3 minutes.
7. In the curry, add roasted vegetables, toss to coat.
8. Serve.

NUTRITION: Calories 321 Total fat: 12 g Total carbs: 13.5 g Fiber: 8.9 g Sugar: 4.5 g Protein: 5.6 g Sodium: 109 mg

272. Creamy Polenta with Mushrooms

Preparation time: 15 minutes
Cooking time: 30 minutes
Servings: 2

INGREDIENTS:
- ½ ounce (14 g) dried porcini mushrooms (optional but recommended)
- 2 tablespoons olive oil
- 1 pound (454 g) baby bella (cremini) mushrooms, quartered
- 1 large shallot, minced
- 1 garlic clove, minced
- 1 tablespoon flour
- 2 teaspoons tomato paste
- ½ cup red wine
- 1 cup mushroom stock (or reserved liquid from soaking the porcini mushrooms, if using)
- ½ teaspoon dried thyme
- 1 fresh rosemary sprig
- 1½ cups water
- ½ teaspoon salt
- 1/3 cup instant polenta

DIRECTIONS:
1. If using the dried porcini mushrooms, soak them in 1 cup of hot water for about 15 minutes to soften them.
2. When they're softened, scoop them out of the water, reserving the soaking liquid. Mince the porcini mushrooms.
3. Heat the olive oil in a large sauté pan over medium-high heat. Add the mushrooms, shallot, and garlic, and sauté for 10 minutes, or until the vegetables are wilted and starting to caramelize.
4. Add the flour and tomato paste, and cook for another 30 seconds. Add the red wine, mushroom stock or porcini soaking liquid, thyme, and rosemary.

5. Bring the mixture to a boil, stirring constantly until it thickens. Reduce the heat and let it simmer for 10 minutes. Meanwhile, bring the water to a boil in a saucepan and add salt.
6. Add the instant polenta and stir quickly while it thickens. Taste and add additional salt, if needed. Serve warm.

NUTRITION: Calories: 450 Fat: 16.0g Protein: 14.1g Carbs: 57.8g

273. Roasted Vegetables and Chickpeas

Preparation time: 15 minutes
Cooking time: 30 minutes
Servings: 2

INGREDIENTS:
- 4 cups cauliflower florets (about ½ small head)
- 2 medium carrots, peeled, halved, and then sliced into quarters lengthwise
- 2 tablespoons olive oil, divided
- ½ teaspoon garlic powder, divided
- ½ teaspoon salt, divided
- 2 teaspoons za'atar spice mix, divided
- 1 (15-ounce / 425-g) can chickpeas, drained, rinsed, and patted dry
- 1 teaspoon harissa spice paste

DIRECTIONS:
1. Preheat the oven to 400°f (205°c). Line a sheet pan with foil or parchment paper. Place the cauliflower and carrots in a large bowl.
2. Drizzle with 1 tablespoon olive oil and sprinkle with ¼ teaspoon of garlic powder, ¼ teaspoon of salt, and 1 teaspoon of za'atar.
3. Toss well to combine. Spread the vegetables onto one half of the sheet pan in a single layer.
4. Place the chickpeas in the same bowl and season with the remaining 1 tablespoon of oil, ¼ teaspoon of garlic powder, and ¼ teaspoon of salt, and the remaining za'atar. Toss well to combine.
5. Spread the chickpeas onto the other half of the sheet pan.
6. Roast for 30 minutes, or until the vegetables are tender and the chickpeas start to turn golden. Flip the vegetables halfway through the cooking time, and give the chickpeas a stir so they cook evenly.
7. The chickpeas may need an extra few minute if you like them crispy. If so, remove the vegetables and leave the chickpeas in until they're cooked to desired crispiness.
8. Taste and add harissa as desired, then serve.

NUTRITION: Calories: 468 Fat: 23.0g Protein: 18.1g Carbs: 54.1g

274. Mexican Roasted Cauliflower

Preparation Time: 15 Minutes
Cooking Time: 30 Minutes
Servings: 4

INGREDIENTS:
- 2 tablespoon of avocado oil
- 1/4 cup of cilantro
- Half teaspoon of garlic powder
- 1 cauliflower, large head, broken into florets
- Half teaspoon of onion powder
- 1/4 teaspoon of cumin

- 1/4 cup of green onion sliced
- 1 teaspoon of chili powder
- 3/4 teaspoon of salt
- 1/4 teaspoon of pepper
- Half avocado, sliced
- 3 lime wedges

DIRECTIONS:

1. Let the oven preheat to 425 F.
2. In a bowl, add all ingredients except for onion, avocado, cilantro and wedges. Toss well, spread on a parchment-lined baking sheet.
3. Bake for 20 minutes, flip the florets and roast for 10 to 12 minutes.
4. Serve with onion, avocado, cilantro and wedges on top.

NUTRITION: Calories 50 Total fat: 4.0 g Total carbs: 5.0 g Fiber: 8.9 g Sugar: 1.4 g Protein: 1.2 g Sodium: 340 mg

275. Roasted Leeks with red onion

Preparation time: 15 minutes
Cooking time: 8 minutes
Servings: 2
INGREDIENTS:

- 3 tablespoons olive oil
- 2 garlic cloves, crushed
- 2 leeks, chopped
- 2 red onions, chopped
- 9 ounces (255 g) fresh spinach
- 1 teaspoon kosher salt

DIRECTIONS:

1. Coat the bottom of the large skillet with the olive oil. Add the garlic, leek, and onions and stir-fry for about 5 minutes.
2. Stir in the spinach. Sprinkle with the salt and sauté for an additional 3 minutes, stirring constantly. Transfer to a plate and serve.

NUTRITION: Calories: 447 Fat: 31.2g Protein: 14.6g Carbs: 28.7g

276. Crispy Plantains With Garlic Sauce

Preparation Time: 20 Minutes
Cooking Time: 25 Minutes
Servings: 2-4
INGREDIENTS:

Plantains

- 1 to 2 tablespoons of cooking oil
- Water, as needed
- 1 tablespoon of salt
- 2 green plantains

Garlic Sauce

- 1/3 cup of olive oil
- 1/4 teaspoon of salt, cumin seeds & red pepper flakes, each
- 1 scallion
- 2 cloves of garlic
- Half lime's juice

DIRECTIONS

1. Peel and slice the plantains into one" thick slice.
2. In a pan, add plantain slices, water to cover them and salt.

3. Cover the pan, let it come to a boil, turn the heat low and simmer for 10 to 15 minutes.
4. In a food processor, add all ingredients of the sauce, pulse until smooth.
5. Drain the plantain and mash lightly in between paper towels, but do not mash them completely.
6. In a skillet, add oil, cook plantain on one side for 3 to 5 minutes. Add salt to taste.
7. Serve with garlic sauce.

NUTRITION: Calories 78 Total fat: 1.3 g Total carbs: 3.1 g Fiber: 8 g Sugar: 1 g Protein: 2.4 g Sodium: 165 mg

277. Paleo Pizza Crust

Preparation Time: 15 Minutes
Cooking Time: 20 Minutes
Servings: 2-4
INGREDIENTS:

- 1 teaspoon of avocado oil
- 2 tablespoons of palm shortening
- 2 cups of mashed yuca
- Dried mixed herbs to taste
- 2 tablespoons of coconut flour
- Half teaspoon of sea salt

DIRECTIONS:

1. Let the oven preheat to 375 F.
2. In a food processor, add all ingredients except flour, mix well.
3. Take it out on parchment paper, and add coconut flour.
4. Cut the dough into 2 pieces.
5. Roll each piece into a crust into half' thickness.
6. Bake for 15 to 20 minutes, flip and bake until it is browned.
7. Add desired sauce, vegan cheese, melt and serve.

NUTRITION: Calories 86 Total fat: 1 g Total carbs: 4 g Fiber: 5 g Sugar: 2 g Protein: 2 g Sodium: 121 mg

278. Zucchini Crisp

Preparation time: 15 minutes
Cooking time: 20 minutes
Servings: 2
INGREDIENTS:

- 4 zucchinis, sliced into ½-inch rounds
- ½ cup unsweetened almond milk
- 1 teaspoon fresh lemon juice
- 1 teaspoon arrowroot powder
- ½ teaspoon salt, divided
- ½ cup whole wheat bread crumbs
- ¼ cup nutritional yeast
- ¼ cup hemp seeds
- ½ teaspoon garlic powder
- ¼ teaspoon crushed red pepper
- ¼ teaspoon black pepper

DIRECTIONS:

1. Preheat the oven to 375°f (190°c). Line two baking sheets with parchment paper and set aside.

2. Put the zucchini in a medium bowl with the almond milk, lemon juice, arrowroot powder, and ¼ teaspoon of salt. Stir to mix well.
3. In a large bowl with a lid, thoroughly combine the bread crumbs, nutritional yeast, hemp seeds, garlic powder, crushed red pepper and black pepper. Add the zucchini in batches and shake until the slices are evenly coated.
4. Arrange the zucchini on the prepared baking sheets in a single layer. Bake in the preheated oven for about 20 minutes, or until the zucchini slices are golden brown.
5. Season with the remaining ¼ teaspoon of salt before serving.

NUTRITION: Calories: 255 Fat: 11.3g Protein: 8.6g Carbs: 31.9g

279. Creamy Sweet Potatoes and Collards

Preparation time: 15 minutes
Cooking time: 35 minutes
Servings: 2
INGREDIENTS:
- 1 tablespoon avocado oil
- 3 garlic cloves, chopped
- 1 yellow onion, diced
- ½ teaspoon crushed red pepper flakes
- 1 large sweet potato, peeled and diced
- 2 bunches collard greens (about 2 pounds/907 g), stemmed, leaves chopped into 1-inch squares
- 1 (14.5-ounce / 411-g) can diced tomatoes with juice
- 1 (15-ounce / 425-g) can red kidney beans or chickpeas, drained and rinsed
- 1½ cups water
- ½ cup unsweetened coconut milk
- Salt and black pepper, to taste

DIRECTIONS:
1. In a large, deep skillet over medium heat, melt the avocado oil. Add the garlic, onion, and red pepper flakes and cook for 3 minutes. Stir in the sweet potato and collards.
2. Add the tomatoes with their juice, beans, water, and coconut milk and mix well. Bring the mixture just to a boil.
3. Reduce the heat to medium-low, cover, and simmer for about 30 minutes, or until softened. Season to taste with salt and pepper and serve.

NUTRITION: Calories: 445 Fat: 9.6g Protein: 18.1g Carbs: 73.1g

280. Mediterranean Romaine Wedge Salad

Preparation time: 15 minutes
Cooking time: 0 minutes
Servings: 4
INGREDIENTS:
- 1 English cucumber, chopped
- 1 cup quartered cherry tomatoes
- 1 cup chopped fennel
- ½ cup chopped roasted red peppers
- ¼ cup pitted, halved Kalamata olives
- 1 scallion, both white and green parts, chopped
- ½ cup Pesto Vinaigrette, divided
- 2 romaine lettuce heads, cut in half lengthwise
- 2 tablespoons chopped fresh basil

DIRECTIONS:
1. In a large bowl, stir together the cucumber, tomatoes, fennel, roasted red peppers, olives, scallion, and ¼ cup of pesto vinaigrette.
2. Place each romaine half on a large plate. Evenly divide the vegetable mixture onto each wedge. Drizzle the remaining dressing over the romaine wedges. Serve topped with basil.

NUTRITION: Calories: 336 Fat: 27g Carbs: 23g Protein: 11g

281. Roasted Brussels Sprouts and Halloumi Salad

Preparation time: 15 minutes
Cooking time: 35 minutes
Servings: 4
INGREDIENTS:
- For the dressing:
- ¼ cup olive oil
- 1/3 cup freshly squeezed lemon juice
- 2 tablespoons honey
- 1 teaspoon mustard
- Sea salt
- Freshly ground black pepper
- For the salad:
- 2 pounds Brussels sprouts, trimmed and halved
- 2 tablespoons olive oil
- 1 teaspoon sea salt
- 1½ cups baby spinach
- ½ cup baby arugula
- 1 shallot, halved and thinly sliced
- 3 tablespoons dried cranberries
- ½ cup blanched almonds, toasted
- ¼ cup shredded halloumi cheese

DIRECTIONS:
1. To Make the Dressing:
2. In a small bowl, whisk together the olive oil, lemon juice, and mustard. Season with salt and pepper and set aside.
3. To Make the Salad:
4. Preheat the oven to 425°F. Put the Brussels sprouts in a large mixing bowl. Drizzle with olive oil and season with salt. Toss to combine.
5. Spread the Brussels sprouts on a large baking sheet. Roast for 25 to 30 minutes, stirring once about halfway through, until crispy on the outside and tender on the inside.
6. While the Brussels sprouts are roasting, in a large mixing bowl, combine the spinach, arugula, shallot, cranberries, and almonds. Once cooked, add the roasted Brussels sprouts to the bowl.
7. Pour the dressing on the salad and toss to combine. Transfer the salad to a large serving platter.

NUTRITION: Calories: 475 Fat: 34g Carbs: 41g Protein: 14g

282. Roasted Vegetable Mélange

Preparation time: 15 minutes
Cooking time: 25 minutes
Servings: 4

INGREDIENTS:

- ½ cauliflower head, cut into small florets
- ½ broccoli head, cut into small florets
- 2 zucchinis, cut into ½-inch pieces
- 2 cups halved mushrooms
- 2 red, orange, or yellow bell peppers, cut into 1-inch pieces
- 1 sweet potato, cut into 1-inch pieces
- 1 red onion, cut into wedges
- 3 tablespoons olive oil
- 2 teaspoons minced garlic
- 1 teaspoon chopped fresh thyme
- Sea salt
- Freshly ground black pepper

DIRECTIONS:

1. Preheat the oven to 400°F. Line a baking sheet with parchment paper and set aside.
2. In a large bowl, toss the cauliflower, broccoli, zucchini, mushrooms, bell peppers, sweet potato, onion, olive oil, garlic, and thyme until well mixed.
3. Spread the vegetables on the baking sheet and season lightly with salt and pepper. Roast until the vegetables are tender and lightly caramelized, stirring occasionally, 20 to 25 minutes. Serve.

NUTRITION: Calories: 183 Fat: 11g Carbs: 20g Protein: 5g

283. Couscous-Avocado Salad

Preparation time: 15 minutes
Cooking time: 10 minutes
Servings: 4

INGREDIENTS:

- For the dressing:
- ¼ cup olive oil
- 2 tablespoons red wine vinegar
- 1 teaspoon minced garlic
- 1 teaspoon chopped fresh oregano
- Pinch red pepper flakes
- Sea salt
- Freshly ground black pepper
- For the salad:
- 1 cup couscous
- 2 cups halved cherry tomatoes
- ½ English cucumber, chopped
- 1 cup chopped marinated artichoke hearts
- 1 avocado, pitted, peeled, and chopped
- 2 tablespoons pine nuts

DIRECTIONS:

1. To Make the Dressing:
2. In a small bowl, whisk together the olive oil, vinegar, garlic, oregano, and red pepper flakes. Season with salt and pepper and set aside.
3. To Make the Salad:
4. In a pot, bring 1½ cups of water to a boil. Stir the couscous into the boiling water and remove from the heat. Cover and let sit for 10 minutes. Fluff with a fork.
5. In a large bowl, toss together the couscous, cherry tomatoes, cucumber, artichoke hearts, avocado, and pine nuts. Add the dressing and toss to combine. Refrigerate for 1 hour and serve.

NUTRITION: Calories: 489 Fat: 30g Carbs: 46g Protein: 11g

284. Paprika Cauliflower Steaks with Walnut Sauce

Preparation time: 15 minutes
Cooking time: 30 minutes
Servings: 2

INGREDIENTS:

- Walnut Sauce:
- ½ cup raw walnut halves
- 2 tablespoons virgin olive oil, divided
- 1 clove garlic, chopped
- 1 small yellow onion, chopped
- ½ cup unsweetened almond milk
- 2 tablespoons fresh lemon juice
- Salt and pepper, to taste
- Paprika Cauliflower:
- 1 medium head cauliflower
- 1 teaspoon sweet paprika
- 1 teaspoon minced fresh thyme leaves (about 2 sprigs)

DIRECTIONS:

1. Preheat the oven to 350°f (180°c). Make the walnut sauce: Toast the walnuts in a large, ovenproof skillet over medium heat until fragrant and slightly darkened, about 5 minutes. Transfer the walnuts to a blender.
2. Heat 1 tablespoon of olive oil in the skillet. Add the garlic and onion and sauté for about 2 minutes, or until slightly softened.
3. Transfer the garlic and onion into the blender, along with the almond milk, lemon juice, salt, and pepper. Blend the ingredients until smooth and creamy. Keep the sauce warm while you prepare the cauliflower.
4. Make the paprika cauliflower: Cut two 1-inch-thick "steaks" from the center of the cauliflower. Lightly moisten the steaks with water and season both sides with paprika, thyme, salt, and pepper.
5. Heat the remaining 1 tablespoon of olive oil in the skillet over medium-high heat. Add the cauliflower steaks and sear for about 3 minutes until evenly browned. Flip the cauliflower steaks and transfer the skillet to the oven.
6. Roast in the preheated oven for about 20 minutes until crisp-tender. Serve the cauliflower steaks warm with the walnut sauce on the side.

NUTRITION: Calories: 367 Fat: 27.9g Protein: 7.0g Carbs: 22.7g

285. Stir-Fried Eggplant

Preparation time: 15 minutes
Cooking time: 15 minutes
Servings: 2

INGREDIENTS:

- 1 cup water, plus more as needed
- ½ cup chopped red onion
- 1 tablespoon finely chopped garlic
- 1 tablespoon dried Italian herb seasoning
- 1 teaspoon ground cumin
- 1 small eggplant (about 8 ounces / 227 g), peeled and cut into ½-inch cubes
- 1 medium carrot, sliced
- 2 cups pinto beans, cut into 1-inch pieces
- 2 ribs celery, sliced
- 1 cup corn kernels
- 2 tablespoons almond butter
- 2 medium tomatoes, chopped

DIRECTIONS:

1. Heat 1 tablespoon of water in a large soup pot over medium-high heat until it sputters. Cook the onion for 2 minutes, adding a little more water as needed.
2. Add the garlic, Italian seasoning, cumin, and eggplant and stir-fry for 2 to 3 minutes, adding a little more water as needed.
3. Add the carrot, pinto beans, celery, corn kernels, and ½ cup of water and stir well. Reduce the heat to medium, cover, and cook for 8 to 10 minutes, stirring occasionally, or until the vegetables are tender. Meanwhile, in a bowl, stir together the almond butter and ½ cup of water.
4. Remove the vegetables from the heat and stir in the almond butter mixture and chopped tomatoes. Cool for a few minutes before serving.

NUTRITION: Calories: 176 Fat: 5.5g Protein: 5.8g Carbs: 25.4g

286. Carrots with dill

Preparation time: 15 minutes
Cooking time: 6 minutes
Servings: 2

INGREDIENTS:

- 2/3 cup water
- 1½ pounds (680 g) baby carrots
- 4 tablespoons almond butter
- 1 teaspoon dried thyme
- 1½ teaspoons dried dill
- Salt, to taste

DIRECTIONS:

1. Pour the water into the Instant Pot and add a steamer basket. Place the baby carrots in the basket. Secure the lid. Select the Manual mode and set the cooking time for 4 minutes at High Pressure.
2. Once cooking is complete, do a quick pressure release. Carefully open the lid. Transfer the carrots to a plate and set aside. Pour the water out of the Instant Pot and dry it.
3. Press the Sauté button on the Instant Pot and heat the almond butter. Stir in the thyme, and dill.
4. Return the carrots to the Instant Pot and stir until well coated. Sauté for another 1 minute. Taste and season with salt as needed. Serve warm.

NUTRITION: Calories: 575 Fat: 23.5g Protein: 2.8g Carbs: 90.6g

287. Quick Steamed Broccoli

Preparation time: 15 minutes
Cooking time: 5 minutes
Servings: 2

INGREDIENTS:

- ¼ cup water
- 3 cups broccoli florets
- Salt and ground black pepper, to taste

DIRECTIONS:

1. Pour the water into the deep pot. Place the broccoli florets in the pot.
2. Close the lid. Cook at high heat for about 5 minutes. Carefully open the lid.
3. Transfer the broccoli florets to a bowl with cold water to keep bright green color. Season the broccoli with salt and pepper to taste, then serve.

NUTRITION: Calories: 16 Fat: 0.2g Protein: 1.9g Carbs: 1.7g

288. Tempeh Lettuce Wraps

Preparation Time: 20 Minutes
Cooking Time: 15 Minutes
Servings: 4

INGREDIENTS:

- 1 cup of vegetable broth
- 1/4 teaspoon of ground coriander
- 1 teaspoon of gluten-free tamari
- 8 ounces of tempeh
- 1/4 cups of red cabbage, sliced thin
- 8 leaves of butter lettuce
- 1 teaspoon of maple syrup
- 1/8 teaspoon of garlic powder
- 1 sliced red bell pepper
- 1 peeled carrot, julienned
- Peanut sauce, for serving

DIRECTIONS:

1. In a food processor, add broken tempeh and pulse until it becomes crumbly.
2. In a bowl, add the rest of the ingredients except for lettuce, vegetables and tempeh.
3. In a pan, add tempeh and the mixture. Stirring, cook for 8-9 minutes; even if it looks dry, it will have some moisture.
4. Turn the heat off when all the liquid is absorbed.
5. In each lettuce wrap, add the vegetables with tempeh. Drizzle peanut sauce, roll and serve.

NUTRITION FOR 2 WRAPS: Calories 201 fat: 7.2 g carbs: 23.6 g Fiber: 8.3 g Sugar: 11.2 g Protein: 2 g Sodium: 539 mg

289. Cucumber Salad with lemon

Preparation time: 10 minutes
Cooking time: 10 minutes
Servings: 6
INGREDIENTS:

- For salad:
- ¼ cup fresh basil leaves, chopped
- ¼ cup fresh mint leaves, chopped
- 1 cucumber, cubed
- For dressing:
- 1 tbsp olive oil
- 2 tbsp fresh lime juice
- Pinch of salt

DIRECTIONS:

1. In a small bowl, mix together all dressing ingredients and set aside. Add all salad ingredients into the mixing bowl and mix well.
2. Pour dressing over salad and toss well. Serve and enjoy.

NUTRITION: Calories: 130 Fat: 7.6g Protein: 3.5g Carbs: 13.9g

290. Potatoes with Lemon Kale & White Beans

Preparation Time: 20 Minutes
Cooking Time: 60 Minutes
Servings: 2-4
INGREDIENTS:

- 1 tablespoon of olive oil
- 1 to 2 minced garlic cloves
- 4 sweet potatoes
- Half-1 teaspoon of red pepper flakes
- 1 teaspoon of lemon zest
- sea salt, to taste
- 1 bunch of kale, chopped without thick stems
- 1 chopped shallot
- Half a lemon's juice
- 1 can of (15 ounces) Cannellini beans

DIRECTIONS:

1. Let the oven preheat to 350 F.
2. With a fork, pierce the sweet potato all over and bake for 45-60 minutes, until soft.
3. In a pan, heat oil and sauté shallots for 2 minutes.
4. Add lemon zest, garlic and salt; cook for 60 seconds.
5. Add beans, pepper flakes and kale; cook for 2-3 minutes.
6. Add lemon juice, adjust the taste. Turn the heat off.
7. Cool the sweet potatoes slightly, cut the potatoes in half and top with the rest of the mixture on top.
8. Serve.

NUTRITION: Calories 295 Total fat: 8.5 g Total carbs: 46 g Fiber: 5 g Sugar: 2 g Protein: 12 g Sodium: 529 mg

291. Creamy Kale and Mushrooms

Preparation time: 15 minutes
Cooking time: 15 minutes
Servings: 3
INGREDIENTS:

- 3 tablespoons coconut oil
- 3 cloves of garlic, minced
- 1 onion, chopped
- 1 bunch kale, stems removed and leaves chopped
- 5 white button mushrooms, chopped
- 1 cup of coconut milk
- Salt and pepper to taste

DIRECTIONS:

8. Heat oil in a pot. Sauté the garlic and onion until fragrant for 2 minutes. Stir in mushrooms. Season with pepper and salt. Cook for 8 minutes.
9. Stir in kale and coconut milk. Simmer for 5 minutes. Adjust seasoning to taste.

NUTRITION: Calories: 365 Fat: 33.5 g Carbs: 17.9 g Protein: 6 g

292. Mediterranean Cauliflower Rice

Preparation Time: 15 Minutes
Cooking Time: 15 Minutes
Servings: 2-3
INGREDIENTS:

- 1/4 teaspoon of red chili flakes
- 1/4 cup of diced onion
- 3 cups riced cauliflower
- half lemon's zest
- 1 tablespoon of olive oil
- 2 minced garlic cloves
- 1 tablespoon of lemon juice
- 2 tablespoons of pine nuts

DIRECTIONS:

1. Sauté onion in hot oil for 4-5 minutes.
2. Add garlic and cook for 1-2 minutes.
3. Turn the flame to high, add chili flakes, cauliflower, pine nuts, zest and lemon juice. Cook for 1 minute or cook to your desired consistency.
4. Turn the heat off and add parsley. Season to taste and serve.
5. Fourth, remove from heat and stir in the parsley. Then, season with salt and pepper to taste and serve.

NUTRITION: Calories 216 Total fat: 3 g Total carbs: 8 g Fiber: 6 g Sugar: 5.6 g Protein: 5 g Sodium: 109 mg

293. Sautéed Dark Leafy Greens

Preparation time: 15 minutes
Cooking time: 10 minutes
Servings: 4
INGREDIENTS:

- 2 tablespoons olive oil
- 8 cups stemmed and coarsely chopped spinach, kale, collard greens, or Swiss chard
- Juice of ½ lemon
- Sea salt
- Freshly ground black pepper

DIRECTIONS:

1. In a large skillet, heat the olive oil over medium-high heat. Add the greens and toss with tongs until wilted and tender, 8 to 10 minutes.
2. Remove the skillet from the heat and squeeze in the lemon juice, tossing to coat evenly. Season with salt and pepper and serve.

NUTRITION: Calories: 129 Fat: 7g Carbs: 14g

294. Tomato salad with olive oil

Preparation time: 15 minutes
Cooking time: 8 minutes
Servings: 4

INGREDIENTS:

- 4 large tomatoes, cut in half horizontally
- 1 tablespoon olive oil
- 1 teaspoon minced garlic
- 1 tablespoon chopped fresh basil
- Sea salt
- Freshly ground black pepper

DIRECTIONS:

1. Preheat the oven to broil. Place the tomato halves, cut-side up, in a 9-by-13-inch baking dish and drizzle them with the olive oil. Rub the garlic into the tomatoes.
2. Broil the tomatoes for about 5 minutes, until softened. Sprinkle with basil and season with salt and pepper. Serve.

NUTRITION: Calories: 113 Fat: 8g Carbs: 8g Protein: 4g

295. Wild Rice with Grapes

Preparation time: 15 minutes
Cooking time: 50 minutes
Servings: 4

INGREDIENTS:

- 1 cup wild rice blend
- 1¾ cups water
- 1 teaspoon olive oil
- 2 cups red seedless grapes
- 2 teaspoons chopped fresh thyme
- Sea salt
- Freshly ground black pepper

DIRECTIONS:

1. In a pot, combine the rice and water and bring to a boil. Cover, reduce the heat to low, and simmer for 45 minutes. Remove from the heat and let stand, covered, for 10 minutes. Fluff with a fork.
2. In a large skillet, heat the olive oil over medium-high heat. Add the grapes and thyme and sauté until the grapes begin to burst, about 5 minutes. Stir in the wild rice mixture and season with salt and pepper. Serve.

NUTRITION: Calories: 146 Fat: 2g Carbs: 31g Protein: 3g

296. Traditional Falafel

Preparation time: 15 minutes
Cooking time: 10 minutes
Servings: 4

INGREDIENTS:

- 1 (15-ounce) can low-sodium chickpeas, drained and rinsed
- ½ sweet onion, chopped
- ¼ cup whole-wheat flour
- ¼ cup coarsely chopped fresh parsley
- ¼ cup coarsely chopped fresh cilantro
- Juice from 1 lemon
- 1 tablespoon minced garlic
- 2 teaspoon ground cumin
- Sea salt
- Freshly ground black pepper
- 2 tablespoons olive oil

DIRECTIONS:

1. In a food processor, pulse the chickpeas, onion, flour, parsley, cilantro, lemon juice, garlic, and cumin until the mixture just holds together. Season with salt and pepper and mix again.
2. Scoop out about 2 tablespoons of the mixture, roll into a ball, and flatten it out slightly to form a thick patty. Repeat with the remaining chickpea mixture.
3. In a large skillet, heat the olive oil over medium-high heat and pan-fry the patties until golden brown, about 4 minutes per side. Serve alone or stuffed into pita bread.

NUTRITION: Calories: 245 Fat: 9g Carbs: 36g Protein: 7g

297. Spicy Split Pea Tabbouleh

Preparation time: 1 hour & 15 minutes
Cooking time: 45 minutes
Servings: 6

INGREDIENTS:

- 1½ cups split peas
- 4 cups water
- 2 large tomatoes, seeded and chopped
- 1 English cucumber, chopped
- 1 yellow bell pepper, chopped
- 1 orange bell pepper, chopped
- ½ red onion, finely chopped
- ¼ cup chopped fresh cilantro
- Juice of 1 lime
- 1 teaspoon ground cumin
- ½ teaspoon ground coriander
- Pinch red pepper flakes
- Sea salt
- Freshly ground black pepper

DIRECTIONS:

1. In a large saucepan, combine the split peas and water over medium-high heat and bring to a boil. Reduce the heat to low and simmer, uncovered, until the peas are tender, 40 to 45 minutes. Drain the peas and rinse them in cold water to cool.
2. Transfer the peas to a large bowl and add the tomatoes, cucumber, bell peppers, onion, cilantro, lime juice, cumin, coriander, and red pepper flakes. Toss to mix well.
3. Place the mixture in the refrigerator for at least 1 hour to let the flavors mesh. Season with salt and pepper and serve.

NUTRITION: Calories: 208 Fat: 1g Carbs: 38g Protein: 14g

298. Mashed Avocado with fresh parsley

Preparation time: 15 minutes
Cooking time: 0 minutes
Servings: 4

INGREDIENTS:

- 1 avocado, peeled and pitted
- 1 celery stalk, chopped
- Juice and zest of ½ lemon
- 1 teaspoon chopped fresh parsley
- 4 whole-wheat bread slices, toasted
- 2 tomatoes, thinly sliced
- Sea salt
- Freshly ground black pepper

DIRECTIONS:

1. In a medium bowl, mash the avocado until well blended but still chunky. Stir in the celery, lemon juice, lemon zest, and parsley until well mixed.
2. Generously spread the mixture on the toast and arrange the tomato slices on top. Season with salt and pepper and serve.

NUTRITION: Calories: 248 Fat: 14g Carbs: 18g Protein: 13g

299. Sweet Potato & Brussel Sprout Vegan Tacos

Preparation Time: 15 Minutes
Cooking Time: 20 Minutes
Servings: 8

INGREDIENTS:

- 3 tablespoon of olive oil
- Half diced yellow onion
- 1 lb. of peeled & cubed sweet potatoes
- 1 diced green bell pepper
- gluten-free tortillas
- 2 crushed garlic cloves
- 1 teaspoon of salt
- 1 lb. of sliced Brussel sprouts
- 2 teaspoon of apple cider vinegar
- 1 teaspoon of hot sauce
- 2 tablespoon of maple syrup
- ¼ teaspoon of ground sage

DIRECTIONS:

1. In a skillet, heat oil and sauté onion, bell pepper for 2-3 minutes.
2. Add sweet potatoes and cook for 6 to 8 minutes.
3. Add sprouts and cook, covered for 3 to 4 minutes.
4. In a bowl, add the rest of the ingredients except tortillas and mix. Add to the pan, cook for 2 to 3 minutes.
5. In each tortilla, add the mixture and serve.

NUTRITION: Calories 283 Total fat: 13 g Total carbs: 39 g Fiber: 6 g Sugar: 7 g Protein: 3 g Sodium: 303 mg

300. Mediterranean Brussels Sprouts

Preparation time: 15 minutes
Cooking time: 23 minutes
Servings: 4

INGREDIENTS:

- 2 cups Brussels sprouts, cut in half
- ¼ cup olive oil
- 1 bay leaf
- 2 teaspoons pine nuts, roasted
- ½ cup olives
- 2 tablespoons sun-dried tomatoes, chopped
- Pepper
- Salt

DIRECTIONS:

1. Preheat the oven to 3500 F. Heat 1 tablespoon of oil in a pan over medium heat. Add Brussels sprouts and salt and cook for 7-8 minutes. Place pan in oven and bake sprouts of 10 minutes.
2. Meanwhile, in separate pan heat remaining oil over medium heat. Add sun-dried tomatoes and olives and cook for 5 minutes.
3. Remove sprouts from oven and mix with tomato olive mixture. Top with pine nuts. Serve and enjoy.

NUTRITION: Calories: 182 Fat: 17.5 g Carbs: 5.9 g Protein: 3.2 g

301. Eggplant with Italian seasoning

Preparation time: 15 minutes
Cooking time: 10 minutes
Servings: 4

INGREDIENTS:

- 1 eggplant, cut into 1-inch pieces
- ½ cup of water
- ¼ cup Can tomato, crushed
- ½ teaspoon Italian seasoning
- 1 teaspoon paprika
- ½ teaspoon chili powder
- 1 teaspoon garlic powder
- 2 tablespoons olive oil
- Salt

DIRECTIONS:

1. Add water and eggplant into the deep pot. Seal pot with lid and cook on high for 5 minutes.
2. Drain eggplant well and clean the pot. Add oil into the pot.
3. Add eggplant along with remaining ingredients and stir well and cook for 5 minutes. Serve and enjoy.

NUTRITION: Calories: 97 Fat: 7.5 g Carbs: 8.2 g Protein: 1.5 g

302. Indian Bell Peppers and Potato Stir Fry

Preparation time: 15 minutes
Cooking time: 10 minutes
Servings: 2

INGREDIENTS:

- 1 tablespoon oil
- ½ teaspoon cumin seeds
- 4 cloves of garlic, minced
- 4 potatoes, scrubbed and halved

- Salt and pepper to taste
- 5 tablespoons water
- 2 bell peppers, seeded and julienned
- Chopped cilantro for garnish

DIRECTIONS:

1. Heat oil in a skillet over medium flame and toast the cumin seeds until fragrant. Add the garlic until fragrant. Stir in the potatoes, salt, pepper, water, and bell peppers.
2. Close the lid and allow to simmer for at least 10 minutes. Garnish with cilantro before cooking time ends. Place in individual containers.
3. Put a label and store it in the fridge. Allow thawing at room temperature before heating in the microwave oven.

NUTRITION: Calories: 83 Fat: 6.4 g Carbs: 7.3 g Protein: 2.8 g

303. Carrot Potato with chopped onion

Preparation time: 15 minutes
Cooking time: 15 minutes
Servings: 6
INGREDIENTS:

- 4 lbs. Baby potatoes, clean and cut in half
- 1 ½ lb. Carrots, cut into chunks
- 1 teaspoon Italian seasoning
- 1 ½ cups vegetable broth
- 1 tablespoon garlic, chopped
- 1 onion, chopped
- 2 tablespoons olive oil
- Pepper
- Salt

DIRECTIONS:

1. Add oil into the large saucepan. Add onion and sauté for 5 minutes. Add carrots and cook for 5 minutes.
2. Add remaining ingredients and stir well. Cover saucepan with lid and cook on high for 5 minutes.
3. Remove lid. Stir and serve.

NUTRITION: Calories: 283 Fat: 5.6 g Carbs: 51.3 g Protein: 10.2 g

304. Potatoes with paprika

Preparation time: 15 minutes
Cooking time: 35 minutes
Servings: 8
INGREDIENTS:

- 4 large sweet potatoes, peel and cut into 1-inch cubes
- ¼ teaspoon paprika
- 2 tablespoons olive oil
- 8 sage leaves
- 2 teaspoons vinegar
- ½ teaspoon of sea salt

DIRECTIONS:

1. Preheat the oven to 375 F. Add sweet potato, olive oil, sage, and salt in a large bowl and toss well. Roast for 35 minutes.
2. Add vinegar, and paprika and mix well. Serve and enjoy.

NUTRITION: Calories: 90 Fat: 3.5 g Carbs: 14 g Protein: 1 g

305. Eggplant with fresh basil

Preparation time: 15 minutes
Cooking time: 10 minutes
Servings: 8
INGREDIENTS:

- 1 small eggplant, cut into cubes
- 1 cup fresh basil
- 2 cups grape tomatoes
- 1 onion, chopped
- 2 summer squash, sliced
- 2 zucchinis, sliced
- 2 tablespoons vinegar
- 2 tablespoons tomato paste
- 1 tablespoon garlic, minced
- 1 fresh lemon juice
- ¼ cup olive oil
- Salt

DIRECTIONS:

1. Add basil, vinegar, tomato paste, garlic, lemon juice, oil, and salt into the blender and blend until smooth. Add eggplant, tomatoes, onion, squash, and zucchini into the saucepan.
2. Pour blended basil mixture over vegetables and stir well. Seal saucepan with lid and cook on high for 10 minutes. Remove lid. Stir well and serve.

NUTRITION: Calories: 103 Fat: 6.8 g Carbs: 10.6 g Protein: 2.4 g

306. Roasted Vinegar Cauliflower

Preparation time: 15 minutes
Cooking time: 30 minutes
Servings: 4
INGREDIENTS:

- 8 cups cauliflower florets
- 1 teaspoon dried marjoram
- 2 tablespoons olive oil
- 2 tablespoons vinegar
- ¼ teaspoon pepper
- ¼ teaspoon salt

DIRECTIONS:

1. Preheat the oven to 450 F. Toss cauliflower, marjoram, oil, pepper, and salt. Toss well. Spread cauliflower onto the baking tray and roast for 15-20 minutes.
2. Toss cauliflower with and vinegar. Return cauliflower to the oven and roast for 5-10 minutes more. Serve and enjoy.

NUTRITION: Calories: 196 Fat: 13 g Carbs: 11 g Protein: 11 g

307. Cauliflower Walnut Taco Meat

Preparation Time: 20 Minutes
Cooking Time: 30 Minutes
Servings: 6-8
INGREDIENTS:

- Taco Meat
- 12 oz. of cauliflower florets
- 1 cup of walnuts
- 2 tablespoons of nutritional yeast
- to 10 oz. button mushrooms, sliced
- 2 teaspoons of olive oil

- Spice Mixture
- 2 teaspoon of chili powder
- 3/4 teaspoon of cumin
- 1 teaspoon of dried oregano
- 1 teaspoon of garlic powder
- 1 tablespoon of coconut sugar
- 2 1/2 teaspoon of smoked paprika
- 1 1/2 teaspoon of onion powder
- Sea salt & black pepper, to taste

DIRECTIONS:

1. Let the oven preheat to 350 F. roast the walnuts on a baking tray for 8-10 minutes.
2. Take them out in a bowl, change the oven temperature to 400 F.
3. Add mushroom and cauliflower on a parchment-lined baking tray, toss with oil.
4. Roast for 20 minutes.
5. In a food processor, add spice mixture (1/4 cup), yeast and walnuts, pulse until just combined.
6. Add the roasted vegetables to the food processor, pulse until just combined.
7. Adjust seasoning with the spice mixture.
8. Serve in tortillas or with gluten-free rice.

NUTRITION: Calories 234 Total fat: 8 g Total carbs: 4 g Fiber: 7 g Sugar: 6.5 g Protein: 6 g Sodium: 102 mg

308. Brussels Sprouts with Cranberries

Preparation time: 15 minutes
Cooking time: 10 minutes
Servings: 6
INGREDIENTS:

- 1 lb. Brussels sprouts, cut in half
- ½ cup dried cranberries
- ½ pecans, toasted

- 1 tablespoon vinegar
- 3 tablespoons olive oil
- Pepper
- Salt

DIRECTIONS:

1. Heat oil in a pan over medium-high heat. Add Brussels sprouts and cook for 5 minutes. Season with pepper and salt and cook for 5 minutes more.
2. Drizzle with vinegar and stir well. Remove pan from heat. Transfer Brussels sprouts to a large bowl and tosses in the pecans, and cranberries. Serve and enjoy.

NUTRITION: Calories: 170 Fat: 13.8 g Carbs: 8.7 g Protein: 5.5 g

309. Asparagus Salad with lemon

Preparation time: 10 minutes
Cooking time: 10 minutes
Servings: 4
INGREDIENTS:

- 2 lb. Asparagus, ends trimmed
- 1 tbsp. lemon juice
- 1 lemon zest
- 3 tbsp olive oil
- ¼ tsp pepper
- ¼ tsp salt

DIRECTIONS:

1. Preheat the grill to high. Arrange asparagus on a foil-lined baking sheet. Drizzle with 2 tablespoons of oil and season with pepper and salt.
2. Place asparagus on the grill and cook for 3-4 minutes. Chop grilled asparagus and transfer to the mixing bowl.
3. Add remaining ingredients to the mixing bowl and toss well. Serve and enjoy.

NUTRITION: Calories: 211 Fat: 16.8g Protein: 9g Carbs: 10.1g

FISH & SEAFOODS

310. Fast Seafood Paella

Preparation time: 15 minutes
Cooking time: 20 minutes
Servings: 4

INGREDIENTS:

- ¼ cup plus 1 tablespoon extra-virgin olive oil
- 1 large onion, finely chopped
- 2 tomatoes, peeled and chopped
- 1½ tablespoons garlic powder
- 1½ cups medium-grain Spanish paella rice or arborio rice
- 2 carrots, finely diced
- Salt, to taste
- 1 tablespoon sweet paprika
- 8 ounces (227 g) lobster meat or canned crab
- ½ cup frozen peas
- 3 cups chicken stock, plus more if needed
- 1 cup dry white wine
- 6 jumbo shrimp, unpeeled
- 1/3 pound (136 g) calamari rings
- 1 lemon, halved

DIRECTIONS:

1. In a large sauté pan or skillet (16-inch is ideal), heat the oil over medium heat until small bubbles start to escape from oil.
2. Add the onion and cook for about 3 minutes, until fragrant, then add tomatoes and garlic powder. Cook for 5 to 10 minutes, until the tomatoes are reduced by half and the consistency is sticky.
3. Stir in the rice, carrots, salt, paprika, lobster, and peas and mix well. In a pot or microwave-safe bowl, heat the chicken stock to almost boiling, then add it to the rice mixture. Bring to a simmer, then add the wine.
4. Smooth out the rice in the bottom of the pan. Cover and cook on low for 10 minutes, mixing occasionally, to prevent burning.
5. Top the rice with the shrimp, cover, and cook for 5 more minutes. Add additional broth to the pan if the rice looks dried out.
6. Right before removing the skillet from the heat, add the calamari rings. Toss the ingredients frequently.
7. In about 2 minutes, the rings will look opaque. Remove the pan from the heat immediately—you don't want the paella to overcook). Squeeze fresh lemon juice over the dish.

NUTRITION: Calories: 632 Fat: 20g Protein: 34g Carbs: 71g

311. Crispy Fried Sardines

Preparation time: 15 minutes
Cooking time: 5 minutes
Servings: 4

INGREDIENTS:

- Avocado oil, as needed
- 1½ pounds (680 g) whole fresh sardines, scales removed
- 1 teaspoon salt
- 1 teaspoon freshly ground black pepper
- 2 cups flour

DIRECTIONS:

1. Preheat a deep skillet over medium heat. Pour in enough oil so there is about 1 inch of it in the pan. Season the fish with the salt and pepper.
2. Dredge the fish in the flour so it is completely covered. Slowly drop in 1 fish at a time, making sure not to overcrowd the pan.
3. Cook for about 3 minutes on each side or just until the fish begins to brown on all sides. Serve warm.

NUTRITION: Calories: 794 Fat: 47g Protein: 48g Carbs: 44g

312. Orange Roasted Salmon

Preparation time: 15 minutes
Cooking time: 25 minutes
Servings: 4

INGREDIENTS:

- ½ cup extra-virgin olive oil, divided
- 2 tablespoons balsamic vinegar
- 2 tablespoons garlic powder, divided
- 1 tablespoon cumin seeds
- 1 teaspoon sea salt, divided
- 1 teaspoon freshly ground black pepper, divided
- 2 teaspoons smoked paprika
- 4 (8-ounce / 227-g) wild salmon fillets, skinless
- 2 small red onions, thinly sliced
- ½ cup halved Campari tomatoes
- 1 small fennel bulb, thinly sliced lengthwise
- 1 large carrot, thinly sliced
- 8 medium portobello mushrooms
- 8 medium radishes, sliced 1/8 inch thick
- ½ cup dry white wine
- ½ lime, zested
- Handful cilantro leaves
- ½ cup halved pitted Kalamata olives
- 1 orange, thinly sliced
- 4 roasted sweet potatoes, cut in wedges lengthwise

DIRECTIONS:

1. Preheat the oven to 375°f (190°c). In a medium bowl, mix 6 tablespoons of olive oil, the balsamic vinegar, 1 tablespoon of garlic powder, the cumin seeds, ¼ teaspoon of sea salt, ¼ teaspoon of pepper, and the paprika.
2. Put the salmon in the bowl and marinate while preparing the vegetables, about 10 minutes.
3. Heat an oven-safe sauté pan or skillet on medium-high heat and sear the top of the salmon for about 2 minutes, or until lightly brown. Set aside.
4. Add the remaining 2 tablespoons of olive oil to the same skillet. Once it's hot, add the onion, tomatoes, fennel, carrot, mushrooms, radishes, the remaining 1 teaspoon of garlic powder, ¾ teaspoon of salt, and ¾ teaspoon of pepper.
5. Mix well and cook for 5 to 7 minutes, until fragrant. Add wine and mix well. Place the salmon on top of the vegetable mixture, browned-side up.

6. Sprinkle the fish with lime zest and cilantro and place the olives around the fish. Put orange slices over the fish and cook for about 7 additional minutes.

7. While this is baking, add the sliced sweet potato wedges on a baking sheet and bake this alongside the skillet. Remove from the oven, cover the skillet tightly, and let rest for about 3 minutes.

NUTRITION: Calories: 841 Fat: 41g Protein: 59g Carbs: 60g

313. Lemon Rosemary Branzino

Preparation time: 15 minutes
Cooking time: 30 minutes
Servings: 4
INGREDIENTS:

- 4 tablespoons extra-virgin olive oil, divided
- 2 (8-ounce / 227-g) branzino fillets, preferably at least 1 inch thick
- 1 garlic clove, minced
- 1 bunch scallions, white part only, thinly sliced
- ½ cup sliced pitted Kalamata or other good-quality black olives
- 1 large carrot, cut into ¼-inch rounds
- 10 to 12 small cherry tomatoes, halved
- ½ cup dry white wine
- 2 tablespoons paprika
- 2 teaspoons kosher salt
- ½ tablespoon ground chili pepper, preferably Turkish or Aleppo
- 2 rosemary sprigs or 1 tablespoon dried rosemary
- 1 small lemon, very thinly sliced

DIRECTIONS:

1. Warm a large, oven-safe sauté pan or skillet over high heat until hot, about 2 minutes. Carefully add 1 tablespoon of olive oil and heat until it shimmers, 10 to 15 seconds.

2. Brown the branzino fillets for 2 minutes, skin-side up. Carefully flip the fillets skin-side down and cook for another 2 minutes, until browned. Set aside.

3. Swirl 2 tablespoons of olive oil around the skillet to coat evenly. Add the garlic, scallions, kalamata olives, carrot, and tomatoes, and let the vegetables sauté for 5 minutes, until softened.

4. Add the wine, stirring until all ingredients are well integrated. Carefully place the fish over the sauce. Preheat the oven to 450°f (235°c).

5. While the oven is heating, brush the fillets with 1 tablespoon of olive oil and season with paprika, salt, and chili pepper.

6. Top each fillet with a rosemary sprig and several slices of lemon. Scatter the olives over fish and around the pan. Roast until lemon slices are browned or singed, about 10 minutes.

NUTRITION: calories: 725 fats: 43g protein: 58g carbs: 25g

314. Almond-Crusted Swordfish

Preparation time: 15 minutes
Cooking time: 15 minutes
Servings: 4
INGREDIENTS:

- ½ cup almond flour
- ¼ cup crushed Marcona almonds
- ½ to 1 teaspoon salt, divided
- 2 pounds (907 g) Swordfish, preferably 1 inch thick
- 1 large egg, beaten (optional)

- ¼ cup pure apple cider
- ¼ cup extra-virgin olive oil, plus more for frying
- 3 to 4 sprigs flat-leaf parsley, chopped
- 1 lemon, juiced
- 1 tablespoon Spanish paprika
- 5 medium baby portobello mushrooms, chopped (optional)
- 4 or 5 chopped scallions, both green and white parts
- 3 to 4 garlic cloves, peeled
- ¼ cup chopped pitted Kalamata olives

DIRECTIONS:

1. On a dinner plate, spread the flour and crushed Marcona almonds and mix in the salt. Alternately, pour the flour, almonds, and ¼ teaspoon of salt into a large plastic food storage bag.

2. Add the fish and coat it with the flour mixture. If a thicker coat is desired, repeat this step after dipping the fish in the egg (if using).

3. In a measuring cup, combine the apple cider, ¼ cup of olive oil, parsley, lemon juice, paprika, and ¼ teaspoon of salt. Mix well and set aside.

4. In a large, heavy-bottom sauté pan or skillet, pour the olive oil to a depth of ⅛ inch and heat on medium heat.

5. Once the oil is hot, add the fish and brown for 3 to 5 minutes, then turn the fish over and add the mushrooms (If using), scallions, garlic, and olives.

6. Cook for an additional 3 minutes. Once the other side of the fish is brown, remove the fish from the pan and set aside.

7. Pour the cider mixture into the skillet and mix well with the vegetables. Put the fried fish into the skillet on top of the mixture and cook with sauce on medium-low heat for 10 minutes, until the fish flakes easily with a fork.

8. Carefully remove the fish from the pan and plate. Spoon the sauce over the fish. Serve with white rice or home-fried potatoes.

NUTRITION: Calories: 620 Fat: 37g Protein: 63g Carbs: 10g

315. Sea Bass Crusted with Moroccan Spices

Preparation time: 15 minutes
Cooking time: 40 minutes
Servings: 4
INGREDIENTS:

- 1½ teaspoons ground turmeric, divided
- ¾ teaspoon saffron
- ½ teaspoon ground cumin
- ¼ teaspoon kosher salt
- ¼ teaspoon freshly ground black pepper
- 1½ pounds (680 g) sea bass fillets, about ½ inch thick
- 8 tablespoons extra-virgin olive oil, divided
- 8 garlic cloves, divided (4 minced cloves and 4 sliced)
- 6 medium baby portobello mushrooms, chopped
- 1 large carrot, sliced on an angle
- 2 sun-dried tomatoes, thinly sliced (optional)
- 2 tablespoons tomato paste
- 1 (15-ounce / 425-g) can chickpeas, drained and rinsed
- 1½ cups low-sodium vegetable broth
- ¼ cup white wine

- 1 tablespoon ground coriander (optional)
- 1 cup sliced artichoke hearts marinated in olive oil
- ½ cup pitted Kalamata olives
- ½ lemon, juiced
- ½ lemon, cut into thin rounds
- 4 to 5 rosemary sprigs or 2 tablespoons dried rosemary
- Fresh cilantro, for garnish

DIRECTIONS:

1. In a small mixing bowl, combine 1 teaspoon turmeric and the saffron and cumin. Season with salt and pepper. Season both sides of the fish with the spice mixture.
2. Add 3 tablespoons of olive oil and work the fish to make sure it's well coated with the spices and the olive oil.
3. In a large sauté pan or skillet, heat 2 tablespoons of olive oil over medium heat until shimmering but not smoking. Sear the top side of the sea bass for about 1 minute, or until golden. Remove and set aside.
4. In the same skillet, add the minced garlic and cook very briefly, tossing regularly, until fragrant. Add the mushrooms, carrot, sun-dried tomatoes (if using), and tomato paste.
5. Cook for 3 to 4 minutes over medium heat, tossing frequently, until fragrant. Add the chickpeas, broth, wine, coriander (if using), and the sliced garlic.
6. Stir in the remaining ½ teaspoon ground turmeric. Raise the heat, if needed, and bring to a boil, then lower heat to simmer. Cover part of the way and let the sauce simmer for about 20 minutes, until thickened.
7. Carefully add the seared fish to the skillet. Ladle a bit of the sauce on top of the fish. Add the artichokes, olives, lemon juice and slices, and rosemary sprigs.
8. Cook another 10 minutes or until the fish is fully cooked and flaky. Garnish with fresh cilantro.

NUTRITION: Calories: 696 Fat: 41g Protein: 48g Carbs: 37g

316. Cilantro Lemon Shrimp

Preparation time: 20 minutes
Cooking time: 10 minutes
Servings: 4
INGREDIENTS:

- 1/3 cup lemon juice
- 4 garlic cloves
- 1 cup fresh cilantro leaves
- ½ teaspoon ground coriander
- 3 tablespoons extra-virgin olive oil
- 1 teaspoon salt
- 1½ pounds (680 g) large shrimp (21 to 25), deveined and shells removed

DIRECTIONS:

1. In a food processor, pulse the lemon juice, garlic, cilantro, coriander, olive oil, and salt 10 times. Put the shrimp in a bowl or plastic zip-top bag, pour in the cilantro marinade, and let sit for 15 minutes.
2. Preheat a skillet on high heat. Put the shrimp and marinade in the skillet. Cook the shrimp for 3 minutes on each side. Serve warm.

NUTRITION: Calories: 225 Fat: 12g Protein: 28g Carbs: 5g

317. Shrimp with Garlic and Mushrooms

Preparation time: 15 minutes
Cooking time: 15 minutes
Servings: 4
INGREDIENTS:

- 1 pound (454 g) peeled and deveined fresh shrimp
- 1 teaspoon salt
- 1 cup extra-virgin olive oil
- 8 large garlic cloves, thinly sliced
- 4 ounces (113 g) sliced mushrooms (shiitake, baby bella, or button)
- ½ teaspoon red pepper flakes
- ¼ cup chopped fresh flat-leaf Italian parsley
- Zucchini noodles or riced cauliflower, for serving

DIRECTIONS:

1. Rinse the shrimp and pat dry. Place in a small bowl and sprinkle with the salt. In a large rimmed, thick skillet, heat the olive oil over medium-low heat.
2. Add the garlic and heat until very fragrant, 3 to 4 minutes, reducing the heat if the garlic starts to burn.
3. Add the mushrooms and sauté for 5 minutes, until softened. Add the shrimp and red pepper flakes and sauté until the shrimp begins to turn pink, another 3 to 4 minutes.
4. Remove from the heat and stir in the parsley. Serve over zucchini noodles or riced cauliflower.

NUTRITION: Calories: 620 Fat: 56g Protein: 24g Carbs: 4g

318. Pistachio-Crusted Whitefish

Preparation Time: 10 minutes
Cooking Time: 20 minutes
Servings: 2
INGREDIENTS:

- ¼ cup shelled pistachios
- 1 tablespoon fresh parsley
- 1 tablespoon panko bread crumbs
- 2 tablespoons olive oil
- ¼ teaspoon salt
- 10 ounces' skinless whitefish (1 large piece or 2 smaller ones)

DIRECTIONS:

1. Preheat the oven to 350°F and set the rack to the middle position. Line a sheet pan with foil or parchment paper.
2. Combine all of the ingredients except the fish in a mini food processor, and pulse until the nuts are finely ground.
3. Alternatively, you can mince the nuts with a chef's knife and combine the ingredients by hand in a small bowl.
4. Place the fish on the sheet pan. Spread the nut mixture evenly over the fish and pat it down lightly.
5. Bake the fish for 20 to 30 minutes, depending on the thickness, until it flakes easily with a fork.
6. Keep in mind that a thicker cut of fish takes a bit longer to bake. You'll know it's done when it's opaque, flakes apart easily with a fork, or reaches an internal temperature of 145°F

NUTRITION: Calories 185, Carbs - 23.8 g, Protein - 10.1 g, Fat - 5.2 g

319. Seafood Risotto

Preparation time: 15 minutes
Cooking time: 30 minutes
Servings: 4

INGREDIENTS:

- 6 cups vegetable broth
- 3 tablespoons extra-virgin olive oil
- 1 large onion, chopped
- 3 cloves garlic, minced
- ½ teaspoon saffron threads
- 1½ cups arborio rice
- 1½ teaspoons salt
- 8 ounces (227 g) shrimp (21 to 25), peeled and deveined
- 8 ounces (227 g) scallops

DIRECTIONS:

1. In a large saucepan over medium heat, bring the broth to a low simmer. In a large skillet over medium heat, cook the olive oil, onion, garlic, and saffron for 3 minutes.
2. Add the rice, salt, and 1 cup of the broth to the skillet. Stir the ingredients together and cook over low heat until most of the liquid is absorbed.
3. Repeat steps with broth, adding ½ cup of broth at a time, and cook until all but ½ cup of the broth is absorbed.
4. Add the shrimp and scallops when you stir in the final ½ cup of broth. Cover and let cook for 10 minutes. Serve warm.

NUTRITION: Calories: 460 Fat: 12g Protein: 24g Carbs: 64g

320. Crispy Homemade Fish Sticks Recipe

Preparation Time: 10 minutes
Cooking Time: 15 minutes
Servings: 2

INGREDIENTS:

- ½ cup of flour
- 1 beaten egg
- 1 cup of flour
- ½ cup of bread crumbs.
- Zest of 1 lemon juice
- Parsley
- Salt
- 1 teaspoon of black pepper
- 1 tablespoon of sweet paprika
- 1 teaspoon of oregano
- 1 ½ lb. Of wild salmon
- Extra virgin olive oil

DIRECTIONS:

1. Preheat your oven to about 450 degrees F. Get a bowl, dry your salmon and season its two sides with the salt.
2. Then chop into small sizes of 1½ inch length each. Get a bowl and mix black pepper with oregano.
3. Add paprika to the mixture and blend it. Then spice the fish stick with the mixture you have just made. Get another dish and pour your flours.
4. You will need a different bowl again to pour your egg wash into. Pick yet the fourth dish, mix your breadcrumb with your cheese and add lemon zest to the mixture.

5. Return to the fish sticks and dip each fish into flour such that both sides are coated with flour. As you dip each fish into flour, take it out and dip it into egg wash and lastly, dip it in the breadcrumb mixture.
6. Do this for all fish sticks and arrange on a baking sheet. Ensure you oil the baking sheet before arranging the stick thereon and drizzle the top of the fish sticks with extra virgin olive oil.
7. Caution: allow excess flours to fall off a fish before dipping it into other ingredients.
8. Also ensure that you do not let the coating peel while you add extra virgin olive oil on top of the fishes.
9. Fix the baking sheet in the middle of the oven and allow it to cook for 13 min. By then, the fishes should be golden brown and you can collect them from the oven, and you can serve immediately.
10. Top it with your lemon zest, parsley and fresh lemon juice.

NUTRITION: 119 Cal, 3.4g fat, 293mg sodium, 9.3g carbs, 13.5g protein.

321. Sauced Shellfish in White Wine

Preparation Time: 10 minutes
Cooking Time: 10 minutes
Servings: 2

INGREDIENTS:

- 2-lbs fresh cuttlefish
- ½-cup olive oil
- 1-pc large onion, finely chopped
- 1-cup of Robola white wine
- ¼-cup lukewarm water
- 1-pc bay leaf
- ½-bunch parsley, chopped
- 4-pcs tomatoes, grated
- Salt and pepper

DIRECTIONS:

1. Take out the hard centerpiece of cartilage (cuttlebone), the bag of ink, and the intestines from the cuttlefish.
2. Wash the cleaned cuttlefish with running water. Slice it into small pieces, and drain excess water.
3. Heat the oil in a saucepan placed over medium-high heat and sauté the onion for 3 minutes until tender.
4. Add the sliced cuttlefish and pour in the white wine. Cook for 5 minutes until it simmers.
5. Pour in the water, and add the tomatoes, bay leaf, parsley, tomatoes, salt, and pepper. Simmer the mixture over low heat until the cuttlefish slices are tender and left with their thick sauce. Serve them warm with rice.
6. Be careful not to overcook the cuttlefish as its texture becomes very hard. A safe rule of thumb is grilling the cuttlefish over a ragingly hot fire for 3 minutes before using it in any recipe.

NUTRITION: Calories: 308, Fats: 18.1g, Dietary Fiber: 1.5g, Carbs: 8g, Protein: 25.6g

322. Pistachio Sole Fish

Preparation Time: 5 minutes
Cooking Time: 10 minutes
Servings: 2

INGREDIENTS:

- 4 (5 ounces) boneless sole fillets
- ½ cup pistachios, finely chopped
- Juice of 1 lemon
- Teaspoon extra virgin olive oil

DIRECTIONS:

1. Pre-heat your oven to 350 degrees Fahrenheit
2. Wrap baking sheet using parchment paper and keep it on the side
3. Pat fish dry with kitchen towels and lightly season with salt and pepper
4. Take a small bowl and stir in pistachios
5. Place sol on the prepped sheet and press 2 tablespoons of pistachio mixture on top of each fillet
6. Rub the fish with lemon juice and olive oil
7. Bake for 10 minutes until the top is golden and fish flakes with a fork

NUTRITION: 166 Calories 6g Fat 2g Carbs

323. Speedy Tilapia with Red Onion and Avocado

Preparation time: 10 minutes
Cooking time: 5 minutes
Servings: 2

INGREDIENTS:

- 1 tablespoon extra-virgin olive oil
- 1 tablespoon freshly squeezed orange juice
- ¼ teaspoon kosher or sea salt
- 4 (4-ounces) tilapia fillets, more oblong than square, skin-on or skinned
- ¼ cup chopped red onion (about 1/8 onion)
- 1 avocado, pitted, skinned, and sliced

DIRECTIONS:

1. In a 9-inch glass pie dish, use a fork to mix together the oil, orange juice, and salt. Working with one fillet at a time, place each in the pie dish and turn to coat on all sides.
2. Arrange the fillets in a wagon-wheel formation, so that one end of each fillet is in the center of the dish and the other end is temporarily draped over the edge of the dish.
3. Top each fillet with 1 tablespoon of onion, then fold the end of the fillet that's hanging over the edge in half over the onion.
4. When finished, you should have 4 folded-over fillets with the fold against the outer edge of the dish and the ends all in the center.
5. Cover the dish with plastic wrap, leaving a small part open at the edge to vent the steam. Microwave on high for about 3 minutes.
6. The fish is done when it just begins to separate into flakes (chunks) when pressed gently with a fork. Top the fillets with the avocado and serve.

NUTRITION: 4 g Carbs, 3 g fiber, 22 g protein

324. Steamed Mussels in white Wine Sauce

Preparation time: 5 minutes
Cooking time: 10 minutes
Servings: 2

INGREDIENTS:

- 2 pounds' small mussels
- 1 tablespoon extra-virgin olive oil
- 1 cup thinly sliced red onion
- 3 garlic cloves, sliced
- 1 cup dry white wine
- 2 (¼-inch-thick) lemon slices
- ¼ teaspoon freshly ground black pepper
- ¼ teaspoon kosher or sea salt
- Fresh lemon wedges, for serving (optional)

DIRECTIONS:

1. In a large colander in the sink, run cold water over the mussels (but don't let the mussels sit in standing water).
2. All the shells should be closed tight; discard any shells that are a little bit open or any shells that are cracked. Leave the mussels in the colander until you're ready to use them.
3. In a large skillet over medium-high heat, heat the oil. Add the onion and cook for 4 minutes, stirring occasionally.
4. Add the garlic and cook for 1 minute, stirring constantly. Add the wine, lemon slices, pepper, and salt, and bring to a simmer. Cook for 2 minutes.
5. Add the mussels and cover. Cook for 3 minutes, or until the mussels open their shells. Gently shake the pan two or three times while they are cooking.
6. All the shells should now be wide open. Using a slotted spoon, discard any mussels that are still closed. Spoon the opened mussels into a shallow serving bowl, and pour the broth over the top. Serve with additional fresh lemon slices, if desired.

NUTRITION: Calories 22, 7 g fat, 1 g fiber, 18 g protein

325. Orange and Garlic Shrimp

Preparation time: 20 minutes
Cooking time: 10 minutes
Servings: 2

INGREDIENTS:

- 1 large orange
- 3 tablespoons extra-virgin olive oil, divided
- 1 tablespoon chopped fresh Rosemary
- 1 tablespoon chopped fresh thyme
- 3 garlic cloves, minced (about 1½ teaspoons)
- ¼ teaspoon freshly ground black pepper
- ¼ teaspoon kosher or sea salt
- 1½ pounds fresh raw shrimp, shells, and tails removed

DIRECTIONS:

1. Zest the entire orange using a citrus grater. In a large zip-top plastic bag, combine the orange zest and 2 tablespoons of oil with the Rosemary, thyme, garlic, pepper, and salt.
2. Add the shrimp, seal the bag, and gently massage the shrimp until all the ingredients are combined and the shrimp is completely covered with the seasonings. Set aside.
3. Heat a grill, grill pan, or a large skillet over medium heat. Brush on or swirl in the remaining 1 tablespoon of oil.

4. Add half the shrimp, and cook for 4 to 6 minutes, or until the shrimp turn pink and white, flipping halfway through if on the grill or stirring every minute if in a pan. Transfer the shrimp to a large serving bowl.
5. Repeat with the remaining shrimp, and add them to the bowl.
6. While the shrimp cook, peel the orange and cut the flesh into bite-size pieces. Add to the serving bowl, and toss with the cooked shrimp. Serve immediately or refrigerate and serve cold.

NUTRITION: Calories 190, 8 g fat, 1 g fiber, 24 g protein

326. Roasted Shrimp-Gnocchi Bake

Preparation time: 10 minutes
Cooking time: 20 minutes
Servings: 2

INGREDIENTS:
- 1 cup chopped fresh tomato
- 2 tablespoons extra-virgin olive oil
- 2 garlic cloves, minced
- ½ teaspoon freshly ground black pepper
- ¼ teaspoon crushed red pepper
- 1 (12-ounces) jar roasted red peppers
- 1-pound fresh raw shrimp, shells and tails removed
- 1-pound frozen gnocchi (not thawed)
- ½ cup cubed feta cheese
- 1/3 cup fresh torn basil leaves

DIRECTIONS:
1. Preheat the oven to 425°F. In a baking dish, mix the tomatoes, oil, garlic, black pepper, and crushed red pepper. Roast in the oven for 10 minutes.
2. Stir in the roasted peppers and shrimp. Roast for 10 more minutes, until the shrimp turn pink and white.
3. While the shrimp cooks, cook the gnocchi on the stovetop according to the package directions.
4. Drain in a colander and keep warm. Remove the dish from the oven. Mix in the cooked gnocchi, feta, and basil, and serve.

NUTRITION: Calories 227, 7 g fat, 1 g fiber, 20 g protein

327. Spicy Shrimp Puttanesca

Preparation time: 5 minutes
Cooking time: 15 minutes
Servings: 2

INGREDIENTS:
- 2 tablespoons extra-virgin olive oil
- 3 anchovy fillets, drained and chopped
- 3 garlic cloves, minced
- ½ teaspoon crushed red pepper
- 1 (14.5-ounces) can low-sodium or no-salt-added diced tomatoes, undrained
- 1 (2.25-ounces) can sliced black olives, drained
- 2 tablespoons capers
- 1 tablespoon chopped fresh oregano
- 1-pound fresh raw shrimp, shells and tails removed

DIRECTIONS:
1. In a large skillet over medium heat, heat the oil. Mix in the anchovies, garlic, and crushed red pepper.

2. Cook for 3 minutes, stirring frequently and mashing up the anchovies with a wooden spoon until they have melted into the oil.
3. Stir in the tomatoes with their juices, olives, capers, and oregano. Turn up the heat to medium-high, and bring to a simmer.
4. When the sauce is lightly bubbling, stir in the shrimp. Reduce the heat to medium, and cook the shrimp for 6 to 8 minutes, or until they turn pink and white, stirring occasionally, and serve.

NUTRITION: Calories 214, 10 g fat, 2 g fiber, 26 g protein

328. Baked Cod with Vegetables

Preparation Time: 15 minutes
Cooking Time: 25 minutes
Serving: 2

INGREDIENTS:
- 1 pound (454 g) thick cod fillet, cut into 4 even portions
- ¼ teaspoon onion powder (optional)
- ¼ teaspoon paprika
- 3 tablespoons extra-virgin olive oil
- 4 medium scallions
- ½ cup fresh chopped basil, divided
- 3 tablespoons minced garlic (optional)
- 2 teaspoons salt
- 2 teaspoons freshly ground black pepper
- ¼ teaspoon dry marjoram (optional)
- 6 sun-dried tomato slices
- ½ cup dry white wine
- ½ cup crumbled feta cheese
- 1 (15-ounce / 425-g) can oil-packed artichoke hearts, drained
- 1 lemon, sliced
- 1 cup pitted kalamata olives
- 1 teaspoon capers (optional)
- 4 small red potatoes, quartered

DIRECTION:
1. Set oven to 375°f (190°c).
2. Season the fish with paprika and onion powder (if desired).
3. Heat an ovenproof skillet over medium heat and sear the top side of the cod for about 1 minute until golden. Set aside.
4. Heat the olive oil in the same skillet over medium heat. Add the scallions, ¼ cup of basil, garlic (if desired), salt, pepper, marjoram (if desired), tomato slices, and white wine and stir to combine. Boil then removes from heat.
5. Evenly spread the sauce on the bottom of skillet. Place the cod on top of the tomato basil sauce and scatter with feta cheese. Place the artichokes in the skillet and top with the lemon slices.
6. Scatter with the olives, capers (if desired), and the remaining ¼ cup of basil. Pullout from the heat and transfer to the preheated oven. Bake for 15 to 20 minutes
7. Meanwhile, place the quartered potatoes on a baking sheet or wrapped in aluminum foil. Bake in the oven for 15 minutes.
8. Cool for 5 minutes before serving.

NUTRITION: Calories 1168, 60g fat, 64g protein

329. Slow Cooker Salmon in Foil

Preparation Time: 5 minutes
Cooking Time: 2 hours
Serving: 2

INGREDIENTS:

- 2 (6-ounce / 170-g) wild salmon fillets
- 1 tablespoon olive oil
- 2 cloves garlic, minced
- ½ tablespoon lime juice
- 1 teaspoon finely chopped fresh parsley
- ¼ teaspoon black pepper

DIRECTION

1. Spread a length of foil onto a work surface and place the salmon fillets in the middle.
2. Blend olive oil, garlic, lime juice, parsley, and black pepper. Brush the mixture over the fillets. Fold the foil over and crimp the sides to make a packet.
3. Place the packet into the slow cooker, cover, and cook on High for 2 hours
4. Serve hot.

NUTRITION: Calories 446, 21g fat, 65g protein

330. Crispy Fish Tacos With Grapefruit Salsa

Preparation Time: 15 Minutes
Cooking Time: 20 minutes
Servings: 4

INGREDIENTS:

- 1/4 cup of tapioca flour
- Half cup of cassava flour
- Paleo Tortillas
- 3/4 cup of sparkling water
- 1 1/2 lb. of cod
- 1 teaspoon of sea salt

Grapefruit Salsa

- 1 chopped avocado
- 3 tablespoons of chopped white onion
- 2 diced grapefruits, without skin
- Sea salt, to taste
- 2 tablespoons of chopped Fresh cilantro
- 1 tablespoon of Lime juice

DIRECTIONS:

1. Slice the fish into 8 pieces, and coat in tapioca lightly.
2. In a bowl, whisk water, salt and cassava.
3. In a pan, add enough oil to fry the cod.
4. Coat the fish in batter, and fry in oil for 3 to 4 minutes on one side.
5. Take it out on a paper towel.
6. Add all the ingredients of salsa in a bowl and mix.
7. In warmed/ grilled tortillas, add fish and salsa, serve.

NUTRITION: Calories 265 Total fat: 12.1 g Total carbs: 14.9 g Fiber: 5.4 g Sugar: 8 g Protein: 21 g Sodium: 145 mg

331. Garlic-Butter Salmon and Asparagus

Preparation Time: 10 minutes
Cooking Time: 15 minutes
Serving: 2

INGREDIENTS:

- 2 (6-ounce / 170-g) wild salmon fillets, skin on and patted dry
- Pink Himalayan salt
- Freshly ground black pepper, to taste
- 1 pound (454 g) fresh asparagus, ends snapped off
- 3 tablespoons almond butter
- 2 garlic cloves, minced

DIRECTION:

1. Prep oven to 400°f (205°c). Line a baking sheet with aluminum foil.
2. Season both sides of the salmon fillets.
3. Situate salmon in the middle of the baking sheet and arrange the asparagus around the salmon.
4. Heat the almond butter in a small saucepan over medium heat.
5. Cook minced garlic
6. Drizzle the garlic-butter sauce over the salmon and asparagus.
7. Bake in the preheated oven for about 12 minutes. You can switch the oven to broil at the end of cooking time for about 3 minutes to get a nice char on the asparagus.
8. Let cool for 5 minutes before serving.

NUTRITION: Calories 435, 26g fat, 42g protein

332. Lemon Rosemary Roasted Branzino

Preparation Time: 15 minutes
Cooking Time: 30 minutes
Serving: 2

INGREDIENTS:

- 4 tablespoons extra-virgin olive oil, divided
- 2 (8-ounce) Branzino fillets
- 1 garlic clove, minced
- 1 bunch scallions
- 10 to 12 small cherry tomatoes, halved
- 1 large carrot, cut into ¼-inch rounds
- ½ cup dry white wine
- 2 tablespoons paprika
- 2 teaspoons kosher salt
- ½ tablespoon ground chili pepper
- 2 rosemary sprigs or 1 tablespoon dried rosemary
- 1 small lemon, thinly sliced
- ½ cup sliced pitted kalamata olives

DIRECTION:

1. Heat a large ovenproof skillet over high heat until hot, about 2 minutes. Add 1 tablespoon of olive oil and heat
2. Add the Branzino fillets, skin-side up, and sear for 2 minutes. Flip the fillets and cook. Set aside.
3. Swirl 2 tablespoons of olive oil around the skillet to coat evenly.
4. Add the garlic, scallions, tomatoes, and carrot, and sauté for 5 minutes
5. Add the wine, stirring until all ingredients are well combined. Carefully place the fish over the sauce.
6. Preheat the oven to 450°f (235°c).

7. Brush the fillets with the remaining 1 tablespoon of olive oil and season with paprika, salt, and chili pepper. Top each fillet with a rosemary sprig and lemon slices. Scatter the olives over fish and around the skillet.
8. Roast for about 10 minutes until the lemon slices are browned. Serve hot.

NUTRITION: Calories 724, 43g fat, 57g protein

333. Grilled Lemon Pesto Salmon

Preparation Time: 5 minutes
Cooking Time: 10 minutes
Serving: 2
INGREDIENTS:

- 10 ounces (283 g) wild salmon fillet
- 2 tablespoons prepared pesto sauce
- 1 large fresh lemon, sliced
- Cooking spray

DIRECTION:
1. Preheat the grill to medium-high heat. Spray the grill grates with cooking spray.
2. Season the salmon well. Spread the pesto sauce on top.
3. Make a bed of fresh lemon slices about the same size as the salmon fillet on the hot grill, and place the salmon on top of the lemon slices. Put any additional lemon slices on top of the salmon.
4. Grill the salmon for 10 minutes.
5. Serve hot.

NUTRITION: Calories 316, 21g fat, 29g protein

334. Paleo Crumbed Fish

Preparation Time: 15 Minutes
Cooking Time: 25 minutes
Servings: 5
INGREDIENTS:

- 2 egg whites, whisked
- 12-14 ounces of white fish fillets
- 2.8 ounces of almond meal
- Salt, pepper, mixed dried herbs to taste
- Chopped walnuts, as needed

DIRECTIONS:
1. In a bowl, add almond meal.
2. In a separate bowl, add whisked egg white.
3. Coat the fish in almond meal, then in egg.
4. Sprinkle with walnuts, salt, pepper and herbs.
5. Bake for 8-10 minutes at 375 F, until flaky.
6. Serve.

NUTRITION: Calories 331 fat: 23 g carbs: 3.9 g Fiber: 5.4 g Sugar: 8 g Protein: 25.8 g Sodium: 145 mg

335. Roasted Trout Stuffed with Veggies

Preparation Time: 10 minutes
Cooking Time: 25 minutes
Serving: 2
INGREDIENT:

- 2 (8-ounce) whole trout fillets
- 1 tablespoon extra-virgin olive oil
- ¼ teaspoon salt

- 1/8 teaspoon black pepper
- 1 small onion, thinly sliced
- ½ red bell pepper
- 1 poblano pepper
- 2 or 3 shiitake mushrooms, sliced
- 1 lemon, sliced

DIRECTION:
1. Set oven to 425°f (220°c). Coat baking sheet with nonstick cooking spray.
2. Rub both trout fillets, inside and out, with the olive oil. Season with salt and pepper.
3. Mix together the onion, bell pepper, poblano pepper, and mushrooms in a large bowl. Stuff half of this mix into the cavity of each fillet. Top the mixture with 2 or 3 lemon slices inside each fillet.
4. Place the fish on the prepared baking sheet side by side. Roast in the preheated oven for 25 minutes
5. Pullout from the oven and serve on a plate.

NUTRITION: Calories 453, 22g fat, 49g protein

336. Lemony Trout with Caramelized Shallots

Preparation Time: 10 minutes
Cooking Time: 20 minutes
Serving: 2
INGREDIENTS:

- Shallots:
- 1 teaspoon almond butter
- 2 shallots, thinly sliced
- Dash salt
- Trout:
- 1 tablespoon almond butter
- 2 (4-ounce / 113-g) trout fillets
- 3 tablespoons capers
- ¼ cup freshly squeezed lemon juice
- ¼ teaspoon salt
- Dash freshly ground black pepper
- 1 lemon, thinly sliced

DIRECTION:
1. For Shallots
2. Situate skillet over medium heat, cook the butter, shallots, and salt for 20 minutes, stirring every 5 minutes.
3. For Trout
4. Meanwhile, in another large skillet over medium heat, heat 1 teaspoon of almond butter.
5. Add the trout fillets and cook each side for 3 minutes, or until flaky. Transfer to a plate and set aside.
6. In the skillet used for the trout, stir in the capers, lemon juice, salt, and pepper, then bring to a simmer. Whisk in the remaining 1 tablespoon of almond butter. Spoon the sauce over the fish.
7. Garnish the fish with the lemon slices and caramelized shallots before serving.

NUTRITION: Calories 344, 18g fat, 21g protein

337. Easy Tomato Tuna Melts

Preparation Time: 5 minutes
Cooking Time: 4 minutes
Serving: 2

INGREDIENTS:

- 1 (5-oz) can chunk light tuna packed in water
- 2 tablespoons plain Greek yogurt
- 2 tablespoons finely chopped celery
- 1 tablespoon finely chopped red onion
- 2 teaspoons freshly squeezed lemon juice
- 1 large tomato, cut into ¾-inch-thick rounds

DIRECTION:

1. Preheat the broiler to High.
2. Stir together the tuna, yogurt, celery, red onion, lemon juice, and cayenne pepper in a medium bowl.
3. Place the tomato rounds on a baking sheet. Top each with some tuna salad.
4. Broil for 3 to 4 minutes. Cool for 5 minutes before serving.

NUTRITION: Calories 244, 10g fat, 30g protein

338. Mackerel and Pinto Bean Salad

Preparation Time: 10 minutes
Cooking Time: 10 minutes
Serving: 2

INGREDIENTS:

- 2 cups pinto beans
- 1 tablespoon avocado oil
- 2 mackerel fillets
- 4 cups mixed salad greens
- 2 hard-boiled eggs, sliced
- 1 avocado, sliced
- 2 tablespoons lemon juice
- 2 tablespoons olive oil
- 1 teaspoon Dijon mustard
- Salt and black pepper, to taste

DIRECTION:

1. Cook the pinto beans in pot of boiling water for about 3 minutes. Drain and set aside.
2. Melt the avocado oil in a pan over medium heat. Add the mackerel fillets and cook each side for 4 minutes.
3. Divide the greens between two salad bowls. Top with the mackerel, sliced egg, and avocado slices.
4. Scourge lemon juice, olive oil, mustard, salt, and pepper, and drizzle over the salad. Add the cooked pinto beans and toss to combine, then serve.

NUTRITION: Calories 737, 57g fat, 34g protein

339. Hazelnut Crusted Sea Bass

Preparation Time: 10 minutes
Cooking Time: 15 minutes
Serving: 2

INGREDIENTS:

- 2 tablespoons almond butter
- 2 sea bass fillets
- 1/3 cup roasted hazelnuts
- A pinch of cayenne pepper

DIRECTION

1. Ready oven to 425°f (220°c). Line a baking dish with waxed paper.
2. Brush the almond butter over the fillets.
3. Pulse the hazelnuts and cayenne in a food processor. Coat the sea bass with the hazelnut mixture, then transfer to the baking dish.
4. Bake in the preheated oven for about 15 minutes. Cool for 5 minutes before serving.

NUTRITION: Calories 468, 31g fat, 40g protein

340. Salmon Baked in Foil

Preparation time: 5 minutes
Cooking time: 25 minutes
Servings: 4

INGREDIENTS:

- 2 cups cherry tomatoes
- 3 tablespoons extra-virgin olive oil
- 3 tablespoons lemon juice
- 3 tablespoons almond butter
- 1 teaspoon oregano
- ½ teaspoon salt
- 4 (5-ounce / 142-g) wild salmon fillets

DIRECTIONS:

1. Preheat the oven to 400°f (205°c). Cut the tomatoes in half and put them in a bowl. Add the olive oil, lemon juice, butter, oregano, and salt to the tomatoes and gently toss to combine.
2. Cut 4 pieces of foil, about 12-by-12 inches each. Place the salmon fillets in the middle of each piece of foil.
3. Divide the tomato mixture evenly over the 4 pieces of salmon. Bring the ends of the foil together and seal to form a closed pocket.
4. Place the 4 pockets on a baking sheet. Bake in the preheated oven for 25 minutes. Remove from the oven and serve on a plate.

NUTRITION: Calories: 410 Fat: 32.0g Protein: 30.0g Carbs: 4.0g

341. Sheet Pan Fish Fajitas

Preparation Time: 10 Minutes
Cooking Time: 25 minutes
Servings: 4

INGREDIENTS:

- 3 sliced bell peppers
- 4 tablespoon of lime juice
- 1 pound of cod, cut into strips
- 1 teaspoon of cumin
- 1 teaspoon of chipotle powder
- 2 tablespoons of avocado oil
- 1 sliced sweet onion
- 1 tablespoon of minced garlic
- 1/4 teaspoon of pepper
- Half teaspoon of coriander
- Half teaspoon of salt
- 2 teaspoon of chili powder
- 1 teaspoon of dried parsley
- Half teaspoon of onion powder

DIRECTIONS:

1. Let the oven preheat to 400 F.
2. In a bowl, add all dried seasoning and mix.
3. Toss peppers and onion with oil (2 tbsp.), lime juice(half) and minced garlic, mix with hands.
4. Spread on a foil-lined baking sheet, spread half of the dried seasoning and toss well.
5. Bake for 12 minutes.
6. In a bowl, add cod and rub with dried seasoning, oil (1 tbsp.) and lime juice. Coat the fish,
7. Take the baking sheet out and place fish on the pan bake for 10 to 12 minutes.
8. Serve.

NUTRITION: Calories 266 Total fat: 12.9 g Total carbs: 8 g Fiber: 7 g Sugar: 5 g Protein: 22 g Sodium: 141 mg

342. Balsamic-Honey Glazed Salmon

Preparation time: 5 minutes
Cooking time: 8 minutes
Servings: 4

INGREDIENTS:

- ½ cup balsamic vinegar
- 1 tablespoon honey
- 4 (8-ounce / 227-g) wild salmon fillets
- Sea salt and freshly ground pepper, to taste
- 1 tablespoon olive oil

DIRECTIONS:

1. Heat a skillet over medium-high heat. Combine the vinegar and honey in a small bowl. Season the salmon fillets with the sea salt and freshly ground pepper; brush with the honey-balsamic glaze.
2. Add olive oil to the skillet, and sear the salmon fillets, cooking for 3 to 4 minutes on each side until lightly browned and medium rare in the center. Let sit for 5 minutes before serving.

NUTRITION: Calories: 454 Fat: 17.3g Protein: 65.3g Carbs: 9.7g

343. Seared Salmon with Lemon Cream Sauce

Preparation time: 10 minutes
Cooking time: 20 minutes
Servings: 4

INGREDIENTS:

- 4 (5-ounce / 142-g) wild salmon fillets
- Sea salt and freshly ground black pepper, to taste
- 1 tablespoon extra-virgin olive oil
- ½ cup low-sodium vegetable broth
- Juice and zest of 1 lemon
- 1 teaspoon chopped fresh thyme
- ½ cup fat-free sour cream
- 1 teaspoon honey
- 1 tablespoon chopped fresh chives

DIRECTIONS:

1. Preheat the oven to 400°f (205°c). Season the salmon lightly on both sides with salt and pepper. Place a large ovenproof skillet over medium-high heat and add the olive oil.
2. Sear the salmon fillets on both sides until golden, about 3 minutes per side. Transfer the salmon to a baking dish and bake

in the preheated oven until just cooked through, about 10 minutes.
3. Meanwhile, whisk together the vegetable broth, lemon juice and zest, and thyme in a small saucepan over medium-high heat until the liquid reduces by about one-quarter, about 5 minutes.
4. Whisk in the sour cream and honey. Stir in the chives and serve the sauce over the salmon.

NUTRITION: Calories: 310 Fat: 18.0g Protein: 29.0g Carbs: 6.0g

344. Tuna and Zucchini Patties

Preparation time: 15 minutes
Cooking time: 12 minutes
Servings: 4

INGREDIENTS:

- 3 slices whole-wheat sandwich bread, toasted
- 2 (5-ounce / 142-g) cans tuna in olive oil, drained
- 1 cup shredded zucchini
- 1 large egg, lightly beaten
- ¼ cup diced red bell pepper
- 1 tablespoon dried oregano
- 1 teaspoon lemon zest
- ¼ teaspoon freshly ground black pepper
- ¼ teaspoon kosher or sea salt
- 1 tablespoon extra-virgin olive oil
- Salad greens or 4 whole-wheat rolls, for serving (optional)

DIRECTIONS:

1. Crumble the toast into bread crumbs with your fingers (or use a knife to cut into ¼-inch cubes) until you have 1 cup of loosely packed crumbs.
2. Pour the crumbs into a large bowl. Add the tuna, zucchini, beaten egg, bell pepper, oregano, lemon zest, black pepper, and salt. Mix well with a fork.
3. With your hands, form the mixture into four (½-cup-size) patties. Place them on a plate, and press each patty flat to about ¾-inch thick.
4. In a large skillet over medium-high heat, heat the oil until it's very hot, about 2 minutes. Add the patties to the hot oil, then reduce the heat down to medium.
5. Cook the patties for 5 minutes, flip with a spatula, and cook for an additional 5 minutes. Serve the patties on salad greens or whole-wheat rolls, if desired.

NUTRITION: Calories: 757 Fat: 72.0g Protein: 5.0g Carbs: 26.0g

345. Fennel Poached Cod with Tomatoes

Preparation time: 15 minutes
Cooking time: 20 minutes
Servings: 4

INGREDIENTS:

- 1 tablespoon olive oil
- 1 cup thinly sliced fennel
- ½ cup thinly sliced onion
- 1 tablespoon minced garlic
- 1 (15-ounce / 425-g) can diced tomatoes
- 2 cups chicken broth
- ½ cup white wine
- Juice and zest of 1 orange
- 1 pinch red pepper flakes

- 1 bay leaf
- 1 pound (454 g) cod

DIRECTIONS:

1. Heat the olive oil in a large skillet. Add the onion and fennel and cook for 6 minutes, stirring occasionally, or until translucent. Add the garlic and cook for 1 minute more.
2. Add the tomatoes, chicken broth, wine, orange juice and zest, red pepper flakes, and bay leaf, and simmer for 5 minutes to meld the flavors.
3. Carefully add the cod in a single layer, cover, and simmer for 6 to 7 minutes. Transfer fish to a serving dish, ladle the remaining sauce over the fish, and serve.

NUTRITION: Calories: 336 Fat: 12.5g Protein: 45.1g Carbs: 11.0g

346. Baked Fish with Pistachio Crust

Preparation time: 15 minutes
Cooking time: 15-20 minutes
Servings: 4

INGREDIENTS:

- ½ cup extra-virgin olive oil, divided
- 1 pound (454 g) flaky white fish (such as cod, haddock, or halibut), skin removed
- ½ cup shelled finely chopped pistachios
- ½ cup ground flaxseed
- Zest and juice of 1 lemon, divided
- 1 teaspoon ground cumin
- 1 teaspoon ground allspice
- ½ teaspoon salt
- ¼ teaspoon freshly ground black pepper

DIRECTIONS:

1. Preheat the oven to 400°f (205°c). Line a baking sheet with parchment paper or aluminum foil and drizzle 2 tablespoons of olive oil over the sheet, spreading to evenly coat the bottom.
2. Cut the fish into 4 equal pieces and place on the prepared baking sheet.
3. In a small bowl, combine the pistachios, flaxseed, lemon zest, cumin, allspice, salt, and pepper. Drizzle in ¼ cup of olive oil and stir well.
4. Divide the nut mixture evenly on top of the fish pieces. Drizzle the lemon juice and remaining 2 tablespoons of olive oil over the fish and bake until cooked through, 15 to 20 minutes, depending on the thickness of the fish. Cool for 5 minutes before serving.

NUTRITION: Calories: 509 Fat: 41.0g Protein: 26.0g Carbs: 9.0g

347. Dill Baked Sea Bass

Preparation time: 15 minutes
Cooking time: 10-15 minutes
Servings: 6

INGREDIENTS:

- ¼ cup olive oil
- 2 pounds (907 g) sea bass
- Sea salt and freshly ground pepper, to taste
- 1 garlic clove, minced
- ¼ cup dry white wine
- 3 teaspoons fresh dill
- 2 teaspoons fresh thyme

DIRECTIONS:

1. Preheat the oven to 425°f (220°c). Brush the bottom of a roasting pan with the olive oil. Place the fish in the pan and brush the fish with oil.
2. Season the fish with sea salt and freshly ground pepper. Combine the remaining ingredients and pour over the fish.
3. Bake in the preheated oven for 10 to 15 minutes, depending on the size of the fish. Serve hot.

NUTRITION: Calories: 224 Fat: 12.1g Protein: 28.1g Carbs: 0.9g

348. Sole Piccata with Capers

Preparation time: 15 minutes
Cooking time: 17 minutes
Servings: 4

INGREDIENTS:

- 1 teaspoon extra-virgin olive oil
- 4 (5-ounce / 142-g) sole fillets, patted dry
- 3 tablespoons almond butter
- 2 teaspoons minced garlic
- 2 tablespoons all-purpose flour
- 2 cups low-sodium chicken broth
- Juice and zest of ½ lemon
- 2 tablespoons capers

DIRECTIONS:

1. Place a large skillet over medium-high heat and add the olive oil. Sear the sole fillets until the fish flakes easily when tested with a fork, about 4 minutes on each side. Transfer the fish to a plate and set aside.
2. Return the skillet to the stove and add the butter. Sauté the garlic until translucent, about 3 minutes.
3. Whisk in the flour to make a thick paste and cook, stirring constantly, until the mixture is golden brown, about 2 minutes.
4. Whisk in the chicken broth, lemon juice and zest. Cook for about 4 minutes until the sauce is thickened. Stir in the capers and serve the sauce over the fish.

NUTRITION: Calories: 271 Fat: 13.0g Protein: 30.0g Carbs: 7.0g

349. Haddock with Cucumber Sauce

Preparation time: 15 minutes
Cooking time: 10 minutes
Servings: 4

INGREDIENTS:

- ¼ cup plain Greek yogurt
- ½ scallion, white and green parts, finely chopped
- ½ English cucumber, grated, liquid squeezed out
- 2 teaspoons chopped fresh mint
- 1 teaspoon honey
- Sea salt and freshly ground black pepper, to taste
- 4 (5-ounce / 142-g) haddock fillets, patted dry
- Nonstick cooking spray

DIRECTIONS:

1. In a small bowl, stir together the yogurt, cucumber, scallion, mint, honey, and a pinch of salt. Set aside. Season the fillets lightly with salt and pepper.
2. Place a large skillet over medium-high heat and spray lightly with cooking spray. Cook the haddock, turning once, until it is just cooked through, about 5 minutes per side.

3. Remove the fish from the heat and transfer to plates. Serve topped with the cucumber sauce.

NUTRITION: Calories: 164 Fat: 2.0g Protein: 27.0g Carbs: 4.0g

350. Crispy Herb Crusted Halibut

Preparation time: 15 minutes
Cooking time: 20 minutes
Servings: 4
INGREDIENTS:

- 4 (5-ounce / 142-g) halibut fillets, patted dry
- Extra-virgin olive oil, for brushing
- ½ cup coarsely ground unsalted pistachios
- 1 tablespoon chopped fresh parsley
- 1 teaspoon chopped fresh basil
- 1 teaspoon chopped fresh thyme
- Pinch sea salt
- Pinch freshly ground black pepper

DIRECTIONS:

1. Preheat the oven to 350°f (180°c). Line a baking sheet with parchment paper. Place the fillets on the baking sheet and brush them generously with olive oil.
2. In a small bowl, stir together the pistachios, parsley, basil, thyme, salt, and pepper. Spoon the nut mixture evenly on the fish, spreading it out so the tops of the fillets are covered.
3. Bake in the preheated oven until it flakes when pressed with a fork, about 20 minutes. Serve immediately.

NUTRITION: Calories: 262 Fat: 11.0g Protein: 32.0g Carbs: 4.0g

351. Mussels with Tomatoes & Chili

Preparation time: 15 minutes
Cooking time: 12 minutes
Servings: 4
INGREDIENTS:

- 2 ripe tomatoes
- 2 tbsps. Olive oil
- 1 tsp. Tomato paste
- 1 garlic clove, chopped
- 1 shallot, chopped
- 1 chopped red or green chili
- A small glass of dry white wine
- Salt and pepper to taste
- 2 lbs./900 g. Mussels, cleaned
- Basil leaves, fresh

DIRECTIONS:

1. Add tomatoes to boiling water for 3 minutes then drain. Peel the tomatoes and chop the flesh. Add oil to an iron skillet and heat to sauté shallots and garlic for 3 minutes.
2. Stir in wine along with tomatoes, chili, salt/pepper and tomato paste. Cook for 2 minutes then add mussels. Cover and let it steam for 4 minutes. Garnish with basil leaves and serve warm.

NUTRITION: Calories 483 Fat 15.2 g Carbs 20.4 g Protein 62.3 g

352. Lemon Garlic Shrimp

Preparation time: 15 minutes
Cooking time: 10 minutes
Servings: 6
INGREDIENTS:
4 tsps. Extra-virgin olive oil, divided

- 2 red bell peppers, diced
- 2 lbs./900 g. Fresh asparagus, sliced
- 2 tsps. Lemon zest, freshly grated
- ½ tsp. Salt, divided
- 5 garlic cloves, minced
- 1 lb./450 g. Peeled raw shrimp, deveined
- 1 c. Reduced-sodium chicken broth or water
- 1 tsp. Cornstarch
- 2 tbsps. Lemon juice
- 2 tbsps. Fresh parsley, chopped

DIRECTIONS:

1. Add 2 teaspoon oil to a large skillet and heat for a minute. Stir in asparagus, lemon zest, bell pepper and salt. Sauté for 6 minutes.
2. Keep the sautéed veggies in a separate bowl. Add remaining oil in the same pan and add garlic. Sauté for 30 seconds then add shrimp. Cook for 1 minute.
3. Mix cornstarch with broth in a bowl and pour this mixture into the pan. Add salt and stir cook for 2 minutes. Turn off flame then add parsley and lemon juice. Serve warm with sautéed vegetables.

NUTRITION: Calories 204 Fat 4 g Carbs 23.6 g Protein 17. 1 g

353. Pepper Tilapia with Spinach

Preparation time: 15 minutes
Cooking time: 27 minutes
Servings: 4
INGREDIENTS:

- 4 tilapia fillets, 8 oz./ 227 g. Each
- 4 cups fresh spinach
- 1 red onion, sliced
- 3 garlic cloves, minced
- 2 tbsps. Extra virgin olive oil
- 3 lemons
- 1 tbsp. Ground black pepper
- 1 tbsp. Ground white pepper
- 1 tbsp. Crushed red pepper

DIRECTIONS:

1. Set the oven to preheat at 350°F/176.6°C. Place the fish in a shallow baking dish and juice two of the lemons.
2. Cover the fish in the lemon juice and then sprinkle the three types of pepper over the fish. Slice the remaining lemon and cover the fish. Bake in the oven for 20 minutes.
3. While the fish cooks, sauté the garlic and onion in the olive oil. Add the spinach and sauté for 7 more minutes. Top the fish with spinach and serve.

NUTRITION: Calories 323 Fat 11.4 g Carbs 10.4 g Protein 50 g

354. Spicy Shrimp Salad

Preparation time: 15 minutes
Cooking time: 0 minutes
Servings: 2

INGREDIENTS:

- ½ lb. Salad shrimp, chopped
- 2 stalks celery, chopped
- ¼ cup red onion, diced
- 1 tsp. Black pepper
- 1 tsp. Red pepper
- 1 tbsp. Lemon juice
- Dash of cayenne pepper
- 1 tbsp. Olive oil
- 2 cucumbers, sliced

DIRECTIONS:

1. Combine the shrimp, celery, and onion in a bowl and mix together. In a separate bowl, whisk the oil and the lemon juice, then add red pepper, black pepper, and cayenne pepper.
2. Pour over the shrimp and mix. Serve with slices of thickly cut cucumber on it and enjoy.

NUTRITION: Calories: 245 Fat: 9g Carbs: 18.2g Protein: 27.3g

355. Baked Cod in Parchment

Preparation time: 15 minutes
Cooking time: 0 minutes
Servings: 1

INGREDIENTS:

- 1-2 potatoes, sliced
- 5 cherry tomatoes, halved
- 5 pitted olives
- Juice of ½ lemon
- ½ tbsp. Olive oil
- 4 oz. Cod
- 20 inches long parchment
- Sea salt and black pepper

DIRECTIONS:

1. Set your oven to preheat at 350°F/176.6°C. Spread the olive oil on parchment and arrange potato on it.
2. In separate bowl combine the tomatoes, olives, and lemon juice. Put the fish fillet on potatoes and top with tomato mixture. Add salt and pepper. Fold the filled parchment squares and bake for 20 minutes.

NUTRITION: Calories 330 Fat 8 g Carbs 35 g Protein 25 g

356. Roasted Fish & New Potatoes

Preparation time: 15 minutes
Cooking time: 35 minutes
Servings: 4

INGREDIENTS:

- 3 tbsps. Extra-virgin olive oil
- 3 tbsps. Orange juice
- 3 tbsps. White vinegar
- ½ tsp. Orange peel, grated
- ¼ tsp. Dried dillweed
- 12 new potatoes, cubed
- 4 wild salmon fillets, skin removed

DIRECTIONS:

1. Preheat oven to 420°F/215°C. Blend first five ingredients. Sprinkle potato with 2 tbsps. Of this mixture. Bake for 20 minutes.
2. Sprinkle fillets with remaining mixture and add to the potatoes. Cook for about 15 minutes and serve.

NUTRITION: Calories 289 Fat 8.2 g Carbs 23.4 g Protein 29 g

MEAT & POULTRY

357. BBQ Chicken & Vegetables Sheet Pan

Preparation Time: 45 Minutes
Cooking Time: 50 minutes
Servings: 4

INGREDIENTS:

- ⅓ cup of sugar-free BBQ sauce
- 1 teaspoon of salt
- 2 heads of broccoli, broken into florets
- 4 lemon slices
- Half tablespoon of oil
- chicken thighs, boneless & skinless
- 2 cups of russet potatoes, diced
- Half teaspoon of thyme
- 1 teaspoon of garlic powder

DIRECTIONS:

1. Coat the chicken thighs in BBQ sauce, mix well. Keep in the fridge for half an hour.
2. Let the oven preheat to 350 F.
3. Add potatoes to one side of the foil-lined baking sheet, toss with half the garlic powder and salt (half) and oil.
4. Oil spray the broccoli and add broccoli to one side of the pan and toss with the rest of the garlic and oil.
5. On one side of the same tray, place the chicken and brush with more BBQ sauce.
6. Bake for 40 to 50 minutes.
7. Serve.

NUTRITION: Calories 378 Total fat: 14 g Total carbs: 6.9 g Fiber: 9 g Sugar: 4 g Protein: 32 g Sodium: 487 mg

358. Korean Beef Bowl

Preparation Time: 15 Minutes
Cooking Time: 15 minutes
Servings: 4

INGREDIENTS:

- 2" of peeled fresh ginger, grated
- 1 teaspoon of onion powder
- 1 tablespoon of sesame oil, toasted
- 2 pounds of ground beef
- 1 diced shallot
- 1 teaspoon of red pepper flakes
- 1 teaspoon of garlic powder
- Half cup of coconut aminos
- 2 cups of mixed greens
- 2 tablespoons of fish sauce
- 4 cups of cauliflower rice

DIRECTIONS:

1. In a skillet, heat oil on medium flame.
2. Add beef and break it into small pieces.
3. Add ginger, onion, garlic powder, red pepper and shallots. Cook for 8 minutes.
4. Add fish sauce, coconut aminos and cook for 3 to 4 minutes.
5. Serve beef with cauliflower rice and mixed greens.

NUTRITION: Calories 392 Total fat: 12 g Total carbs: 7 g Fiber: 6.9 g Sugar: 4.1 g Protein: 38 g Sodium: 397 mg

359. Beef and Chili Mix

Preparation time: 15 minutes
Cooking Time: 16 Minutes
Servings: 4

INGREDIENTS:

- 2 green chili peppers
- 8 oz beef flank steak
- 1 teaspoon salt
- 2 tablespoons olive oil
- 1 teaspoon apple cider vinegar

DIRECTIONS:

1. Pour olive oil in the skillet. Place the flank steak in the oil and roast it for 3 minutes from each side. Then sprinkle the meat with salt and apple cider vinegar.
2. Chop the chili peppers and add them in the skillet. Fry the beef for 10 minutes more. Stir it from time to time.

NUTRITION: Calories 166 Fat 10.5g Carbs 0.2g Protein17.2g

360. Creamy Tuscan Chicken

Preparation Time: 15 Minutes
Cooking Time: 30 minutes
Servings: 6

INGREDIENTS:

- 1 tablespoon of coconut oil
- 4 minced garlic cloves
- Sea salt & pepper
- 1/4 teaspoon of garlic powder
- 1 cup of chicken broth
- 1.5 lbs. of boneless & skinless chicken thighs
- 1/4 teaspoon of onion powder
- 1 chopped onion
- 1 tablespoon of tapioca flour
- 1 1/2 cups of chopped baby spinach
- Half cup of coconut milk
- Half tablespoon of ground mustard
- 1 1/2 tablespoon of nutritional yeast
- Salt & pepper, to taste
- 1 teaspoon of Italian seasoning blend
- 2/3 cup of chopped sun-dried tomatoes

DIRECTIONS:

1. Season the chicken with onion powder, salt, garlic and pepper.
2. In a skillet, add oil on medium heat. Cook chicken for 5 to 7 minutes on one side, take it out on a plate.
3. Add onions and cook until tender; add garlic and cook for 45 seconds.
4. Add tapioca and coconut milk, and broth. Whisk well.
5. Add Italian seasoning, mustard, salt, pepper and yeast. Cook till it starts to thicken.
6. Add tomatoes and spinach and cook until spinach wilts; add the chicken back in the pan.
7. Cook for 2 minutes, serve.

NUTRITION: Calories 368 Total fat: 25 g Total carbs: 12 g Fiber: 2 g Sugar: 5 g Protein: 23 g Sodium: 253 mg

361. Mediterranean Lamb Bowl

Preparation time: 15 minutes
Cooking time: 15 minutes
Servings: 2
INGREDIENTS:

- 2 tablespoons extra-virgin olive oil
- ¼ cup diced yellow onion
- 1-pound ground lamb
- 1 teaspoon dried mint
- 1 teaspoon dried parsley
- ½ teaspoon red pepper flakes
- ¼ teaspoon garlic powder
- 1 cup cooked rice
- ½ teaspoon za'atar seasoning
- ½ cup halved cherry tomatoes
- 1 cucumber, peeled and diced
- 1 cup store-bought hummus or Garlic-Lemon Hummus
- 1 cup crumbled feta cheese
- 2 pita breads, warmed (optional)

DIRECTIONS:

1. In a large sauté pan or skillet, heat the olive oil over medium heat and cook the onion for about 2 minutes, until fragrant.
2. Add the lamb and mix well, breaking up the meat as you cook. Once the lamb is halfway cooked, add mint, parsley, red pepper flakes, and garlic powder.
3. In a medium bowl, mix together the cooked rice and za'atar, then divide between individual serving bowls. Add the seasoned lamb, then top the bowls with the tomatoes, cucumber, hummus, feta, and pita (if using).

NUTRITION: Calories: 1,312 Protein: 62g Carbs: 62g Fat: 96g

362. Lamb Burger

Preparation time: 15 minutes
Cooking time: 15 minutes
Servings: 4
INGREDIENTS:

- 1-pound ground lamb
- ½ small red onion, grated
- 1 tablespoon dried parsley
- 1 teaspoon dried oregano
- 1 teaspoon ground cumin
- 1 teaspoon garlic powder
- ½ teaspoon dried mint
- ¼ teaspoon paprika
- ¼ teaspoon kosher salt
- 1/8 teaspoon freshly ground black pepper
- Extra-virgin olive oil, for panfrying
- 4 pita breads, for serving (optional)
- Tzatziki Sauce, for serving (optional)
- Pickled Onions, for serving (optional)

DIRECTIONS:

1. In a bowl, combine the lamb, onion, parsley, oregano, cumin, garlic powder, mint, paprika, salt, and pepper. Divide the meat into 4 small balls and work into smooth discs.
2. In a large sauté pan or skillet, heat a drizzle of olive oil over medium heat or brush a grill with oil and set it too medium.
3. Cook the patties for 4 to 5 minutes on each side, until cooked through and juices run clear. Enjoy lamb burgers in pitas, topped with tzatziki sauce and pickled onions (if using).

NUTRITION: Calories: 328 Protein: 19g Carbs: 2g Fat: 27g

363. Marinated Lamb Kebabs with Crunchy Yogurt Dressing

Preparation time: 15 minutes
Cooking time: 15 minutes
Servings: 4
INGREDIENTS:

- ½ cup plain, unsweetened, full-fat Greek yogurt
- ¼ cup extra-virgin olive oil
- ¼ cup freshly squeezed lemon juice
- 1 teaspoon grated lemon zest
- 2 garlic cloves, minced
- 2 tablespoons honey
- 2 tablespoons balsamic vinegar
- 1½ teaspoons oregano, fresh, minced
- 1 teaspoon thyme, fresh, minced
- 1 bay leaf
- 1 teaspoon kosher salt
- ½ teaspoon freshly ground black pepper
- ½ teaspoon red pepper flakes
- 2 pounds' leg of lamb, trimmed, cleaned and cut into 1-inch pieces
- 1 large red onion, diced large
- 1 recipe Crunchy Yogurt Dip
- Parsley, chopped, for garnish
- Lemon wedges, for garnish

DIRECTIONS:

1. In a bowl or large resealable bag, combine the yogurt, olive oil, lemon juice and zest, garlic, honey, balsamic vinegar, oregano, thyme, bay leaf, salt, pepper, and red pepper flakes. Mix well.
2. Add the lamb pieces and marinate, refrigerated, for 30 minutes. Preheat the oven to 375°F. Thread the lamb onto the skewers, alternating with chunks of red onion as desired.
3. Put the skewers onto a baking sheet and roast for 10 to 15 minutes, rotating every 5 minutes to ensure that they cook evenly.

4. Plate the skewers and allow them to rest briefly. Top or serve with the yogurt dressing. To finish, garnish with fresh chopped parsley and a lemon wedge.

NUTRITION: Calories: 578 Protein: 56g Carbs: 20g Fat: 30g

364. Garlic Pork Tenderloin and Lemony Orzo

Preparation time: 15 minutes
Cooking time: 20 minutes
Servings: 6

INGREDIENTS:
- 1-pound pork tenderloin
- ½ teaspoon Shawarma Spice Rub
- 1 tablespoon salt
- ½ teaspoon coarsely ground black pepper
- ½ teaspoon garlic powder
- 6 tablespoons extra-virgin olive oil
- 3 cups Lemony Orzo

DIRECTIONS:
1. Preheat the oven to 350°F. Rub the pork with shawarma seasoning, salt, pepper, and garlic powder and drizzle with the olive oil.
2. Put the pork on a baking sheet and roast for 20 minutes, or until desired doneness. Remove the pork from the oven and let rest for 10 minutes. Assemble the pork on a plate with the orzo and enjoy.

NUTRITION: Calories: 579 Protein: 33g Carbs: 37g Fat: 34g

365. Roasted Pork with Apple-Dijon Sauce

Preparation time: 15 minutes
Cooking time: 40 minutes
Servings: 8

INGREDIENTS:
- 1½ tablespoons extra-virgin olive oil
- 1 (12-ounce) pork tenderloin
- ¼ teaspoon kosher salt
- ¼ teaspoon freshly ground black pepper
- ¼ cup apple jelly
- ¼ cup apple juice
- 2 to 3 tablespoons Dijon mustard
- ½ tablespoon cornstarch
- ½ tablespoon cream

DIRECTIONS:
1. Preheat the oven to 325°F. In a large sauté pan or skillet, heat the olive oil over medium heat.
2. Add the pork to the skillet, using tongs to turn and sear the pork on all sides. Once seared, sprinkle pork with salt and pepper, and set it on a small baking sheet.
3. In the same skillet, with the juices from the pork, mix the apple jelly, juice, and mustard into the pan juices. Heat thoroughly over low heat, stirring consistently for 5 minutes. Spoon over the pork.
4. Put the pork in the oven and roast for 15 to 17 minutes, or 20 minutes per pound. Every 10 to 15 minutes, baste the pork with the apple-mustard sauce.

5. Once the pork tenderloin is done, remove it from the oven and let it rest for 15 minutes. Then, cut it into 1-inch slices.
6. In a small pot, blend the cornstarch with cream. Heat over low heat. Add the pan juices into the pot, stirring for 2 minutes, until thickened. Serve the sauce over the pork.

NUTRITION: Calories: 146 Protein: 13g Carbs: 8g Fat: 7g

366. Moroccan Pot Roast

Preparation time: 15 minutes
Cooking time: 50 minutes
Servings: 4

INGREDIENTS:
- 8 ounces' mushrooms, sliced
- 4 tablespoons extra-virgin olive oil
- 3 small onions, cut into 2-inch pieces
- 2 tablespoons paprika
- 1½ tablespoons garam masala
- 2 teaspoons salt
- ¼ teaspoon ground white pepper
- 2 tablespoons tomato paste
- 1 small eggplant, peeled and diced
- 1¼ cups low-sodium beef broth
- ½ cup halved apricots
- 1/3 cup golden raisins
- 3 pounds' beef chuck roast
- 2 tablespoons honey
- 1 tablespoon dried mint
- 2 cups cooked brown rice

DIRECTIONS:
1. Set an electric pressure cooker to Sauté and put the mushrooms and oil in the cooker. Sauté for 5 minutes, then add the onions, paprika, garam masala, salt, and white pepper. Stir in the tomato paste and continue to sauté.
2. Add the eggplant and sauté for 5 more minutes, until softened. Pour in the broth. Add the apricots and raisins. Sear the meat for 2 minutes on each side. Close and lock the lid and set the pressure cooker too high for 50 minutes.
3. When cooking is complete, quick release the pressure. Carefully remove the lid, then remove the meat from the sauce and break it into pieces. While the meat is removed, stir honey and mint into the sauce.
4. Assemble plates with ½ cup of brown rice, ½ cup of pot roast sauce, and 3 to 5 pieces of pot roast.

NUTRITION: Calories: 829 Protein: 69g Carbs: 70g Fat: 34g

367. Shawarma Pork Tenderloin with Pitas

Preparation time: 15 minutes
Cooking time: 35 minutes
Servings: 8

INGREDIENTS:
- For the shawarma spice rub:
- 1 teaspoon ground cumin
- 1 teaspoon ground coriander
- 1 teaspoon ground turmeric
- ¾ teaspoon sweet Spanish paprika
- ½ teaspoon ground cloves

- ¼ teaspoon salt
- ¼ teaspoon freshly ground black pepper
- 1/8 teaspoon ground cinnamon
- For the shawarma:
- 1½ pounds pork tenderloin
- 3 tablespoons extra-virgin olive oil
- 1 tablespoon garlic powder
- Salt
- Freshly ground black pepper
- 1½ tablespoons Shawarma Spice Rub
- 4 pita pockets, halved, for serving
- 1 to 2 tomatoes, sliced, for serving
- ¼ cup Pickled Onions, for serving
- ¼ cup Pickled Turnips, for serving
- ¼ cup store-bought hummus or Garlic-Lemon Hummus

DIRECTIONS:

1. To Make the Shawarma Seasoning:
2. In a small bowl, combine the cumin, coriander, turmeric, paprika, cloves, salt, pepper, and cinnamon and set aside.
3. To Make the Shawarma:
4. Preheat the oven to 400°F. Put the pork tenderloin on a plate and cover with olive oil and garlic powder on each side.
5. Season with salt and pepper and rub each side of the tenderloin with a generous amount of shawarma spices.
6. Place the pork tenderloin in the center of a roasting pan and roast for 20 minutes per pound, or until the meat begins to bounce back as you poke it.
7. If it feels like there's still fluid under the skin, continue cooking. Check every 5 to 7 minutes until it reaches the desired tenderness and juices run clear.
8. Remove the pork from the oven and let rest for 10 minutes. Serve the pork tenderloin shawarma with pita pockets, tomatoes, Pickled Onions (if using), Pickled Turnips (if using), and hummus.

NUTRITION: Calories: 316 Protein: 29g Carbs: 17g Fat: 15g

368. Flank Steak with Artichokes

Preparation time: 15 minutes
Cooking time: 60 minutes
Servings: 4-6
INGREDIENTS:

- 4 tablespoons grapeseed oil, divided
- 2 pounds' flank steak
- 1 (14-ounce) can artichoke hearts, drained and roughly chopped
- 1 onion, diced
- 8 garlic cloves, chopped
- 1 (32-ounce) container low-sodium beef broth
- 1 (14.5-ounce) can diced tomatoes, drained
- 1 cup tomato sauce
- 2 tablespoons tomato paste
- 1 teaspoon dried oregano
- 1 teaspoon dried parsley
- 1 teaspoon dried basil
- ½ teaspoon ground cumin
- 3 bay leaves
- 2 to 3 cups cooked couscous (optional)

DIRECTIONS:

1. Preheat the oven to 450°f. In an oven-safe sauté pan or skillet, heat 3 tablespoons of oil on medium heat.
2. Sear the steak for 2 minutes per side on both sides. Transfer the steak to the oven for 30 minutes, or until desired tenderness.
3. Meanwhile, in a large pot, combine the remaining 1 tablespoon of oil, artichoke hearts, onion, and garlic.
4. Pour in the beef broth, tomatoes, tomato sauce, and tomato paste. Stir in oregano, parsley, basil, cumin, and bay leaves.
5. Cook the vegetables, covered, for 30 minutes. Remove bay leaf and serve with flank steak and ½ cup of couscous per plate, if using.

NUTRITION: Calories: 577 Protein: 55g Carbs: 22g Fat: 28g

369. Easy Honey-Garlic Pork Chops

Preparation time: 15 minutes
Cooking time: 25 minutes
Servings: 4
INGREDIENTS:

- 4 pork chops, boneless or bone-in
- ¼ teaspoon salt
- 1/8 teaspoon freshly ground black pepper
- 3 tablespoons extra-virgin olive oil
- 5 tablespoons low-sodium chicken broth, divided
- 6 garlic cloves, minced
- ¼ cup honey
- 2 tablespoons apple cider vinegar

DIRECTIONS:

1. Season the pork chops with salt and pepper and set aside.
2. In a large sauté pan or skillet, heat the oil over medium-high heat. Add the pork chops and sear for 5 minutes on each side, or until golden brown.
3. Once the searing is complete, move the pork to a dish and reduce the skillet heat from medium-high to medium.
4. Add 3 tablespoons of chicken broth to the pan; this will loosen the bits and flavors from the bottom of the skillet.
5. Once the broth has evaporated, add the garlic to the skillet and cook for 15 to 20 seconds, until fragrant.
6. Add the honey, vinegar, and the remaining 2 tablespoons of broth. Bring the heat back up to medium-high and continue to cook for 3 to 4 minutes.
7. Stir periodically; the sauce is ready once it's thickened slightly. Add the pork chops back into the pan, cover them with the sauce, and cook for 2 minutes. Serve.

NUTRITION: Calories: 302 Protein: 22g Carbs: 19g Fat: 16g

370. Moussaka

Preparation time: 15 minutes
Cooking time: 40 minutes
Servings: 6-8
INGREDIENTS:

- For the eggplant:
- 2 pounds' eggplant, cut into ¼-inch-thick slices
- 1 teaspoon salt
- 2 to 3 tablespoons extra-virgin olive oil
- For the filling:
- 1 tablespoon extra-virgin olive oil

- 2 shallots, diced
- 1 tablespoon dried, minced garlic
- 1-pound ground lamb
- 4 ounces portobello mushrooms, diced
- 1 (14.5-ounce) can crushed tomatoes, drained
- ¼ cup tomato paste
- 1 cup low-sodium beef broth
- 2 bay leaves
- 2 teaspoons dried oregano
- ¾ teaspoon salt
- 2½ cups store-bought béchamel sauce
- 1/3 cup panko bread crumbs

DIRECTIONS:

1. To Make the Eggplant
2. Preheat the oven to 450°F. Line large baking sheets with paper towels and arrange the eggplant slices in a single layer and sprinkle with salt.
3. Place another layer of paper towel on the eggplant slices. Continue until all eggplant slices are covered.
4. Let the eggplant sweat for 30 minutes to remove excess moisture. While this is happening, make the meat sauce.
5. Pat the eggplant dry. Dry the baking sheets and brush with oil and place the eggplant slices onto the baking sheets.
6. Bake for 15 to 20 minutes, or until lightly browned and softened. Remove from the oven and cool slightly before assembling the moussaka.
7. To Make the Filling
8. In a large, oven-safe sauté pan or skillet, heat the olive oil over high heat. Cook the shallots and garlic for 2 minutes, until starting to soften.
9. Add the ground lamb and brown it with the garlic and onions, breaking it up as it cooks. Add the mushrooms and cook for 5 to 7 minutes, or until they have dehydrated slightly.
10. Add the tomatoes and paste, beef broth, bay leaves, oregano, and salt and stir to combine.
11. Once the sauce is simmering, lower to medium-low and cook for 15 minutes, or until it reduces to a thick sauce. Remove the sauce to a separate bowl before assembly.
12. Reduce the oven temperature to 350°F. Place half the eggplant slices in the bottom of the skillet used to make the sauce. Top the slices with all the meat filling.
13. Place the remaining eggplant on top of the meat filling and pour the jarred béchamel sauce over the eggplant. Sprinkle with the bread crumbs.
14. Bake for 30 to 40 minutes or until golden brown. Let stand for 10 minutes before serving.

NUTRITION: Calories: 491 Protein: 23g Carbs: 30g Fat: 33g

371. Herbed Lamb Leg

Preparation time: 15 minutes
Cooking Time: 50 Minutes
Servings: 4

INGREDIENTS:

- 1 1/2-pound lamb leg, trimmed, meat only
- 1 tablespoon Provance herbs
- 1 teaspoon salt
- 1 tablespoon olive oil

DIRECTIONS:

1. Rub the lamb led with Provance herbs and salt. Then brush it carefully with olive oil and wrap in the foil.
2. Bake the meat for 50 minutes at 360F. Then discard the foil and chill the lamb meat little. Slice it.

NUTRITION: Calories 336 Fat 14.9g Carbs 0g Protein 47.9g

372. Baked Pork Chops

Preparation time: 15 minutes
Cooking Time: 30 Minutes
Servings: 4

INGREDIENTS:

- 4 pork loin chops, boneless
- A pinch of salt and black pepper
- 1 tablespoon sweet paprika
- 2 tablespoons Dijon mustard
- Cooking spray

DIRECTIONS:

1. In a bowl, mix the pork chops with salt, pepper, paprika and the mustard and rub well.
2. Grease a baking sheet with cooking spray, add the pork chops, cover with tin foil, introduce in the oven and bake at 400 degrees F for 30 minutes.
3. Divide the pork chops between plates and serve with a side salad.

NUTRITION: Calories 167 Fat 5g Carbs 2g Protein 25g

373. Coconut Pork Steaks

Preparation time: 15 minutes
Cooking Time: 10 Minutes
Servings: 4

INGREDIENTS:

- 4 pork steaks (3.5 oz each steak)
- 1 tablespoon ground turmeric
- 1 teaspoon salt
- 1 tablespoon coconut oil
- 1 teaspoon apple cider vinegar

DIRECTIONS:

1. Rub the pork steaks with ground turmeric, salt, and apple cider vinegar. Melt the coconut oil in the skillet and add pork steaks.
2. Roast the pork steaks for 5 minutes from each side. Serve.

NUTRITION: Calories 366 Fat 28.6g Carbs 2.1g Protein 25.1g

374. Sweet & Spicy Chicken Fingers

Preparation Time: 15 Minutes
Cooking Time: 35 minutes
Servings: 6

INGREDIENTS:

- Half teaspoon of sea salt
- Half cup of honey
- ¼ teaspoon of black pepper
- 1 1/2 cups of almond flour
- Half teaspoon of garlic powder
- 1/4 cup of tapioca
- 1 lb. of chicken tenders
- 2 eggs

- ⅓ cup of hot sauce

DIRECTIONS:
1. Let the oven preheat to 425 F.
2. In a bowl, add flour, salt and pepper, mix.
3. In a different bowl, whisk eggs with 1 teaspoon of water.
4. Coat the chicken in tapioca starch, then in eggs and lastly in a flour mixture. Place the breaded chicken tenders on a parchment-lined baking tray.
5. Bake for 25 minutes.
6. In a pan, add garlic powder, honey and hot sauce, whisk on high flame.
7. Toss the chicken tenders in sauce, bake for 2 to 5 minutes more.
8. Serve with sauce.

NUTRITION: Calories 287 Total fat: 13.7 g Total carbs: 11 g Fiber: 4 g Sugar: 12.8 g Protein: 27 g Sodium: 214 mg

375. Classic Chicken Cooking with Tomatoes & Tapenade

Preparation Time: 25 minutes
Cooking Time: 25 minutes
Servings: 2

INGREDIENTS:
- 4-5 oz. Chicken breasts, boneless and skinless
- ¼-tsp salt (divided)
- 3-tbsp fresh basil leaves, chopped (divided)
- 1-tbsp olive oil
- 1½-cups cherry tomatoes, halved
- ¼-cup olive tapenade

DIRECTIONS:
1. Arrange the chicken on a sheet of glassine or waxed paper. Sprinkle half of the salt and a third of the basil evenly over the chicken.
2. Press lightly, and flip over the chicken pieces. Sprinkle the remaining salt and another third of the basil. Cover the seasoned chicken with another sheet of waxed paper.
3. By using a meat mallet or rolling pin, pound the chicken to a half-inch thickness.
4. Heat the olive oil in a 12-inch skillet placed over medium-high heat. Add the pounded chicken breasts.
5. Cook for 6 minutes on each side until the chicken turns golden brown with no traces of pink in the middle. Transfer the browned chicken breasts in a platter, and cover to keep them warm.
6. In the same skillet, add the olive tapenade and tomatoes. Cook for 3 minutes until the tomatoes just begin to be tender.
7. To serve, pour over the tomato-tapenade mixture over the cooked chicken breasts, and top with the remaining basil.

NUTRITION: Calories: 190, Fats: 7g, Dietary Fiber: 1g, Carbs: 6g, Protein: 26g

376. Grilled Grapes & Chicken Chunks

Preparation Time: 4 to 24 hours
Cooking Time: 6 minutes
Servings: 2

INGREDIENTS:
- 2-cloves garlic, minced
- ¼-cup extra-virgin olive oil
- 1-tbsp rosemary, minced
- 1-tbsp oregano, minced
- 1-tsp lemon zest
- ½-tsp red chili flakes, crushed
- 1-lb. Chicken breast, boneless and skinless
- 1¾-cups green grapes, seedless and rinsed
- ½-tsp salt
- 1-tbsp lemon juice
- 2-tbsp extra-virgin olive oil

DIRECTIONS:
1. Combine and mix all the marinade ingredients in a small mixing bowl. Mix well until fully combined. Set aside.
2. Cut the chicken breast into ¾-inch cubes. Alternately thread the chicken and grapes onto 12 skewers. Place the skewers in a large baking dish to hold them for marinating.
3. Pour the marinade over the skewers, coating them thoroughly. Marinate for 4 to 24 hours.
4. Remove the skewers from the marinade and allow dripping off any excess oil. Sprinkle over with salt.
5. Grill the chicken and grape skewers for 3 minutes on each side until cooked through.
6. To serve, arrange the skewers on a serving platter and drizzle with lemon juice and olive oil.

NUTRITION: Calories: 230, Fats: 20g, Dietary Fiber: 1g, Carbs: 14g, Protein: 1g

377. Turkish Turkey Mini Meatloaves

Preparation Time: 15 minutes
Cooking Time: 20 minutes
Servings: 2

INGREDIENTS:
- 1-lb. Ground turkey breast
- 1-pc egg
- ¼-cup whole-wheat breadcrumbs, crushed
- ¼-cup feta cheese, plus more for topping
- ¼-cup Kalamata olives, halved
- ¼-cup fresh parsley, chopped
- ¼-cup red onion, minced
- ¼-cup + 2-tbsp hummus (refer to Homemade Hummus recipe)
- 2-cloves garlic, minced
- ½-tsp dried basil
- ¼- tsp. Dried oregano
- Salt & pepper
- ½-pc small cucumber, peeled, seeded, and chopped
- 1-pc large tomato, chopped
- 3-tbsp fresh basil, chopped
- ½-lemon, juice
- 1-tsp extra-virgin olive oil
- Salt & pepper

DIRECTIONS:

1. Preheat your oven to 425 °f.
2. Line a 5"x9" baking sheet with foil, and spray the surfaces with non-stick grease. Set aside.
3. Except for the ¼-cup hummus, combine and mix all the turkey meatloaf ingredients in a large mixing bowl. Mix well until fully combined.
4. Divide mixture equally into 4 portions. Form the portions into loaves. Spread a tablespoon of the remaining hummus on each meatloaf. Place the loaves on the greased baking sheet.
5. Bake for 20 minutes until the loaves no longer appear pink in the center. (Ensure the meatloaf cooks through by inserting a meat thermometer and the reading reaches 165 °f.)
6. Combine and mix all the topping ingredients in a small mixing bowl. Mix well until fully combined.
7. To serve, spoon the topping over the cooked meatloaves.

NUTRITION: Calories: 130, Fats: 7g, Dietary Fiber: 4g, Carbs: 14g, Protein: 6g

378. Charred Chicken Souvlaki Skewers

Preparation Time: min 8 hours
Cooking Time: 15 minutes
Servings: 2

INGREDIENTS:

- ½-cup olive oil
- ½-cup fresh squeezed lemon juice
- 1-tbsp red wine vinegar
- 1-tbsp finely minced garlic (or garlic puree from a jar)
- 1-tbsp dried Greek oregano
- 1-tsp dried thyme
- 6-pcs chicken breasts, boneless, skinless, with trimmed off tendons and fats
- Fresh cucumber and cherry tomatoes for garnish

DIRECTIONS:

1. Combine and mix all the marinade ingredients in a small mixing bowl. Mix well until fully combined.
2. Slice each chicken breast crosswise into six 1-inch strips.
3. Place the chicken strips into a large plastic container with a tight-fitting lid.
4. Pour the marinade into the plastic container, and seal with its lid. Gently shake the container and turn it over so that the marinade evenly coats all of the meat. Refrigerate the sealed plastic container to marinate for 8 hours or more.
5. Spray the grill's surfaces with non-stick grease. Preheat your charcoal or gas barbecue grill to medium-high heat.
6. Take the chicken out and let it cool to room temperature. Drain the chicken pieces and thread them onto skewers. (Try to thread six pieces for each skewer and fold over each chicken piece so it will not spin around the skewer.)
7. Grill the chicken souvlaki skewers for 15 minutes, turning once after seeing the appearance of desirable grill marks.
8. To serve, place the souvlaki on a serving plate alongside the cucumber and tomato garnish.

NUTRITION: Calories: 360, Fats: 26g, Dietary Fiber: 0g, Carbs: 3g, Protein: 30g

379. Lemon Caper Chicken

Preparation Time: 10 minutes
Cooking Time: 15 minutes
Servings: 2

INGREDIENTS:

- 2 tablespoon virgin olive oil
- 2 chicken breasts (boneless, skinless, cut in half, pound to ¾ an inch thick)
- ¼ cup capers
- 2 lemons (wedges)
- 1 teaspoon oregano
- 1 teaspoon basil
- ½ teaspoon black pepper

DIRECTIONS:

1. Take a large skillet and place it on your stove and add the olive oil to it. Turn the heat to medium and allow it to warm up.
2. As the oil heats up season your chicken breast with the oregano, basil, and black pepper on each side.
3. Place your chicken breast into the hot skillet and cook on each side for five minutes.
4. Transfer the chicken from the skillet to your dinner plate. Top with capers and serve with a few lemon wedges.

NUTRITION: Calories 182, Carbs - 3.4 g, Protein - 26.6 g, Fat - 8.2 g

380. Herb Roasted Chicken

Preparation Time: 20 minutes
Cooking Time: 1 hour
Servings: 2

INGREDIENTS:

1 tablespoon virgin olive oil

- 1 whole chicken
- 2 rosemary springs
- 3 garlic cloves (peeled)
- 1 lemon (cut in half)
- 1 teaspoon sea salt
- 1 teaspoon black pepper

DIRECTIONS:

1. Turn your oven to 450 degrees F.
2. Take your whole chicken and pat it dry using paper towels. Then rub in the olive oil. Remove the leaves from one of the springs of rosemary and scatter them over the chicken. Sprinkle the sea salt and black pepper over top. Place the other whole sprig of rosemary into the cavity of the chicken. Then add in the garlic cloves and lemon halves.
3. Place the chicken into a roasting pan and then place it into the oven. Allow the chicken to bake for 1 hour, then check that the internal temperature should be at least 165 degrees F. If the chicken begins to brown too much, cover it with foil and return it to the oven to finish cooking.
4. When the chicken has cooked to the appropriate temperature remove it from the oven. Let it rest for at least 20 minutes before carving.
5. Serve with a large side of roasted or steamed vegetables or your favorite salad.

NUTRITION: Calories – 309, Carbs 1.5 g, Protein - 27.2 g, Fat - 21.3 g

381. Italian Chicken Meatballs

Preparation Time: 20 minutes
Cooking Time: 32 minutes
Servings: 20

INGREDIENTS:

- 3 tomatoes
- Kosher salt
- ½ cup of freshly chopped parsley
- 1 teaspoon of dry oregano
- Kosher salt
- ½ teaspoon of fresh thyme
- ¼ teaspoon of sweet paprika
- 1 red onion
- 1 lb. Of ground chicken
- ½ minced garlic cloves
- Black pepper
- 1 raw egg
- Extra virgin olive oil.

DIRECTIONS:

1. Heat the oven to 375 degrees and get a cooking pan. Coat with extra virgin olive oil and set aside.
2. Get a large bowl and mix your tomatoes with kosher salt and thinly chopped onions.
3. Add half of your fresh thyme and sprinkle a little extra virgin olive oil on it again.
4. Transfer this to your cooking and use a spoon to spread. Add ground chicken to the mixing bowl you recently used, and add egg, and oregano.
5. Include paprika, garlic, the other half of thyme, chopped parsley and black pepper.
6. Sprinkle a little amount of extra virgin olive oil on it, and mix till the meatball mixture is combined. Form about 1 ½ inch chicken meatballs with the mixture and cut it all to this size.
7. Get another cooking pan and arrange these meatballs in it. Add tomatoes and onions, and blend them with the meatballs. Bake in your preheated oven for about 30 min.
8. Your meatballs should turn golden brown, you can make them more colorful by removing them and coating them with extra virgin olive oil before you continue baking.
9. But that is not necessary. A couple of minutes after this, your meatballs cam is served.
10. No surprises, your tomatoes are fast falling.

NUTRITION: 79 , 74.7mg sodium, 1.4g sugar, 301.1g potassium, 0.92g fiber, 44.2mg calcium, 0.94g iron, 4.1g carbs, 7.8g protein.

382. Oven Roasted Garlic Chicken Thigh

Preparation time: 10 minutes
Cooking time: 45 minutes
Servings: 2

INGREDIENTS:

- 8 chicken thighs
- Salt and pepper as needed
- 1 tablespoon extra-virgin olive oil
- 6 cloves garlic, peeled and crushed
- 1 jar (10 ounces) roasted red peppers, drained and chopped
- 1 1/2 pounds' potatoes, diced
- 2 cups cherry tomatoes, halved
- 1/3 cup capers, sliced

- 1 teaspoon dried Italian seasoning
- 1 tablespoon fresh basil

DIRECTIONS:

1. Season chicken with kosher salt and black pepper.
2. Take a cast-iron skillet over medium-high heat and heat up olive oil.
3. Sear the chicken on both sides.
4. Add remaining ingredients except for basil and stir well.
5. Remove heat and place cast iron skillet in the oven.
6. Bake for 45 minutes at 400 degrees Fahrenheit until the internal temperature reaches 165 degrees Fahrenheit.
7. Serve and enjoy!

NUTRITION: Calories: 500, Fat: 23g, Carbs: 37g, Protein: 35g

383. Steak & Vegetable Stir-fry

Preparation Time: 15 Minutes
Cooking Time: 20 minutes
Servings: 4-6

Ingredients:

- 2 tablespoons of coconut oil
- 1 cup sliced red onion
- 1 cup sliced red bell pepper
- 1 1/2 cups of chopped broccoli
- 3 tablespoons of sliced green onion
- 1 lb. of skirt steak, ¼-inch strips
- 1 1/2 cups of trimmed green beans
- 1/4 cup of sliced water chestnuts
- 1 tablespoon of sesame seeds

Sauce:

- Half teaspoon of grated ginger
- 2 tablespoons of warm water
- 2 tablespoons of coconut aminos
- 2 minced garlic cloves

DIRECTIONS:

1. Cook steak in hot oil for 2 to 3 minutes, until browned all over, take it out on a plate.
2. Add the vegetables to the same pan and cook for 5 minutes.
3. In a bowl, mix all the sauce's ingredients.
4. Add the meat back to the pan with sauce and the rest of the ingredients, toss and serve.

NUTRITION: Calories 325 Total fat: 14.2 g Total carbs: 8.7 g Fiber: 3.2 g Sugar: 11.7 g Protein: 33.3 g Sodium: 265 mg

384. Grilled Chicken Breasts

Preparation Time: 30 minutes
Cooking Time: 10 minutes
Servings: 2

INGREDIENTS:

- Boneless skinless chicken breast, 4.
- Lemon juice, 3 tbsp.
- Olive oil, 3 tbsp.
- Chopped fresh parsley, 3 tbsp.
- Minced garlic cloves, 3.
- Paprika, 1 tsp.
- Dried oregano, ½ tsp.
- Salt and pepper, to taste.

DIRECTIONS:

1. In a large Ziploc bag, mix well oregano, paprika, garlic, parsley, olive oil, and lemon juice.
2. Pierce chicken with a knife several times and sprinkle with salt and pepper.
3. Add chicken to bag and marinate 20 minutes or up to two days in the fridge.
4. Remove chicken from bag and grill for 5 minutes per side in a 350 F preheated grill.
5. When cooked, transfer to a plate for 5 minutes before slicing.
6. Serve and enjoy with a side of rice or salad

NUTRITION: Calories: 238, Protein: 24 g, Carbs: 2 g, Fats: 19 g

SIDE DISHES

385. Dried Apple Rings

Preparation Time: 20 Minutes
Cooking Time: 5 hours
Servings: 4-6
Ingredients:

- 3 pounds of peeled apples, cut into 0.1-inches of rings
- 1 teaspoon of salt
- 1.7ounces of lemon juice

Directions:

1. In a bowl, add 3 cups of water, lemon juice and salt. Mix well.
2. Add the rings to the lemon water, let it rest for ten minutes.
3. Take the rings out and drain them on a paper towel.
4. Lay 2 layers of cheesecloth on a cooling rack, place the slices on top and place the rack on the cooking grate.
5. Place the entire set up in the cold oven at 125 F. As the temperature reaches, keep the oven door open slightly.
6. Change the temperature to 150 F.
7. Let the apples dry for 5 hours, with the door slightly open. Cool completely before serving.

Nutrition: Calories 21 Total fat: 0 g Total carbs: 2 g Fiber: 2 g Sugar: 3.2 g Protein: 0 g Sodium: 45 mg

386. Chickpea Medley

Preparation time: 5minutes
Cooking Time: 0 minutes
Servings: 4
Ingredients:

- 2 tablespoons tahini
- 2 tablespoons coconut amines
- 1 (15-ounce) can chickpeas or 1.1/2 cups cooked chickpeas, rinsed and drained
- 1 cup finely chopped lightly packed spinach
- Carrot, peeled and grated

Directions:

1. Merge together the tahini and coconut amines in a bowl.
2. Add the chickpeas, spinach, and carrot to the bowl. Stir well and serve at room temperature.
3. Simple Swap: Coconut amines are almost like a sweeter, mellower version of soy sauce. However, if you want to use regular soy sauce or tamari, just use 11/2 tablespoons and add a dash of maple syrup or agave nectar to balance out the saltiness.

Nutrition: Calories: 437 Total fat: 8g Protein: 92g Sodium: 246 Fat: 19g

387. Roasted Pine Nut Orzo

Preparation time: 10minutes
Cooking Time: 15minutes
Servings: 3
Ingredients:

- 16 ounces' orzo
- 1 cup diced roasted red peppers
- 1/4 cup pitted, chopped Klamath olives
- 4 garlic cloves, minced or pressed
- 3 tablespoons olive oil
- 1.1/2 tablespoons squeezed lemon juice
- 2 teaspoons balsamic vinegar
- 1 teaspoon sea salt
- 1/4 cup pine nuts
- 1/4 cup packed thinly sliced or torn fresh basil

Directions:

1. Use a large pot of water to a boil over medium-high heat and add the orzo. Cook, stirring often, for 10 minutes, or until the orzo has a chewy and firm texture. Drain well.
2. While the orzo is cooking, in a large bowl, combine the peppers, olives, garlic, olive oil, lemon juice, vinegar, and salt. Stir well.
3. In a dry skillet toasts the pine nuts over medium-low heat until aromatic and lightly browned, shaking the pan often so that they cook evenly
4. Upon reaching the desired texture and add it to the sauce mixture within a minute or so, to avoid clumping.

Nutrition: Calories: 423 Total fat: 4g Protein: 64g Sodium: 231 Fat: 12g

388. Banana and Almond Butter Oats

Preparation Time: 10 minutes
Cooking Time: 5 minutes
Servings: 2
Ingredients:

- 1 cup gluten-free moved oats
- 1 cup almond milk
- 1 cup of water
- 1 teaspoon cinnamon
- 2 tablespoons almond spread
- 1 banana, cut

Directions:

1. Mix the water and almond milk to a bubble in a little pot. Add the oats and diminish to a stew.
2. Cook until oats have consumed all fluid. Blend in cinnamon. Top with almond spread and banana and serve.

Nutrition: Calories: 112, Fat: 10g Protein: 9g Carbss: 54g

389. Chicken & Mushroom Skewers

Preparation Time: 20 Minutes
Cooking Time: 10 minutes
Servings: 4-6
Ingredients:

- 4 oz. of button mushroom
- Half teaspoon olive oil
- Half bunch of cilantro
- 1 red chili pepper
- Salt, to taste
- 3 oz. of chicken breasts

Directions:

1. 1. Chop the chili without seeds.

2. Onto soaked skewers, thread the mushrooms and chicken pieces alternatively. Season with salt.
3. In a pan, add oil and chilies, cook the skewers until golden brown. Serve with cilantro on top.

Nutrition: Calories 176 Total fat: 4.3 g Total carbs: 4 g Fiber: 1.8 g Sugar: 3 g Protein:21 g Sodium: 155 mg

390. Peas & Pancetta

Preparation Time: 10 Minutes
Cooking Time: 10 minutes
Servings: 4
Ingredients:

- 2 oz. of cooked pancetta
- ¼ cup of dry white wine
- 3 tablespoons of chopped onion
- Salt & pepper to taste
- 1 pound of peas
- 2 tablespoons of olive oil
- 1 ½ tablespoon of fresh thyme, chopped

Directions:
1. In a pan, cook onion and pancetta in hot oil for 5 minutes.
2. Add the rest of the ingredients, stir well.
3. Let it come to a boil, turn the heat low and simmer for 3-5 minutes.
4. Serve.

Nutrition: Calories 189 Total fat: 9.1 Total carbs: 17 g Fiber: 3 g Sugar: 3 g Protein: 7.7 g Sodium: 232.2 mg

391. Green Beans Almondine

Preparation Time: 10 Minutes
Cooking Time: 10 minutes
Servings: 4
Ingredients:

- 1/4 cup of slivered almonds
- 1 tablespoon of minced garlic
- Half teaspoon of Salt & pepper
- 1 lb. of trimmed green beans
- 2 tablespoons of olive oil
- 2 tablespoons of water

Directions:
1. In a pan, heat oil on medium flame.
2. Sauté garlic for 1 minute. Add beans with salt and pepper, cook for 2 minutes.
3. Add water, cover, and cook for 5 minutes.
4. Take the lid off and add almonds; cook for 1 to 2 minutes.

Nutrition: Calories 139 Total fat: 11 g Total carbs: 10 g Fiber: 4 g Sugar: 4 g Protein: 4 g Sodium: 298 mg

392. Paleo Ginger Garlic Zoodles

Preparation Time: 10 Minutes
Cooking Time: 20 minutes
Servings: 2
Ingredients:

- 1/4 cup of coconut oil
- 1 tablespoon of grated ginger
- 4 zucchinis, spiralized
- minced garlic cloves
- 2 cups of broccoli florets
- 1 tablespoon of maple syrup
- Half teaspoon of sea salt
- 1 cup of cauliflower florets
- black pepper, to taste
- 3 tablespoons of coconut aminos
- 1/4 cup sliced green onions

Directions:
1. In a skillet, add zoodles, garlic, ginger, oil and salt; cook for 5 to 10 minutes.
2. Do not overcook or mush the zoodles.
3. Add cauliflower, broccoli, maple syrup and coconut aminos. Cook for 2 to 5 minutes, covered.
4. Turn the heat off and let it rest for few minutes. Serve with black pepper and green onion on top.

Nutrition: Calories 216 Total fat: 6 g Total carbs: 4 g Fiber: 7 g Sugar: 3 g Protein: 3 g Sodium: 121 mg

393. Vegan Avocado Caesar Mix

Preparation Time: 20 Minutes
Cooking Time: 10 minutes
Servings: 4
Ingredients:
Vegan Caesar Dressing

- 1 cup of vegan mayo
- 1 tablespoon of Dijon mustard
- 1 tablespoon of briny green peppercorns, drained
- 1½ teaspoons of capers, drained
- 2 roasted garlic cloves

Cashew Parmesan

- ⅔ cup of nutritional yeast
- 1 tablespoon of salt
- 1⅓ cups of roasted cashews, unsalted

Vegetable Mix

- 2 cups of mixed greens
- ¼ cup of cashew Parmesan
- 2 romaine lettuce, large heads, whole leaves
- 2 avocados
- Half cup of vegan Caesar dressing

Directions:
1. In a bowl, add the dressing ingredients. Blend with a stick blender until smooth.
2. In a food processor, add the cashew parmesan ingredients, pulse until smooth.

3. In a bowl, add vegetable mixture and add dressing and cashew mixture (do not add all the cashew mix or all the dressing, use as per taste).
4. Toss and serve with the main course.

Nutrition: Calories 315 Total fat: 23 g Total carbs: 28 g Fiber: 7 g Sugar: 6 g Protein: 9 g Sodium: 201 mg

394. Cinnamon Maple Glazed Carrots

Preparation Time: 10 Minutes
Cooking Time: 15 minutes
Servings: 4
Ingredients:

- 1 lb. of small mixed colored Carrots
- Sea salt, to taste
- Half cup of Water
- 1 teaspoon of Ground cinnamon
- 1 teaspoon of Coconut oil
- 1 to 2 tablespoons of Maple syrup

Directions:
1. In a pot, sauté carrots in hot oil for 2 minutes.
2. Add water and simmer, partially covered, for ten minutes.
3. As the water is almost evaporated, add rest of the ingredients, mix well.
4. Serve.

Nutrition: Calories 63 Total fat: 1 g Total carbs: 13 g Fiber: 3 g Sugar: 8 g Protein: 0 g Sodium: 299 mg

395. Red Cabbage Mexican Slaw

Preparation Time: 15 Minutes
Cooking Time: 0 minutes
Servings: 8
Ingredients:

- 3 cups of shredded Red cabbage
- Half cup of Pomegranate arils
- 4 shredded Carrots
- 3 cups of shredded White cabbage
- 1/3 cup of chopped Cashews
- 1 Lime's juice
- ¾ cup of chopped Fresh cilantro
- 1/4 cup of oil mayonnaise
- 1 teaspoon of Red chili flakes

Directions:
1. In a bowl, toss the carrots and cabbage. Add lime juice and toss.
2. Add rest of the ingredients, mix and serve.

Nutrition: Calories 122 Total fat: 8 g Total carbs: 11 g Fiber: 3 g Sugar: 5 g Protein: 2 g Sodium: 299 mg

396. Spinach Artichoke Twice Baked Potatoes

Preparation Time: 15 Minutes
Cooking Time: 90 minutes
Servings: 4-8
Ingredients:

- 5 ounces of baby spinach, fresh
- Half diced onion
- 4 russet potatoes
- 2 minced garlic cloves
- 5.3 ounces of canned coconut cream
- 2 tablespoon of coconut oil
- 1.5 Tablespoon of lemon juice
- 3/4 teaspoon of sea salt
- 2 tablespoon of nutritional yeast

Directions:
1. Coat the potatoes in oil and season with salt, bake for 60 minutes at 400 F.
2. Slice the potatoes in half and take the middle part out, leave a layer.
3. In a skillet, heat oil on medium flame and sauté onion until translucent, add garlic and cook for 1 minute.
4. Add spinach and cook until wilted.
5. Add artichokes and cook for 1 minutes, season to taste. Turn the heat off.
6. In a bowl, add potato's inside of only three potatoes with salt, coconut oil, lemon juice and nutritional yeast. Mash and mix with artichoke mixture and stuff the potatoes skin.
7. Bake for 15 to 20 minutes at 400 F.
8. Serve.

Nutrition: Calories 322 Total fat: 6.9 g Total carbs: 12 g Fiber: 3.2 g Sugar: 3.9 g Protein: 2 g Sodium: 191 mg

397. Frijoles De La Olla

Preparation time: 15minutes
Cooking Time: 65minutes
Servings: 4
Ingredients:
- 1-pound dry pinto beans, rinsed
- 1 small yellow onion, diced
- 1 jalapeño pepper, seeded and finely chopped
- 1.1/2 teaspoons minced garlic (3 cloves)
- 1 tablespoon ground cumin
- 1/2 teaspoon Mexican oregano (optional)
- 1 teaspoon red pepper flakes (optional)
- 4 cups water
- 2 tablespoons salt

Directions:
1. Place the beans, onion, jalapeño, garlic, cumin, oregano (if using), red pepper flakes (if using), water, and salt in a slow cooker.
2. Cook on low heat.

Nutrition: Calories: 256 Total fat: 8g Protein: 28g

398. Balsamic Mushrooms

Preparation Time: 30 Minutes
Cooking Time: 20 minutes
Servings: 4
Ingredients:

- 2 tablespoons of balsamic vinegar
- 1 lb. of mushrooms
- Half teaspoon of dried parsley
- 2 tablespoons of olive oil
- 1 teaspoon of minced garlic minced
- 1/4 teaspoon of pepper
- Half teaspoon of dried basil
- Half teaspoon of salt

Directions:

1. In a bowl, add all ingredients, except for mushrooms.
2. Mix and add mushrooms, let it rest for 20 minutes.
3. Spread on a foil lined baking sheet and roast for 20 minutes at 400 F.

Nutrition: Calories 96 Total fat: 7 g Total carbs: 5 g Fiber: 1 g Sugar: 3 g Protein: 4 g Sodium: 299 mg

399. Baked Sweet Potato Fries

Preparation Time: 15 Minutes
Cooking Time: 25 minutes
Servings: 6
Ingredients:

- 2 unpeeled garlic cloves
- Sea salt, to taste
- 3 tablespoons of olive oil
- 3 peeled sweet potatoes
- 2 fresh sprigs of rosemary

Directions:

1. Let the oven preheat to 400 F, oil spray a baking sheet.
2. Slice every potato in 16 wedges.
3. In a bowl, toss the wedges with oil and garlic cloves. spread on a baking sheet, with rosemary and salt.
4. Bake for 20-25 minutes, flip halfway through. serve.

Nutrition: Calories 119 Total fat: 7 g Total carbs: 14 g Fiber: 3 g Sugar: 3 g Protein: 1 g Sodium: 287 mg

400. Jalapeno Deviled Eggs

Preparation Time: 20 Minutes
Cooking Time: 0 minutes
Servings: 12
Ingredients:

- 4 to 5 tablespoons of Avocado mayo
- 3 Jalapeños
- 2 tablespoons of grain mustard
- 12 Hard-boiled eggs
- Sea salt & black pepper, to taste
- 4 slices of Cooked bacon

Directions:

1. Cut the eggs in half lengthwise and take the yolk in a bowl.

2. Add 1 jalapeno, mustard, mayo, bacon slices to the yolks and mix well. Sprinkle salt and pepper.
3. Stuff the egg cavity with mayo mixture, top with jalapenos and bacon, serve.

Nutrition for 2 halves: Calories 127 Total fat: 10 g Total carbs: 0 g Fiber: 0 g Sugar: 3 g Protein: 7 g Sodium: 201 mg

401. Raw Almond Dip

Preparation Time: 6 to 12 hours
Cooking Time: 0 minutes
Servings: 8
Ingredients:

- 1/4 cup of tahini
- 1/4 cup of lemon juiced
- 1/4 cup of olive oil
- 1 cup of raw soaked almonds
- Half teaspoon of salt
- 3/4 teaspoon of turmeric powder
- 3/4 cup of water
- 2 garlic cloves
- 1/4 teaspoon of cumin ground
- Half teaspoon of black pepper

Directions:

1. Soak the almonds for 6-12 hours then drain.
2. In a food processor add all ingredients, pulse until smooth.
3. Adjust seasoning.

Nutrition: Calories 201 Total fat: 4.5 g Total carbs: 6.3 g Fiber: 0 g Sugar: 3 g Protein: 5.1 g Sodium: 154 mg

402. Black Bean Burgers

Preparation Time: 5 Minutes
Cooking Time: 20 Minutes
Servings: 4
Ingredients:

- 1 onion, diced
- 1/2 cup corn nibs
- 2 cloves garlic, minced
- 1/2 teaspoon oregano, dried
- 1/2 cup flour
- 1 jalapeno pepper, small
- 2 cups black beans, mashed & canned
- 1/4 cup breadcrumbs (vegan)
- 2 teaspoons parsley, minced
- 1/4 teaspoon cumin
- 1 tablespoon olive oil
- 2 teaspoons chili powder
- 1/2 red pepper, diced
- Sea salt to taste

Directions:

1. Set your flour on a plate, and then get out your garlic, onion, peppers and oregano, throwing it in a pan.
2. Cook over medium-high heat, and then cook until the onions are translucent.
3. Place the peppers in, and sauté until tender.
4. Cook for two minutes, and then set it to the side.

5. Use a potato masher to mash your black beans, and then stir in the vegetables, cumin, breadcrumbs, parsley, salt and chili powder, and then divide it into six patties.
6. Coat each side, and then cook until it's fried on each side.

Nutrition: Calories: 211 Carbs: 12g Fat: 7g Protein: 12g

403. Cinnamon Mashed Sweet Potatoes

Preparation Time: 15 Minutes
Cooking Time: 35 minutes
Servings: 2-3
Ingredients:

- Half cup of almond milk, Unsweetened
- 1/4 cup of Ghee
- 3/4 teaspoon of Sea salt
- 1 teaspoon of Cinnamon
- 3 peeled Sweet potatoes, cubed
- 1 teaspoon of Vanilla extract

Directions:
1. Boil the potatoes for half an hour.
2. Mash the potatoes with rest of the ingredients expect for ghee, mix.
3. In a skillet melt ghee and cook until it turns to golden color, pour over mashed potatoes and serve.

Nutrition: Calories 130 Total fat: 4 g Total carbs: 20 g Fiber: 3 g Sugar: 3 g Protein: 1 g Sodium: 267 mg

404. Hearty Black Lentil Curry

Preparation Time: 15 Minutes
Cooking Time: 6 Hours
Servings: 7
Ingredients:

- 1 cup of black lentils, rinsed and soaked overnight
- 14 ounces of chopped tomatoes
- 2 large white onions, peeled and sliced
- 1 1/2 teaspoon of minced garlic
- 1 teaspoon of grated ginger
- 1 red chili
- 1 teaspoon of salt
- 1/4 teaspoon of red chili powder
- 1 teaspoon of paprika
- 1 teaspoon of ground turmeric
- 2 teaspoons of ground cumin
- 2 teaspoons of ground coriander
- 1/2 cup of chopped coriander
- 4-ounce of vegetarian butter
- 1 fluid of ounce water
- 2 fluid of ounce vegetarian double cream

Directions:
1. Place a large pan over a moderate heat, add butter and let heat until melt.
2. Add the onion and garlic and ginger and let cook for 10 to 15 minutes or until onions are caramelized.
3. Then stir in salt, red chili powder, paprika, turmeric, cumin, ground coriander, and water.

4. Transfer this mixture to a 6-quarts slow cooker and add tomatoes and red chili.
5. Drain lentils, add to slow cooker and stir until just mix.
6. Plug in slow cooker; adjust cooking time to 6 hours and let cook on low heat setting.
7. When the lentils are done, stir in cream and adjust the seasoning.
8. Serve with boiled rice or whole wheat bread.

Nutrition: Calories: 171 Carbs: 10g Fat: 7g Protein: 12g

405. Flavorful Refried Beans

Preparation Time: 15 Minutes
Cooking Time: 8 Hours
Servings: 8
Ingredients:

- 3 cups of pinto beans, rinsed
- 1 small jalapeno pepper, seeded and chopped
- 1 medium-sized white onion, peeled and sliced
- 2 tablespoons of minced garlic
- 5 teaspoons of salt
- 2 teaspoons of ground black pepper
- 1/4 teaspoon of ground cumin
- 9 cups of water

Directions:
1. Using a 6-quarts slow cooker, place all the Ingredients: and stir until it mixes properly.
2. Cover the top, plug in the slow cooker; adjust the cooking time to 6 hours, let it cook on high heat setting and add more water if the beans get too dry.
3. When the beans are done, drain them and reserve the liquid.
4. Mash the beans using a potato masher and pour in the reserved cooking liquid until it reaches your desired mixture.
5. Serve immediately.

Nutrition: Calories: 198 Carbs: 12g Fat: 7g Protein: 15.5g

406. Smoky Red Beans and Rice

Preparation Time: 15 Minutes
Cooking Time: 5 Hours
Servings: 8
Ingredients:

- 30 ounces of cooked red beans
- 1 cup of brown rice, uncooked
- 1 cup of chopped green pepper
- 1 cup of chopped celery
- 1 cup of chopped white onion
- 1 1/2 teaspoon of minced garlic
- 1/2 teaspoon of salt
- 1/4 teaspoon of cayenne pepper
- 1 teaspoon of smoked paprika
- 2 teaspoons of dried thyme
- 1 bay leaf
- 2 1/3 cups of vegetable broth

Directions:
1. Using a 6-quarts slow cooker, all the Ingredients are except for the rice, salt, and cayenne pepper.
2. Stir until it mixes appropriately and then cover the top.

3. Plug in the slow cooker; adjust the cooking time to 4 hours, and steam on a low heat setting.
4. Then pour in and stir the rice, salt, cayenne pepper and continue cooking for an additional 2 hours at a high heat setting.

Nutrition: Calories: 234 Carbs: 13g Fat: 5g Protein: 6g

407. Spicy Black-Eyed Peas

Preparation Time: 15 Minutes
Cooking Time: 60 Minutes
Servings: 8
Ingredients:

- 32-ounce black-eyed peas, uncooked
- 1 cup of chopped orange bell pepper
- 1 cup of chopped celery
- 8-ounce of chipotle peppers, chopped
- 1 cup of chopped carrot
- 1 cup of chopped white onion
- 1 teaspoon of minced garlic
- 3/4 teaspoon of salt
- 1/2 teaspoon of ground black pepper
- 2 teaspoons of liquid smoke flavoring
- 2 teaspoons of ground cumin
- 1 tablespoon of adobo sauce
- 2 tablespoons of olive oil
- 1 tablespoon of apple cider vinegar
- 4 cups of vegetable broth

Directions:
1. Place a medium-sized non-stick skillet pan over an average temperature of heat; add the bell peppers, carrot, onion, garlic, oil and vinegar.
2. Stir until it mixes properly and let it cook for 5 to 8 minutes or until it gets translucent.
3. Transfer this mixture to a 6-quarts slow cooker and add the peas, chipotle pepper, adobo sauce and the vegetable broth.
4. Stir until mixes properly and cover the top.
5. Plug in the slow cooker; adjust the cooking time to 8 hours and let it cook on the low heat setting or until peas are soft.

Nutrition: Calories: 345 Carbs: 31g Fat: 2.8g Protein: 7g

408. Whole Roasted Radishes

Preparation Time: 10 Minutes
Cooking Time: 30 minutes
Servings: 4
Ingredients:

- 3 tablespoons of olive oil
- 1 tablespoon of lemon juice
- 1 teaspoon of black pepper
- 2 bunches of radishes, trimmed
- 1½ teaspoons of kosher salt

Directions:
1. Let the oven preheat to 400 F.
2. Toss the radishes with lemon juice, olive oil, salt and pepper.
3. Spread on a baking tray, roast for 25-30 minutes, serve.

Nutrition: Calories 101 Total fat: 10 g Total carbs: 3 g Fiber: 3.2 g
Sugar: 1 g Protein: 0 g Sodium: 167 mg

409. Super Radish Avocado Salad

Preparation Time: 5 Minutes
Cooking Time: 0 Minutes
Servings: 2
Ingredients:

- 6 shredded carrots
- 6 ounces diced radishes
- 1 diced avocado
- 1/3 cup ponzu

Directions:
1. Bring all the above ingredients together in a serving bowl and toss.
2. Enjoy!

Nutrition: Calories: 219 Carbs: 9g Fat: 6g Protein: 12g

410. Gingery Cucumbers

Preparation Time: 5 Minutes
Cooking Time: 0 Minutes
Servings: 2
Ingredients:

- 1 sliced cucumber
- 3 teaspoon rice wine vinegar
- 1 1/2 tablespoon sugar
- 1 teaspoon minced ginger

Directions:
1. Bring all of the above ingredients together in a mixing bowl, and toss the ingredients well.
2. Enjoy!

Nutrition: Calories: 202 Carbs: 14g Fat: 5g Protein: 13g

411. Mushroom Salad

Preparation Time: 10 Minutes
Cooking Time: 10 Minutes
Servings: 2
Ingredients:

- 1 tablespoon butter
- 1/2-pound cremini mushrooms, chopped
- 2 tablespoons extra-virgin olive oil
- Salt and black pepper to taste
- 2 bunches arugula
- 4 slices prosciutto
- 1 tablespoon apple cider vinegar
- 4 sundried tomatoes in oil, drained and chopped
- Fresh parsley leaves, chopped

Directions:
1. Heat a pan with butter and half of the oil.
2. Add the mushrooms, salt, and pepper. Stir-fry for 3 minutes. Reduce heat. Stir again, and cook for 3 minutes more.
3. Add rest of the oil and vinegar. Stir and cook for 1 minute.
4. Place arugula on a platter, add prosciutto on top, add the mushroom mixture, sundried tomatoes, more salt and pepper, parsley, and serve.

Nutrition: Calories: 191 Carbs: 6g Fat: 7g Protein: 17g

412. Crispy Roasted Artichokes

Preparation Time: 15 Minutes
Cooking Time: 40 minutes
Servings: 6
Ingredients:

- ⅓ cup of olive oil
- 12 quartered artichokes
- Half cup of vegan mayonnaise
- 2 tablespoons of lemon juice
- 4 garlic cloves
- Salt and black pepper, to taste

Directions:

1. In a pot, add water, lemon juice (1 tbsp.), salt, let it boil.
2. Peel the artichoke tougher leaves and cut the top off and discard any fuzzy part from the center.
3. Add the trimmed artichoke to boiling water, cook for 8-10 minutes. drain and dry the artichoke.
4. Let the oven preheat to 400 F.
5. In a bowl, toss the unpeeled garlic cloves with boiled artichokes, sprinkle with salt and pepper.
6. Roast for 25-30 minutes, tossing occasionally.
7. Peel the garlic and mash with a fork, add mayo with salt, pepper and lemon juice.
8. Serve the artichoke with aioli.

Nutrition: Calories 285 Total fat: 27 g Total carbs: 10 g Fiber: 1 g Sugar: 1 g Protein: 3 g Sodium: 201 mg

413. Cauliflower Rice

Preparation Time: 10 Minutes
Cooking Time: 5 minutes
Servings: 6
Ingredients:

- 1 head of cauliflower
- Salt and black pepper, to taste
- 1-2 tablespoons of olive oil

Directions:

1. In a food processor add florets in batches and pulse till they resemble rice.
2. In a skillet, add oil and toss cauliflower rice on medium flame with salt and pepper.
3. Cook for 2-3 minutes. serve.

Nutrition: Calories 53 Total fat: 4 g Total carbs: 10 g Fiber: 3.2 g Sugar: 2 g Protein: 2 g Sodium: 198 mg

414. Rice with Asparagus and Cauliflower

Preparation Time: 10 Minutes
Cooking Time: 20 Minutes
Servings: 2
Ingredients:

- 3 ounces' asparagus
- 3 ounces' cauliflower, chopped
- 2 ounces' tomato sauce
- 1/2 cup of brown rice
- 3/4 cup of water
- 1/3 teaspoon salt
- 1/4 teaspoon ground black pepper
- 1/4 teaspoon garlic powder
- 1 tablespoon olive oil

Directions:

1. Take a medium saucepan, place it over medium heat, add oil, and add asparagus and cauliflower and then sauté for 5 to 7 minutes until golden brown.
2. Season with garlic powder, salt, and black pepper, stir in tomato sauce, and then cook for 1 minute.
3. Add rice, pour in water, stir until mixed, cover with a lid and cook for 10 to 12 minutes until rice has absorbed all the liquid and become tender.
4. When done, remove the pan from heat, fluff rice with a fork, and then serve.

Nutrition: Calories: 269 Carbs: 4g Fat: 4g Protein: 40g

415. Spaghetti with Tomato Sauce

Preparation Time: 5 Minutes
Cooking Time: 15 Minutes
Servings: 2
Ingredients:

- 4 ounces' spaghetti
- 2 green onions, greens, and whites separated
- 1/8 teaspoon coconut sugar
- 3 ounces' tomato sauce
- 1 tablespoon olive oil
- 1/3 teaspoon salt
- 1/4 teaspoon ground black pepper

Directions:

1. Prepare the spaghetti, and for this, cook it according to the Directions on the packet and then set aside.
2. Then take a skillet pan, place it over medium heat, add oil and when hot, add white parts of green onions and cook for 2 minutes until tender.
3. Add tomato sauce, season with salt and black pepper and bring it to a boil.
4. Switch heat to medium-low level, simmer sauce for 1 minute, then add the cooked spaghetti and toss until mixed.
5. Divide spaghetti between two plates, and then serve.

Nutrition: Calories: 265 Carbs: 8g Fat: 2g Protein: 11g

416. Crispy Cauliflower

Preparation Time: 5 Minutes
Cooking Time: 15 Minutes
Servings: 2
Ingredients:

- 6 ounces of cauliflower florets
- 1/2 of zucchini, sliced
- 1/2 teaspoon of sea salt
- 1/2 tablespoon curry powder
- 1/4 teaspoon maple syrup
- 2 tablespoons olive oil

Directions:

1. Switch on the oven, then set it to 450 degrees F and let it preheat.

2. Meanwhile, take a medium bowl, add cauliflower florets and zucchini slices, add remaining ingredients reserving 1 tablespoon oil, and toss until well coated.
3. Take a medium skillet pan, place it over medium-high heat, add remaining oil and wait until it gets hot.
4. Spread cauliflower and zucchini in a single layer and sauté for 5 minutes, tossing frequently.
5. Then transfer the pan into the oven and then bake for 8 to 10 minutes until vegetables have turned golden brown and thoroughly cooked, stirring halfway.

Nutrition: Calories: 161 Carbs: 2g Fat: 2g Protein: 7g

417. Avocado Toast with Chickpeas

Preparation Time: 5 Minutes
Cooking Time: 5 Minutes
Servings: 2
Ingredients:

- 1/2 of avocado, peeled, pitted
- 4 tablespoons canned chickpeas, liquid reserved
- 1 tablespoon lime juice
- 1 teaspoon apple cider vinegar
- 2 slices of bread, toasted
- 1/4 teaspoon salt
- 1/4 teaspoon paprika
- 1 teaspoon olive oil

Directions:

1. Take a medium skillet pan, place it over medium heat, add oil and when hot, add chickpeas and cook for 2 minutes.
2. Sprinkle 1/8 teaspoon each salt and paprika over chickpeas, toss to coat, and then remove the pan from heat.
3. Place avocado in a bowl, mash by using a fork, drizzle with lime juice and vinegar and stir until well mixed.
4. Spread mashed avocado over bread slices, scatter chickpeas on top and then serve.

Nutrition: Calories: 235 Carbs: 5g Fat: 6g Protein: 31g

418. Cold Lemon Noodles

Preparation Time: 15 Minutes
Cooking Time: 0 minutes
Servings: 4
Ingredients:

- Half teaspoon of Dijon mustard
- 3 zucchinis, spiralized into noodles
- Half teaspoon of garlic powder
- ⅓ cup of olive oil
- 1 tablespoon of fresh thyme, chopped
- Zest and juice of 1 lemon
- Salt and pepper, to taste
- 1 bunch of sliced radishes

Directions:

1. In a bowl, add mustard, garlic powder, lemon juice and zest, whisk well.
2. Slowly add olive oil while whisking, add salt and pepper.
3. Add zucchini Noodles and radishes in a bowl, add the dressing on top.
4. Toss and serve with fresh thyme on top.

Nutrition: Calories 198 Total fat: 19 g Total carbs: 8 g Fiber: 8 g Sugar: 3.4 g Protein: 2 g Sodium: 109 mg

419. Garlicky Roasted Mushrooms

Preparation Time: 10 Minutes
Cooking Time: 12 minutes
Servings: 6
Ingredients:

- 1 tablespoon of Olive Oil
- 1/8 teaspoon of each, Kosher Salt, Garlic Powder & Black Pepper
- 2 minced garlic cloves
- 1 lb. of Mushrooms, trimmed
- 2 tablespoon of sliced Chives

Directions:

1. Let the oven preheat to 400 F.
2. In a bowl, add all ingredients, toss to coat.
3. Spread on an oil sprayed baking sheet, bake for 10 to 12 minutes.
4. Serve.

Nutrition: Calories 59 Total fat: 3 g Total carbs: 4 g Fiber: 1 g Sugar: 3.4 g Protein: 3 g Sodium: 78 mg

420. Teriyaki Eggplant

Preparation Time: 15 Minutes
Cooking Time: 15 Minutes
Servings: 2
Ingredients:

- 1/2-pound eggplant
- 1 green onion, chopped
- 1/2 teaspoon grated ginger
- 1/2 teaspoon minced garlic
- 1/3 cup soy sauce
- 1 tablespoon coconut sugar
- 1/2 tablespoon apple cider vinegar
- 1 tablespoon olive oil

Directions:

1. Prepare vegan teriyaki sauce and for this, take a medium bowl, add ginger, garlic, soy sauce, vinegar, and sugar in it and then whisk until sugar has dissolved completely.
2. Cut eggplant into cubes, add them into vegan teriyaki sauce, toss until well coated and marinate for 10 minutes.
3. When ready to cook, take a grill pan, place it over medium-high heat, grease it with oil, and when hot, add marinated eggplant.
4. Cook for 3 to 4 minutes per side until nicely browned and beginning to charred, drizzling with excess marinade frequently and transfer to a plate.
5. Sprinkle green onion on top of the eggplant and then serve.

Nutrition: Calories: 132 Carbs: 4g Fat: 0.4g Protein: 13g

421. Broccoli Stir-Fry with Sesame Seeds

Preparation Time: 5 Minutes
Cooking Time: 8 Minutes
Servings: 4

Ingredients:

- Two tablespoons extra-virgin olive oil (optional)
- One tablespoon grated fresh ginger
- cups broccoli florets
- ¼teaspoon sea salt (optional)
- Two garlic cloves, minced
- Two tablespoons toasted sesame seeds

Directions:

1. Heat the olive oil (if desired) in a large nonstick skillet over medium-high heat until shimmering.
2. Fold in the ginger, broccoli, and sea salt (if desired) and stir-fry for 5 to 7 minutes, or until the broccoli is browned.
3. Cook the garlic until tender, about 30 seconds.
4. Sprinkle with the sesame seeds and serve warm.

Nutrition: Calories: 135 Fat: 10.9g Carbs: 9.7g Protein: 4.1g Fiber: 3.3g

422. Bream

Preparation time: 10 minutes
Cooking Time: 60 minutes
Servings: 4

Ingredients:

- Olive oil cooking spray
- 2 medium zucchinis, cut into 1/2inch-thick rounds
- 2 gold potatoes, thinly sliced
- 4 tomatoes, sliced
- 1.3/4 cups tomato sauce
- 10 garlic cloves cut into large chunks
- 1.1/2 tablespoons olive oil
- 4 teaspoons dried basil
- 2 teaspoons dried oregano
- Teaspoon sea salt

Directions:

1. In a large bowl, combine the zucchini, potatoes, tomatoes, tomato sauce, garlic, olive oil, basil, oregano, and salt and stir well. Pour the vegetable into the dish.
2. Bake for 30 minutes, stir well, and bake for another 30 minutes, or until the potatoes are tender. Stir again and serve.

Nutrition: Calories: 337 Total fat: 8 Protein: 82g Sodium: 346 Fat: 17.2g

423. Roasted Butternut Squash & Brussels Sprouts

Preparation Time: 10 Minutes
Cooking Time: 30 minutes
Servings: 6

Ingredients:

- 1 lb. of halved Brussels sprouts
- 3 tablespoons of Maple syrup
- slices of diced Bacon
- 12 ounces of peeled Butternut squash, diced
- 3 minced garlic cloves
- 3 tablespoons of Olive oil
- whole peeled cloves of Garlic
- Half teaspoon of each sea salt & Black pepper
- 3 tablespoons of grain mustard
- 1 1/2 teaspoons of Smoked paprika

Directions:

1. Let the oven preheat to 425 F.
2. In a bowl, toss squash with bacon, all garlic, Brussels sprouts.
3. In a bowl, add the rest of the ingredients, whisk and pour over squash bowl; toss well.
4. Spread on a baking sheet and roast for half an hour. Serve.

Nutrition: Calories 267 Total fat: 15 g Total carbs: 24 g Fiber: 9.8 g Sugar: 11 g Protein: 7 g Sodium: 82 mg

424. Rainbow Vegetable Skewers

Preparation Time: 15 Minutes
Cooking Time: 10 minutes
Servings: 4

Ingredients:

Lemon-Parsley Dressing

- 1 lemon's zest
- 1 tablespoon of Dijon mustard
- ¾ teaspoon of garlic powder
- ⅓ cup of lemon juice
- Salt and pepper, to taste
- Half cup of olive oil
- ¼ cup of fresh parsley, chopped
- A pinch of cayenne pepper

Skewers

- 2 sliced summer squash
- 2 sliced zucchinis
- 1 eggplant, large cubed
- 4 orange sweet peppers, cut into squares
- 3 red onions, sliced into large pieces
- Salt & pepper
- 4 cups of cherry tomatoes
- 2 tablespoons of fresh parsley, chopped

Directions:

1. In a bowl, add all ingredients of dressing except olive oil. Whisk well and gradually pour olive oil while whisking until combined. Set it aside.
2. Thread the vegetables onto soaked skewers, alternatively.
3. Pour some sauce over skewers, brush all over, sprinkle salt and pepper.
4. Preheat a grill pan and cook the skewers for 3-5 minutes on each side.
5. Serve with sauce and parsley on top.

Nutrition: Calories 119 Total fat: 1 g Total carbs: 26 g Fiber: 2 g Sugar: 15 g Protein: 5 g

425. Plum Watermelon Fruit Salsa

Preparation Time: 10 Minutes
Cooking Time: 0 minutes
Servings: 10

Ingredients:

- 2 cups of diced Cantaloupe
- 2 chopped Jalapeños
- Half cup of diced Plums
- 2 tablespoons of Lime juice
- 2 cups of diced Watermelon
- half cup of chopped sweet onion
- 1 cup of chopped Fresh cilantro

Directions:

1. In a bowl, add all ingredients toss well.

Nutrition: Calories 28 Total fat: 0 g Total carbs: 7 g Fiber: 0 g Sugar: 5 g Protein: 0 g Sodium: 82 mg

426. Pizza salad Cabbage Slaw

Preparation Time: 30 Minutes
Cooking Time: 0 minutes
Servings: 4

Ingredients:

- 2 teaspoons of sea salt
- Half teaspoon of dried oregano
- Black pepper, to taste
- 1 sliced red onion
- 1 pound of white cabbage
- 1 roasted sliced red bell pepper in oil
- 3 tablespoons of olive oil
- 1 tablespoon of white wine vinegar
- 1 teaspoon of sunflower seeds
- A pinch of red pepper flakes
- 1 teaspoon of poppy seeds

Directions:

1. In a food processor, shred the cabbage finely. Take it out in a bowl, and sprinkle with salt.
2. Let it rest for 20-30 minutes, lightly squeeze to get rid of moisture and shake the salt.
3. Transfer to a bowl, add onion and red pepper. Toss.
4. In a bowl, add the rest of the ingredients, mix and pour over the cabbage bowl.
5. Toss and serve.

Nutrition: Calories 137 Total fat: 11 g Total carbs: 10 g Fiber: 7 g Sugar: 5 g Protein: 2 g Sodium: 210 mg

427. Garlic Crispy Smashed Potatoes

Preparation Time: 20 Minutes
Cooking Time: 1 hour and 30 minutes
Servings: 6

Ingredients:

Potatoes

- 2 tablespoons of Olive oil
- 12 Yukon small gold potatoes
- Sea salt, Fresh parsley & Black pepper, to taste

Cashew Cream

- 1 whole bulb of Garlic
- 2 tablespoons of Fresh chives
- 3/4 cup of soaked Cashews
- 1 tablespoon of Lemon juice

Directions:

1. Let the oven preheat to 400 F.
2. Peel any outer papery layer of garlic, cut the top off the only ¼". Coat in olive oil and wrap in foil.
3. Place in the oven, bake for 40 to 50 minutes.
4. In a food processor, add drained cashews with a little bit of hot water and pulse until smooth. Add the roasted peeled garlic, chives and the rest of the ingredients. Pulse until smooth.
5. Boil potatoes for 8 to 10 minutes. Drain and dry the potatoes, transfer on a baking sheet.
6. Lightly smash with glass, add oil, salt and pepper.
7. Bake for half an hour until crispy and golden. Take the tray out, drizzle with olive oil, broil for 5 minutes.
8. Serve with garlicky cashew cream.

Nutrition: Calories 328 Total fat: 12 g Total carbs: 38 g Fiber: 9 g Sugar: 5 g Protein: 11 g Sodium: 132 mg

428. Tabbouleh Salad

Preparation time: 5minutes
Cooking Time: package direction
Servings: 4

Ingredients:

- 1/4 cup olive oil
- 2 tablespoons freshly squeezed lemon juice
- 2 garlic cloves, minced
- Pinch salt
- Pinch freshly ground black pepper
- 2 tomatoes, diced
- 1/2 cup chopped fresh parsley
- Cup dry bulgur wheat, cooked according to the package directions

Directions:

1. Merge together the olive oil, lemon juice, garlic, salt, and pepper. Gently stir in the tomatoes and parsley.
2. Attach the bulgur and toss to combine everything thoroughly. Taste and season with salt and pepper as needed.

Nutrition: Calories: 110 Fats: 12.1g, Carbs: 15.6g Proteins: 7.6g

429. Caesar Salad

Preparation time: 10 minutes
Cooking Time: 0 minutes
Servings: 4

Ingredients:

- 2 cups chopped romaine lettuce
- 2 tablespoons Caesar Dressing
- 1 serving Herbed Croutons or store-bought croutons
- Vegan cheese, grated (optional)
- Make it a meal
- 1/2 cup canned chickpeas
- 2 additional tablespoons Caesar Dressing

Directions:

1. To make the Caesar salad
2. Merge together the lettuce, dressing, croutons, and cheese (if using).
3. To make it a meal

Nutrition: Calories: 120 Fats: 13.1g, Carbs: 12.6g Proteins: 7.6g

430. Greek Potato Salad

Preparation time: 10 minutes
Cooking Time: 20 minutes
Servings: 3
Ingredients:

- 6 potatoes, scrubbed or peeled and chopped
- Salt
- 1/4 cup olive oil
- 2 tablespoons apple cider vinegar
- 2 tablespoons freshly squeezed lemon juice
- 1 teaspoon dried herbs
- 1/2 cucumber, chopped
- 1/4 red onion, diced
- 1/4 cup chopped pitted black olives
- Freshly ground black pepper

Directions:

1. Set the potatoes in a pot, add a pinch of salt, and pour in enough water to cover. Boil the water. Cook the potatoes for 15 to 20 minutes, until soft. Drain and set aside to cool. (Alternatively, put the potatoes in a large microwave-safe dish with a bit of water. Cover and heat on high power for 10 minutes.)
2. In a large bowl, whisk together the olive oil, vinegar, lemon juice, and dried herbs. Toss the cucumber, red onion, and olives with the dressing.
3. Add the cooked, cooled potatoes, and toss to combine. Taste and season with salt and pepper as needed.

Nutrition: Calories: 110 Fats: 17.1g, Carbs: 19.6g Proteins: 7.6g

431. Garlic Roasted Brussels Sprouts

Preparation Time: 10 Minutes
Cooking Time: 25 minutes
Servings: 4
Ingredients:

- 2 tablespoons of minced garlic
- ¼ teaspoon of salt
- 2 lbs. Brussels sprouts, cut in half
- half tablespoon of fresh chopped rosemary
- 1 tablespoon of olive oil
- Half teaspoon of black pepper

Directions:

1. Let the oven preheat to 400 F.
2. Toss the Brussels sprouts with the rest of the ingredients and spread them on a parchment-lined baking tray.
3. Bake for 15 minutes, flip and bake for 5-10 minutes.

Nutrition: Calories 135 Total fat: 4 g Total carbs: 22 g Fiber: 9 g Sugar: 5 g Protein: 8 g Sodium: 203 mg

432. Shaved Brussels Sprout

Preparation Time: 10 Minutes
Cooking Time: 10 minutes
Servings: 4
Ingredients:

- 3/4 cup of chopped pecans
- Half teaspoon of salt
- 2 tablespoons of balsamic vinegar
- 1/4 cup of hemp seeds
- cups of shaved Brussels sprouts
- 1 tablespoon of olive oil
- 1 teaspoon of black pepper
- Half cup of dried cranberries
- Half teaspoon of rosemary

Directions:

1. Sauté shaved Brussels sprouts in hot oil for 5 minutes.
2. Add the rest of the ingredients, toss and heat it through and serve.

Nutrition: Calories 109 Total fat: 2 g Total carbs: 1 g Fiber: 9.8 g Sugar: 2 g Protein: 3 g Sodium: 76 mg

433. Mashed Cauliflower

Preparation Time: 15 minutes
Cooking time: 15 minutes
Servings: 5
Ingredients:

- 5 cups water
- 2 cups cauliflower florets
- 1 tablespoon ghee
- Salt
- Freshly ground black pepper

Directions:

1. Merge the 5 cups water to a boil. Add the cauliflower florets and boil for 10 to 12 minutes, until very tender. Drain the cauliflower in a colander and return it to the pot.
2. Using a fork or potato masher, mash the florets. Add the ghee and season with salt and pepper. Mash briefly to combine.
3. Evenly divide the mashed cauliflower between 2 single-serving 24-ounce meal prep containers. Refrigerate for up to 3 days.
4. Reheat: Reheat the mashed cauliflower in the microwave in 30-second increments, stirring between each, until it reaches your desired temperature.
5. Freeze: This can be frozen. Cool the mashed cauliflower before transferring to a quart-size resalable freezer bag. Freeze flat for 1 month. Thaw in the refrigerator overnight.

Nutrition: Calories: 345; Fat: 67g; Protein: 15g; Total carbs: 34g

434. Sheet Pan Rainbow Veggies

Preparation Time: 20 minutes
Cooking time: 15 minutes
Servings: 6
Ingredients:

- 2 cups broccoli florets cut into large dice
- 2 cups whole button mushrooms
- 2 cups butternut squash, chopped small
- 1 zucchini, chopped small

- 1 yellow squash, chopped small
- 1 red bell pepper, chopped small
- 1 onion, chopped into 1-inch pieces
- 2 tablespoons olive oil
- 2 tablespoons balsamic vinegar
- 4 garlic cloves, minced
- 2 tablespoons dried thyme
- Salt
- Freshly ground black pepper

Directions:

1. Preheat the oven to 425°F.
2. On the prepared sheet pan, toss together the broccoli, mushrooms, butternut squash, zucchini; yellow squash, red bell pepper, onion, olive oil, vinegar, garlic, and thyme. Season with salt and pepper. Arrange the vegetables in a single layer.
3. . Roast for 12 to 15 minutes and slightly browned.

Nutrition: Calories: 459; Fat: 34g; Protein: 28g; Total carbs: 17g

435. Garlic-Lemon Roasted Broccoli

Preparation Time: 5 minutes
Cooking time: 15 minutes
Servings: 4
Ingredients:

- 4 cups fresh broccoli florets
- 2 to 3 tablespoons olive oil
- 2 garlic cloves, minced
- Juice of 1 lemon
- Salt
- Freshly ground black pepper

Directions:

1. Preheat the oven to 425°F.
2. On the prepared sheet pan, toss together the broccoli, olive oil, garlic and lemon juice. Season with salt and pepper. Spread the broccoli into a single layer on the sheet pan.
3. Bake for 12 to 15 minutes, checking every 5 minutes to shake the pan so it cooks evenly.

Nutrition: Calories: 356; Fat: 17g; Protein: 28g; Total carbs: 21g;

436. Savory Sweet Potatoes

Preparation Time: 10 minutes
Cooking time: 35 minutes
Servings: 4
Ingredients:

- 2 large sweet potatoes cut into bite-size pieces
- 1 tablespoon olive oil
- 1 teaspoon paprika
- 1 teaspoon dried thyme
- 1/2 teaspoon dried parsley
- 1/4 teaspoon salt

Directions:

1. Preheat the oven to 450°F.
2. On the prepared sheet pan, toss together the sweet potatoes and olive oil to coat. Add the paprika, thyme, parsley, and salt and toss again to combine. Roll out the sweet potatoes into a single layer.
3. Bake for 30 to 35 minutes, or until the sweet potatoes are tender.

4. Let cool before dividing among 4 single-serving 24-ounce meal prep containers. Refrigerate for up to 4 days.
5. Reheat: Warm the sweet potatoes in the microwave for 60 seconds.

Nutrition: Calories: 391; Fat: 34g; Protein: 53g; Total carbs: 31g

437. Oven-Roasted Asparagus

Preparation Time: 10 minutes
Cooking time: 8 minutes
Servings: 3
Ingredients:

- 8 ounces' asparagus, rinsed, woody ends trimmed by 1 inch, dried
- 1/2 teaspoon salt
- 1/2 teaspoon freshly ground black pepper
- 3 garlic cloves, minced

Directions:

1. Preheat the oven to 425°F.
2. Scatter the asparagus into a single layer on the prepared sheet pan.
3. In a small bowl, stir together the salt, pepper, and garlic.
4. Lightly coat the asparagus with cooking spray. Sprinkle with the cheese mixture. Using your hands, mix the asparagus with all the ingredients and spread them into an even layer again. Lightly coat once more with cooking spray.
5. Bake for 8 minutes.

Nutrition: Calories: 267; Fat: 56g; Protein: 31g; Total carbs: 23

438. Simple Spaghetti Squash

Preparation Time: 5 minutes
Cooking time: 50 minutes
Servings: 2
Ingredients:

- 1 spaghetti squash, rinsed, ends trimmed, halved lengthwise, seeds and pulp removed
- 2 tablespoons olive oil or avocado oil
- Sea salt
- Freshly ground black pepper

Directions:

1. Preheat the oven to 350°F.
2. Slice the squash halves, cut-side up, on a baking sheet or sheet pan and drizzle with olive oil. Season with salt and pepper. Turn the squash halves cut-side down.
3. Bake for 40 to 50 minutes, until the squash is easily pierced with a fork. Remove from the oven and let cool.

Nutrition: Calories: 191; Fat: 68g; Protein: 42g; Total carbs: 23g

439. Fresh Black Bean Dip

Preparation time: 15 minutes
Cooking time: 5 minutes
Servings: 5
Ingredients:

- 1 small yellow onion, peeled and chopped
- 2 jalapeño peppers
- 1 clove garlic, peeled and chopped
- 1/4 cup red bell pepper
- 2 (15-ounce) cans black beans, drained

- 3 tablespoons water
- 1 teaspoon ground cumin
- 2 teaspoons cocoa powder
- 3 tablespoons fresh lime juice
- 2 tablespoons fresh chopped cilantro
- 4 cherry tomatoes, sliced

Directions:

1. Add onion, jalapeño, garlic, bell pepper, black beans, and water to a food processor bowl. Pulse three times, pushing down contents that go up sides of bowl. Add cumin and cocoa powder and pulse again until smooth.
2. Pour into a medium microwave-safe container and cook 60 seconds. Stir and repeat. Remove from microwave and let cool 1 minute.
3. Stir in lime juice and cilantro. Cover and refrigerate up to 5 days or freeze up to 2 months. To serve, cook in microwave in 30-second intervals until heated through, then garnish with sliced cherry tomatoes.

Nutrition: Calories: 88 Fat: 0.3 g Protein: 5.5 g Carbss: 18.9 g

440. Easy Vegan Quest Dip

Preparation time: 10 minutes
Cooking time: 2 minutes
Servings: 6
Ingredients:

- 1 (8-ounce) package vegan cream cheese
- 1 (10-ounce) can mild green chili enchilada sauce
- 3 tablespoons nutritional yeast flakes
- 1 teaspoon garlic powder
- 1/2 teaspoon salt
- 1/4 teaspoon black pepper

Directions:

1. Scoop vegan cream cheese into a small microwave-safe bowl and microwave about 20 seconds. Remove, stir, and repeat until sauce is smooth and stirs easily.
2. Pour green chili enchilada sauce over cream cheese. Stir to combine. Stir in nutritional yeast flakes, garlic powder, salt, and pepper. Let cool about 5 minutes before covering and refrigerating up to 7 days.
3. To serve, remove from refrigerator and cook in microwave in 30-second intervals until heated through.

Nutrition: Calories: 78 Fat: 0.3 g Protein: 2.5 g Carbss: 19.9 g

441. Vegan Seven-Layer Dip

Preparation time: 15 minutes
Cooking time: 5 minutes
Servings: 10
Ingredients:

- 1 (12-ounce) package vegan meat crumbles
- 1 tablespoon olive oil
- 3 tablespoons taco seasoning
- 1 can black beans
- 1.1/2 cups mild chunky salsa, divided
- 2 cups vegan Cheddar shreds
- 1 cup vegan sour cream
- 1 cup guacamole
- 1 (2.25-ounce) can black olives, chopped

- 1/2 cup chopped tomatoes
- 1/2 cup chopped green onion

Directions:

1. In a large skillet, brown vegan meat crumbles in olive oil over medium heat about 5 minutes. Add taco seasoning. Set aside to cool to room temperature, about 5 minutes.
2. Place beans in a blender or food processor with 1/2 cup salsa. Blend about 20 seconds until beans are consistency of refried beans.
3. Spread beans into bottom of a large serving tray that is about 11/2" deep. Sprinkle shredded cheese on top of beans. Sprinkle vegan meat crumbles on top of cheese. Carefully spread sour cream on top of vegan crumbles, and then spread guacamole on top of sour cream. Pour remaining salsa over guacamole and spread evenly. Sprinkle with olives. Garnish with tomatoes and green onions. Cover and refrigerate up to 3 days.

Nutrition: Calories: 58 Fat: 3.3 g Protein: 2.5 g Carbss: 17.9 g

442. Roasted Broccolini

Preparation Time: 10 Minutes
Cooking Time: 15 minutes
Servings: 4
Ingredients:

- 2 tablespoons of olive oil
- Salt & pepper, to taste
- 2 teaspoons of chopped garlic
- 2 bunches of broccolini
- Half lemon

Directions:

1. Let the oven preheat to 425 F.
2. Toss the broccolini with oil, salt, garlic and pepper. Spread on a parchment-lined baking sheet.
3. Roast for 12 to 15 minutes. Serve.

Nutrition: Calories 102 Total fat: 7 g Total carbs: 7 g Fiber: 1 g Sugar: 2 g Protein: 3 g Sodium: 25 mg

443. Green Chili Hummus with Salsa

Preparation time: 10 minutes
Cooking time: 0 minutes
Servings: 12
Ingredients:

- 1 (15-ounce) can chickpeas, rinsed and drained
- 2 tablespoons tahini
- 2 tablespoons nutritional yeast flakes
- 2 teaspoons garlic powder
- 1 (4-ounce) can green chilies
- 1/2 cup fresh spinach
- 1 (8-ounce) jar mild chunky salsa

Directions:

1. Combine chickpeas, tahini, nutritional yeast flakes, garlic powder, green chilies, and spinach in a food processor. Pulse 3 seconds until coarse and crumbly.
2. Set a colander and pour salsa into colander to strain liquid.
3. Add liquid 1 tablespoon at a time to food processor and pulse until a spreadable consistency is reached.
4. Spoon hummus into a small serving dish and top with strained salsa.

5. Cover and keep refrigerated until ready to serve (up to 4 days). Alternatively, it can be frozen up to 1 month.
6. Serve and enjoy.

Nutrition: Calories: 169 Fat: 8.3 g Protein: 4.5 g Carbss: 20.9 g

444. Crostini with Pecan Basil Pesto

Preparation time: 10 minutes
Cooking time: 10 minutes
Servings: 8

Ingredients:

- 1/3 cup pecans
- 1 cup fresh spinach
- 1/3 cup olive oil
- 1 teaspoon garlic powder
- 5 fresh basil leaves
- 1 baguette, sliced into 24 (1/2"-thick) slices

Directions:

1. Set oven and place pecans on an ungreased baking sheet and toast in oven about 5 minutes. Remove and cool about 2 minutes.
2. Place cooled pecans, spinach, olive oil, vegan cheese, garlic powder, and basil leaves in a food processor. Pulse 3 seconds to combine.
3. Set bread slices in one layer on a large ungreased baking sheet. Place in oven and toast about 5 minutes. Remove from oven and cool about 5 minutes, then transfer to a medium sealed container and refrigerate up to 3 days.
4. To serve, wrap toast with foil and heat in toaster oven at 350°F for 5 minutes, until heated through. Top with Pecan Basil Pesto.

Nutrition: Calories: 65 Fat: 2.3 g Protein: 9.5 g Carbss: 14.9 g

445. Black-Eyed Pea Dip

Preparation time: 25 minutes
Cooking time: 25 minutes
Servings: 6

Ingredients:

- 1 (15-ounce) can black eye peas, drained
- 3 tablespoons finely chopped peeled yellow onion
- 1/4 cup vegan sour cream
- 1/2 (8-ounce) jar mild chunky salsa
- 1 cup vegan Cheddar shred.

Directions:

1. Place black eye peas in an ungreased 8" × 8" casserole dish and use a fork to mash up most of beans.
2. Add in onions, sour cream, salsa, and 1/2 vegan Cheddar shreds. Stir to combine. Top mixture with remaining vegan Cheddar shreds.
3. Bake 25 minutes until top cheese layer melts. Remove from oven and allow to cool 15 minutes.
4. Transfer dip to a large sealable container and refrigerate up to 5 days. To serve, cook in microwave in 30-second intervals until heated through.

Nutrition: Calories: 105 Fat: 2.3 g Protein: 8 g Carbss: 18.9 g

446. Caramelized Onion Hummus

Preparation time: 10 minutes
Cooking time: 15 minutes
Servings: 10

Ingredients:

- 1 small yellow onion
- 3 tablespoons olive oil, divided
- 1 teaspoon agave nectar
- 1 (15-ounce) can chickpeas, rinsed and drained
- 1/4 cup pine nuts
- 3 tablespoons lime juice
- 1/2 teaspoon dried basil
- 1 tablespoon nutritional yeast flakes
- 1 clove garlic, peeled

Directions:

1. Set a skillet on a low heat and add onions. Drizzle with 1 tablespoon olive oil. Cook until tender, about 5 minutes. Then add agave nectar and continue cooking about 10 minutes, until caramelized. Remove from heat and set aside.
2. Add chickpeas into a food processor with pine nuts and pulse 5 seconds. Add remaining tablespoons olive oil, lime juice, basil, nutritional yeast flakes, garlic, and 1/2 caramelized onions. Pulse 3 seconds until smooth. Top with remaining caramelized onions. Transfer to a medium lidded container and refrigerate up to 5 days.

Nutrition: Calories: 79 Fat: 8.3 g Protein: 17.5 g Carbss: 18.9 g

447. Spicy Roasted Chickpeas

Preparation time: 10 minutes
Cooking time: 25 minutes
Servings: 4

Ingredients:

- 1 can chickpeas
- 11/2 teaspoons olive oil
- 1 tablespoon Southwest Chipotle seasoning
- 1/2 teaspoon salt
- 1/8 teaspoon ground black pepper

Directions:

1. Preheat oven to 400°F.
2. Add chickpeas and olive oil to a medium bowl and stir until each chickpea is coated with oil. Place chickpeas on prepared pan.
3. Bake 25 minutes until chickpeas are crispy on outside.
4. Remove from oven and sprinkle seasoning over top. Stir until thoroughly coated. Sprinkle with salt and pepper, then transfer to a small sealed container and refrigerate up to 5 days.

Nutrition: Calories: 167 Fat: 11g Protein: 15.5 g Carbss: 21 g

448. Southwestern Hummus

Preparation time: 5 minutes
Cooking time: 0 minutes
Servings: 10

Ingredients:

- 1 (15-ounce) can chickpeas, rinsed and drained
- 1/4 cup tahini
- 1/4 cup lime juice
- 1 cup mild chunky salsa

- 1 tablespoon Southwest Chipotle seasoning

Directions:
1. Pour all ingredients in bowl of food processor and pulse 3 seconds. Use a spatula to scrape down any ingredients on side of bowl. Pulse again until consistency is smooth.
2. Transfer to a small sealed container and refrigerate up to 5 days.

Nutrition: Calories: 234 Fat: 17 g Protein: 8.8 g Carbss: 23.5 g

449. Vegan Bacon Ricotta Crostini

Preparation time: 15 minutes

Cooking time: 15 minutes

Servings: 10

Ingredients:
- 1 baguette, cut into 24 slices
- 1 tablespoon olive oil
- 1 clove garlic, peeled and chopped
- 8 slices vegan bacon
- 1 cup cashews
- 1/2 cup unsweetened almond milk
- 1 tablespoon nutritional yeast flakes
- 1 teaspoon dried basil
- 1 tablespoon mild miso paste
- 1/4 cup maple syrup

Directions:
1. Preheat oven to 375°F. Set a baking sheet.
2. Set slices on prepared baking sheet and bake 10 minutes until toasted. Transfer to a large sealable bag and refrigerate up to 5 days.
3. Place a medium skillet over medium heat. Add olive oil and garlic. Set aside.
4. In same skillet, cook vegan bacon 3 minutes per side. Take off from skillet and set aside to cool about 5 minutes, and then break into pieces.
5. Add soaked cashews, almond milk, nutritional yeast flakes, basil, and miso paste to bowl of food processor. Pulse 3 seconds. Repeat process until mixture is smooth and leaves no large pieces of cashews.
6. Transfer to a medium sealable container and refrigerate up to 5 days. To serve, top each piece of toasted crostini with one dollop cashew ricotta, followed by divided-out vegan bacon pieces and maple syrup. Toast in toaster oven at 300°F for 5 minutes until crispy.

Nutrition: Calories: 456 Fat: 11.9 g Protein: 17.9 g Carbss: 29.7 g

450. Vegan Beer Brats in a Blanket

Preparation time: 15 minutes

Cooking time: 20 minutes

Servings: 10

Ingredients:
- 1/4 cup yellow mustard
- 1 tablespoon agave nectar
- 1 (12-ounce) bottle pale lager beer
- 4 vegan brats
- 8 dairy-free crescent rolls
- 1 cup dill and garlic sauerkraut
- 1 cup vegan mozzarella cheese
- 4 slices vegan bacon, halved

Directions:
1. Preheat oven to 350F.
2. Combine mustard and agave nectar in a small lidded bowl. Cover and refrigerate up to 7 days.
3. Pour beer into a medium saucepan and bring to a boil over medium heat. Add brats and cook. Once processed, cut each brat in half. Set aside.
4. Arrange dough pieces on prepared baking sheet, adding sauerkraut and vegan cheese evenly over each.
5. Wrap each brat piece in 1/2 slice vegan bacon. Place on piece of dough. Wrap dough tightly around each brat and pinch to seal dough. Bake 15 minutes.
6. Let rolls cool 10 minutes, then transfer to a large lidded container and refrigerate up to 5 days. To serve, remove from refrigerator and heat in microwave in 30-second intervals until heated through. Pour mustard sauce over each roll.

Nutrition: Calories: 278 Fat: 5.9 g Protein: 20.1 g Carbss: 21g

451. Baked Jalapeño Poppers

Preparation time: 10 minutes

Cooking time: 20 minutes

Servings: 10

Ingredients:
- 1/2 (8-ounce) container dairy-free cream cheese, softened
- 1/2 (14.2-ounce) container Diana Jalapeño Garlic Havarti Style Wedge, shredded
- 3/4 cup + 1 tablespoon plain soy milk, divided
- 1/8 teaspoon garlic powder
- 1/2 teaspoon salt
- 10 jalapeños, halved and seeded
- 2 tablespoons ground flaxseed
- 1/2 cup all-purpose flour
- 1/2 cup bread crumbs

Directions:
1. Preheat oven to 350°F.
2. Place vegan cream cheese, shredded vegan cheese, 1 tablespoon soy milk, garlic powder, and salt in a medium bowl and stir until well combined. Stuff each halved jalapeño with an even amount cream cheese mixture.
3. In a separate medium bowl combine flaxseed and remaining soy milk. Set aside.
4. Pour flour into a small dish and bread crumbs into another. Set aside.
5. Roll a stuffed jalapeño in flour, and then dip in flaxseed mixture, followed by a final dip in bread crumbs. Place breaded popper on prepared pan and repeat dipping process with remaining stuffed jalapeños.
6. Take out from oven and let cool. Transfer to a large sealed container and refrigerate up to 5 days. To serve, heat in a toaster oven at 350°F for about 5 minutes.

Nutrition: Calories: 129 Fat: 873 g Protein: 12 g Carbss: 14g

452. Vegan Spinach Cheese Pinwheels

Preparation time: 45 minutes
Cooking time: 20 minutes
Servings: 10

Ingredients:

- 1/2 cup shredded vegan jack cheese
- 2 tablespoons chopped green onion
- 1/4 teaspoon garlic powder
- 1/2 teaspoon salt
- 1/4 cup all-purpose flour
- 1 Pepperidge Farm Puff Pastry Sheet
- 1 tablespoon vegan butter, melted
- 1 tablespoon plain soy milk
- 1 package frozen chopped spinach

Directions:

1. In a medium bowl stir together vegan cheeses, green onions, garlic powder, and salt.
2. Prepare a work area by sprinkling with flour. Lay out pastry sheet on floured surface. Stir together melted vegan butter and soy milk in a small bowl and brush over top of pastry sheet, reserving remaining mixture.
3. Spread cheese mixture over buttered pastry sheet, and then spread drained spinach over cheese mixture.
4. Begin with side closest to you and roll pastry sheet, wrapping ingredients in as you roll. Wrap pastry roll in aluminum foil and freeze about 30 minutes.
5. Preheat oven to 400°F. Grease a baking sheet with vegetable cooking spray.
6. Use a serrated knife to cut pastry roll into 1/2" slices. Place slices on prepared pan and brush with reserved butter mixture.
7. Bake 20 minutes until pinwheels are a golden color.
8. Remove from oven and let cool about 5 minutes before transferring to a large sealed container. Refrigerate up to 5 days. To serve, cook in a toaster oven at 350°F until heated through, about 5 minutes.

Nutrition: Calories: 143 Fat: 8 g Protein: 12g Carbss: 14g

453. Cheesy Kale Chips

Preparation Time: 10 Minutes
Cooking Time: 8-9 hours
Servings: 3-4

Ingredients:

- 1 cup of cashews
- 1/3 cup of water
- 1/4 teaspoon of bell pepper
- chili flake, to taste
- to 8 kale leaves, torn into big pieces without tough stems
- 2 tablespoons of nutritional yeast
- 1 teaspoon of salt

Directions

1. In a food processor, add all the ingredients except for kale. Pulse until smooth.
2. Use water to get the desired consistency.
3. Pour over kale leaves and toss well to get them covered.
4. Place on an oven tray and dehydrate at 140 F for 8 to 9 hours while leaving the oven door slightly open.
5. Serve.

Nutrition: Calories 102 Total fat: 3.4 g Total carbs: 2 g Fiber: 4 g Sugar: 2 g Protein: 2 g Sodium: 87.1 mg

454. Carrot Hummus

Preparation time: 15 minutes
Cooking time: 0 minutes
Servings: 9

Ingredients:

- 1 (15-ounce) can chickpeas, rinsed and drained
- 1 cup roughly chopped peeled carrots
- 1 tablespoon balsamic vinegar
- 2 teaspoons garlic powder
- 1/2 teaspoon ground cumin
- 1/2 teaspoon ground turmeric
- 1 teaspoon dried basil
- 1 tablespoon tamari
- 4 tablespoons water
- 2 tablespoons olive oil

Directions:

1. Place all ingredients except water and olive oil in a food processor and pulse until combined. Remove lid and stir ingredients, adding water 1 tablespoon at a time until desired consistency is reached.
2. Transfer to a medium lidded container and refrigerate up to 7 days. To serve, drizzle olive oil on top of hummus.

Nutrition: Calories: 197 Fat: 20 g Protein: 16g Carbss: 11g

455. Vegan Cheesy Popcorn

Preparation time: 5 minutes
Cooking time: 3 minutes
Servings: 2

Ingredients:

- 1/3 cup popcorn kernels
- 2 teaspoons nutritional yeast flakes
- 1 teaspoon paprika
- 1/2 teaspoon ground turmeric
- 1/8 teaspoon salt

Directions:

1. Place popcorn kernels in a microwave popcorn popper. Place lid on container and microwave about 3 minutes.
2. Place nutritional yeast flakes, paprika, and turmeric in a small bowl. Stir to combine.
3. Use oven mitts to remove popcorn popper from microwave, then carefully remove lid.
4. Pour popcorn into a large sealable container, removing unpeopled kernels. Spray popcorn generously with vegetable cooking spray. Sprinkle nutritional yeast mixture and salt over top and use your hands or a spoon to distribute seasonings evenly throughout popcorn.

Nutrition: Calories: 210 Fat: 19 g Protein: 11g Carbss: 21 g

456. Pico De Gallo Stuffed Avocado

Preparation Time: 10 Minutes

Cooking Time: 0 minutes

Servings: 6

Ingredients:

- 3 tablespoons of diced onions
- 1 tablespoon of lime juice
- 2 Roma tomatoes, diced
- 1 1/2 - 2 tablespoons of chopped cilantro
- 3 avocados
- 1 tablespoon of chopped jalapeno
- Half teaspoon of salt

Directions:

1. In a bowl, add all ingredients except for avocados. Toss.
2. Cut avocados in half and take some of the avocados out.
3. Stuff with pico de gallo. Serve.

Nutrition: Calories 267 Total fat: 18.1 g Total carbs: 8 g Fiber: 2 g Sugar: 2 g Protein: 7 g Sodium: 100 mg

RICE, BEAN, AND GRAIN RECIPES

457. Wild Rice, Celery, and Cauliflower Pilaf

Preparation time: 15 minutes
Cooking time: 45 minutes
Servings: 4

INGREDIENTS:

- 1 tablespoon olive oil, plus more for greasing the baking dish
- 1 cup wild rice
- 2 cups low-sodium chicken broth
- 1 sweet onion, chopped
- 2 stalks celery, chopped
- 1 teaspoon minced garlic
- 2 carrots, peeled, halved lengthwise, and sliced
- ½ cauliflower head, cut into small florets
- 1 teaspoon chopped fresh thyme
- Sea salt, to taste

DIRECTIONS:

1. Preheat the oven to 350°f (180°c). Line a baking sheet with parchment paper and grease with olive oil.
2. Put the wild rice in a saucepan, then pour in the chicken broth. Bring to a boil. Reduce the heat to low and simmer for 30 minutes or until the rice is plump.
3. Meanwhile, heat the remaining olive oil in an oven-proof skillet over medium-high heat until shimmering.
4. Add the onion, celery, and garlic to the skillet and sauté for 3 minutes or until the onion is translucent.
5. Add the carrots and cauliflower to the skillet and sauté for 5 minutes. Turn off the heat and set aside.
6. Pour the cooked rice in the skillet with the vegetables. Sprinkle with thyme and salt. Set the skillet in the preheated oven and bake for 15 minutes or until the vegetables are soft. Serve immediately.

NUTRITION: Calories: 214 Fat: 3.9g Protein: 7.2g Carbs: 37.9g

458. Slow Cooked Turkey and Brown Rice

Preparation time: 15 minutes
Cooking time: 3 hours & 10 minutes
Servings: 6

INGREDIENTS:

- 1 tablespoon extra-virgin olive oil
- 1½ pounds (680 g) ground turkey
- 2 tablespoons chopped fresh sage, divided
- 2 tablespoons chopped fresh thyme, divided
- 1 teaspoon sea salt
- ½ teaspoon ground black pepper
- 2 cups brown rice
- 1 (14-ounce / 397-g) can stewed tomatoes, with the juice
- ¼ cup pitted and sliced Kalamata olives
- 3 medium zucchinis, sliced thinly
- ¼ cup chopped fresh flat-leaf parsley
- 1 medium yellow onion, chopped

- 1 tablespoon plus 1 teaspoon balsamic vinegar
- 2 cups low-sodium chicken stock
- 2 garlic cloves, minced

DIRECTIONS:

1. Heat the olive oil in a nonstick skillet over medium-high heat until shimmering. Add the ground turkey and sprinkle with 1 tablespoon of sage, 1 tablespoon of thyme, salt and ground black pepper.
2. Sauté for 10 minutes or until the ground turkey is lightly browned. Pour them in the slow cooker, then pour in the remaining ingredients. Stir to mix well.
3. Put the lid on and cook on high for 3 hours or until the rice and vegetables are tender. Pour them in a large serving bowl, then spread.

NUTRITION: Calories: 499 Fat: 16.4g Protein: 32.4g Carbs: 56.5g

459. Papaya, Jicama, and Peas Rice Bowl

Preparation time: 15 minutes
Cooking time: 45 minutes
Servings: 4

INGREDIENTS:

- Sauce:
- Juice of ¼ lemon
- 2 teaspoons chopped fresh basil
- 1 tablespoon raw honey
- 1 tablespoon extra-virgin olive oil
- Sea salt, to taste
- Rice:
- 1½ cups wild rice
- 2 papayas, peeled, seeded, and diced
- 1 jicama, peeled and shredded
- 1 cup snow peas, julienned
- 2 cups shredded cabbage
- 1 scallion, white and green parts, chopped

DIRECTIONS:

1. Combine the ingredients for the sauce in a bowl. Stir to mix well. Set aside until ready to use. Pour the wild rice in a saucepan, then pour in enough water to cover. Bring to a boil.
2. Reduce the heat to low, then simmer for 45 minutes or until the wild rice is soft and plump. Drain and transfer to a large serving bowl.
3. Top the rice with papayas, jicama, peas, cabbage, and scallion. Pour the sauce over and stir to mix well before serving.

NUTRITION: Calories: 446 Fat: 7.9g Protein: 13.1g Carbs: 85.8g

460. Italian Baked Beans

Preparation time: 5 minutes
Cooking time: 15 minutes
Servings: 6

INGREDIENTS:

- 2 teaspoons extra-virgin olive oil
- ½ cup minced onion (about ¼ onion)
- 1 (12-ounce) can low-sodium tomato paste
- ¼ cup red wine vinegar
- 2 tablespoons honey
- ¼ teaspoon ground cinnamon
- ½ cup water
- 2 (15-ounce) cans cannellini or great northern beans, undrained

DIRECTIONS:

1. In a medium saucepan over medium heat, heat the oil. Add the onion and cook for 5 minutes, stirring frequently.
2. Add the tomato paste, vinegar, honey, cinnamon, and water, and mix well. Turn the heat to low. Drain and rinse one can of the beans in a colander and add to the saucepan.
3. Pour the entire second can of beans (including the liquid) into the saucepan. Let it cook for 10 minutes, stirring occasionally, and serve.
4. Ingredient tip: Switch up this recipe by making new variations of the homemade ketchup. Instead of the cinnamon, try ¼ teaspoon of smoked paprika and 1 tablespoon of hot sauce. Serve.

NUTRITION: Calories: 236 Fat: 3g Carbs: 42g Protein: 10g

461. Cannellini Bean Lettuce Wraps

Preparation time: 15 minutes
Cooking time: 10 minutes
Servings: 4

INGREDIENTS:

- 1 tablespoon extra-virgin olive oil
- ½ cup diced red onion (about ¼ onion)
- ¾ cup chopped fresh tomatoes (about 1 medium tomato)
- ¼ teaspoon freshly ground black pepper
- 1 (15-ounce) can cannellini or great northern beans, drained and rinsed
- ¼ cup finely chopped fresh curly parsley
- ½ cup Lemony Garlic Hummus or ½ cup prepared hummus
- 8 romaine lettuce leaves

DIRECTIONS:

1. In a large skillet over medium heat, heat the oil. Add the onion and cook for 3 minutes, stirring occasionally.
2. Add the tomatoes and pepper and cook for 3 more minutes, stirring occasionally. Add the beans and cook for 3 more minutes, stirring occasionally. Remove from the heat, and mix in the parsley.
3. Spread 1 tablespoon of hummus over each lettuce leaf. Evenly spread the warm bean mixture down the center of each leaf.
4. Fold one side of the lettuce leaf over the filling lengthwise, then fold over the other side to make a wrap and serve.

NUTRITION: Calories: 211 Fat: 8g Carbs: 28g Protein: 10g

462. Israeli Eggplant, Chickpea, and Mint Sauté

Preparation time: 5 minutes
Cooking time: 20 minutes
Servings: 6

INGREDIENTS:

- Nonstick cooking spray
- 1 medium globe eggplant (about 1 pound), stem removed
- 1 tablespoon extra-virgin olive oil
- 2 tablespoons freshly squeezed lemon juice (from about 1 small lemon)
- 2 tablespoons balsamic vinegar
- 1 teaspoon ground cumin
- ¼ teaspoon kosher or sea salt
- 1 (15-ounce) can chickpeas, drained and rinsed
- 1 cup sliced sweet onion (about ½ medium Walla Walla or Vidalia onion)
- ¼ cup loosely packed chopped or torn mint leaves
- 1 tablespoon sesame seeds, toasted if desired
- 1 garlic clove, finely minced (about ½ teaspoon)

DIRECTIONS:

1. Place one oven rack about 4 inches below the broiler element. Turn the broiler to the highest setting to preheat. Spray a large, rimmed baking sheet with nonstick cooking spray.
2. On a cutting board, cut the eggplant lengthwise into four slabs (each piece should be about ½- to 1/8-inch thick). Place the eggplant slabs on the prepared baking sheet. Set aside.
3. In a small bowl, whisk together the oil, lemon juice, vinegar, cumin, and salt. Brush or drizzle 2 tablespoons of the lemon dressing over both sides of the eggplant slabs. Reserve the remaining dressing.
4. Broil the eggplant directly under the heating element for 4 minutes, flip them, then broil for another 4 minutes, until golden brown.
5. While the eggplant is broiling, in a serving bowl, combine the chickpeas, onion, mint, sesame seeds, and garlic. Add the reserved dressing, and gently mix to incorporate all the ingredients.
6. When the eggplant is done, using tongs, transfer the slabs from the baking sheet to a cooling rack and cool for 3 minutes.
7. When slightly cooled, place the eggplant on a cutting board and slice each slab crosswise into ½-inch strips.
8. Add the eggplant to the serving bowl with the onion mixture. Gently toss everything together, and serve warm or at room temperature.

NUTRITION: Calories: 159 Fat: 4g Carbs: 26g Protein: 6g

463. Mediterranean Lentils and Rice

Preparation time: 5 minutes
Cooking time: 25 minutes
Servings: 4

INGREDIENTS:

- 2¼ cups low-sodium or no-salt-added vegetable broth
- ½ cup uncooked brown or green lentils
- ½ cup uncooked instant brown rice
- ½ cup diced carrots (about 1 carrot)
- ½ cup diced celery (about 1 stalk)

- 1 (2.25-ounce) can sliced olives, drained (about ½ cup)
- ¼ cup diced red onion (about 1/8 onion)
- ¼ cup chopped fresh curly-leaf parsley
- 1½ tablespoons extra-virgin olive oil
- 1 tablespoon freshly squeezed lemon juice (from about ½ small lemon)
- 1 garlic clove, minced (about ½ teaspoon)
- ¼ teaspoon kosher or sea salt
- ¼ teaspoon freshly ground black pepper

DIRECTIONS:
1. In a medium saucepan over high heat, bring the broth and lentils to a boil, cover, and lower the heat to medium-low. Cook for 8 minutes.
2. Raise the heat to medium, and stir in the rice. Cover the pot and cook the mixture for 15 minutes, or until the liquid is absorbed. Remove the pot from the heat and let it sit, covered, for 1 minute, then stir.
3. While the lentils and rice are cooking, mix together the carrots, celery, olives, onion, and parsley in a large serving bowl.
4. In a small bowl, whisk together the oil, lemon juice, garlic, salt, and pepper. Set aside. When the lentils and rice are cooked, add them to the serving bowl.
5. Pour the dressing on top, and mix everything together. Serve warm or cold, or store in a sealed container in the refrigerator for up to 7 days.

NUTRITION: Calories: 230 Fat: 8g Carbs: 34g Protein: 8g

464. Brown Rice Pilaf with Golden Raisins

Preparation time: 5 minutes
Cooking time: 15 minutes
Servings: 6
INGREDIENTS:
- 1 tablespoon extra-virgin olive oil
- 1 cup chopped onion (about ½ medium onion)
- ½ cup shredded carrot (about 1 medium carrot)
- 1 teaspoon ground cumin
- ½ teaspoon ground cinnamon
- 2 cups instant brown rice
- 1¾ cups 100% orange juice
- ¼ cup water
- 1 cup golden raisins
- ½ cup shelled pistachios
- Chopped fresh chives (optional)

DIRECTIONS:
1. In a medium saucepan over medium-high heat, heat the oil. Add the onion and cook for 5 minutes, stirring frequently.
2. Add the carrot, cumin, and cinnamon, and cook for 1 minute, stirring frequently. Stir in the rice, orange juice, and water.
3. Bring to a boil, cover, then lower the heat to medium-low. Simmer for 7 minutes, or until the rice is cooked through and the liquid is absorbed. Stir in the raisins, pistachios, and chives (if using) and serve.

NUTRITION: Calories: 320 Fat: 7g Carbs: 61g Protein: 6g

465. Quinoa and Chickpea Vegetable Bowls

Preparation time: 15 minutes
Cooking time: 15 minutes
Servings: 4
INGREDIENTS:
- 1 cup red dry quinoa, rinsed and drained
- 2 cups low-sodium vegetable soup
- 2 cups fresh spinach
- 2 cups finely shredded red cabbage
- 1 (15-ounce / 425-g) can chickpeas, drained and rinsed
- 1 ripe avocado, thinly sliced
- 1 cup shredded carrots
- 1 red bell pepper, thinly sliced
- 4 tablespoons Mango Sauce
- ½ cup fresh cilantro, chopped
- Mango Sauce:
- 1 mango, diced
- ¼ cup fresh lime juice
- ½ teaspoon ground turmeric
- 1 teaspoon finely minced fresh ginger
- ¼ teaspoon sea salt
- Pinch of ground red pepper
- 1 teaspoon pure maple syrup
- 2 tablespoons extra-virgin olive oil

DIRECTIONS:
1. Pour the quinoa and vegetable soup in a saucepan. Bring to a boil. Reduce the heat to low. Cover and cook for 15 minutes or until tender. Fluffy with a fork.
2. Meanwhile, combine the ingredients for the mango sauce in a food processor. Pulse until smooth.
3. Divide the quinoa, spinach, and cabbage into 4 serving bowls, then top with chickpeas, avocado, carrots, and bell pepper.
4. Dress them with the mango sauce and spread with cilantro. Serve immediately.

NUTRITION: Calories: 366 Fat: 11.1g Protein: 15.5g Carbs: 55.6g

466. Ritzy Veggie Chili

Preparation time: 15 minutes
Cooking time: 5 hours
Servings: 4
INGREDIENTS:
- 1 (28-ounce / 794-g) can chopped tomatoes, with the juice
- 1 (15-ounce / 425-g) can black beans, drained and rinsed
- 1 (15-ounce / 425-g) can redly beans, drained and rinsed
- 1 medium green bell pepper, chopped
- 1 yellow onion, chopped
- 1 tablespoon onion powder
- 1 teaspoon paprika
- 1 teaspoon cayenne pepper
- 1 teaspoon garlic powder
- ½ teaspoon sea salt
- ½ teaspoon ground black pepper
- 1 tablespoon olive oil
- 1 large Hass avocado, pitted, peeled, and chopped, for garnish

DIRECTIONS:

1. Combine all the ingredients, except for the avocado, in the slow cooker. Stir to mix well.
2. Put the slow cooker lid on and cook on high for 5 hours or until the vegetables are tender and the mixture has a thick consistency.
3. Pour the chili in a large serving bowl. Allow to cool for 30 minutes, then spread with chopped avocado and serve.

NUTRITION: Calories: 633 Fat: 16.3g Protein: 31.7g Carbs: 97.0g

467. Spicy Italian Bean Balls with Marinara

Preparation time: 15 minutes
Cooking time: 45 minutes
Servings: 2-4
INGREDIENTS:

- Bean Balls:
- 1 tablespoon extra-virgin olive oil
- ½ yellow onion, minced
- 1 teaspoon fennel seeds
- 2 teaspoons dried oregano
- ½ teaspoon crushed red pepper flakes
- 1 teaspoon garlic powder
- 1 (15-ounce / 425-g) can white beans (cannellini or navy), drained and rinsed
- ½ cup whole-grain bread crumbs
- Sea salt and ground black pepper, to taste
- Marinara:
- 1 tablespoon extra-virgin olive oil
- 3 garlic cloves, minced
- Handful basil leaves
- 1 (28-ounce / 794-g) can chopped tomatoes with juice reserved
- Sea salt, to taste

DIRECTIONS:

1. Preheat the oven to 350°F (180°C). Line a baking sheet with parchment paper. Heat the olive oil in a nonstick skillet over medium heat until shimmering.
2. Add the onion and sauté for 5 minutes or until translucent. Sprinkle with fennel seeds, oregano, red pepper flakes, and garlic powder, then cook for 1 minute or until aromatic.
3. Pour the sautéed mixture in a food processor and add the beans and bread crumbs. Sprinkle with salt and ground black pepper, then pulse to combine well and the mixture holds together.
4. Shape the mixture into balls with a 2-ounce (57-g) cookie scoop, then arrange the balls on the baking sheet.
5. Bake in the preheated oven for 30 minutes or until lightly browned. Flip the balls halfway through the cooking time.
6. While baking the bean balls, heat the olive oil in a saucepan over medium-high heat until shimmering. Add the garlic and basil and sauté for 2 minutes or until fragrant.
7. Fold in the tomatoes and juice. Bring to a boil. Reduce the heat to low. Put the lid on and simmer for 15 minutes. Sprinkle with salt.
8. Transfer the bean balls on a large plate and baste with marinara before serving.

NUTRITION: Calories: 351 Fat: 16.4g Protein: 11.5g Carbs: 42.9g

468. Baked Rolled Oat with Pears and Pecans

Preparation time: 15 minutes
Cooking time: 30 minutes
Servings: 6
INGREDIENTS:

- 2 tablespoons coconut oil, melted, plus more for greasing the pan
- 3 ripe pears, cored and diced
- 2 cups unsweetened almond milk
- 1 tablespoon pure vanilla extract
- ¼ cup pure maple syrup
- 2 cups gluten-free rolled oats
- ½ cup raisins
- ¾ cup chopped pecans
- ¼ teaspoon ground nutmeg
- 1 teaspoon ground cinnamon
- ½ teaspoon ground ginger
- ¼ teaspoon sea salt

DIRECTIONS:

1. Preheat the oven to 350°f (180°c). Grease a baking dish with melted coconut oil, then spread the pears in a single layer on the baking dish evenly.
2. Combine the almond milk, vanilla extract, maple syrup, and coconut oil in a bowl. Stir to mix well.
3. Combine the remaining ingredients in a separate large bowl. Stir to mix well. Fold the almond milk mixture in the bowl, then pour the mixture over the pears.
4. Place the baking dish in the preheated oven and bake for 30 minutes or until lightly browned and set. Serve immediately.

NUTRITION: Calories: 479 Fat: 34.9g Protein: 8.8g Carbs: 50.1g

469. Brown Rice Pilaf with Pistachios and Raisins

Preparation time: 15 minutes
Cooking time: 15 minutes
Servings: 6
INGREDIENTS:

- 1 tablespoon extra-virgin olive oil
- 1 cup chopped onion
- ½ cup shredded carrot
- ½ teaspoon ground cinnamon
- 1 teaspoon ground cumin
- 2 cups brown rice
- 1¾ cups pure orange juice
- ¼ cup water
- ½ cup shelled pistachios
- 1 cup golden raisins
- ½ cup chopped fresh chives

DIRECTIONS:

1. Heat the olive oil in a saucepan over medium-high heat until shimmering. Add the onion and sauté for 5 minutes or until translucent.
2. Add the carrots, cinnamon, and cumin, then sauté for 1 minutes or until aromatic.

3. Pour int the brown rice, orange juice, and water. Bring to a boil. Reduce the heat to medium-low and simmer for 7 minutes or until the liquid is almost absorbed.
4. Transfer the rice mixture in a large serving bowl, then spread with pistachios, raisins, and chives. Serve immediately.

NUTRITION: Calories: 264 Fat: 7.1g Protein: 5.2g Carbs: 48.9g

470. Cherry, Apricot, and Pecan Brown Rice Bowl

Preparation time: 15 minutes
Cooking time: 1 hour & 5 minutes
Servings: 2
INGREDIENTS:

*   2 tablespoons olive oil
*   2 green onions, sliced
*   ½ cup brown rice
*   1 cup low -sodium chicken stock
*   2 tablespoons dried cherries
*   4 dried apricots, chopped
*   2 tablespoons pecans, toasted and chopped
*   Sea salt and freshly ground pepper, to taste

DIRECTIONS:

1. Heat the olive oil in a medium saucepan over medium-high heat until shimmering. Add the green onions and sauté for 1 minutes or until fragrant.
2. Add the rice. Stir to mix well, then pour in the chicken stock. Bring to a boil. Reduce the heat to low. Cover and simmer for 50 minutes or until the brown rice is soft.
3. Add the cherries, apricots, and pecans, and simmer for 10 more minutes or until the fruits are tender.
4. Pour them in a large serving bowl. Fluff with a fork. Sprinkle with sea salt and freshly ground pepper. Serve immediately.

NUTRITION: Calories: 451 Fat: 25.9g Protein: 8.2g Carbs: 50.4g

471. Curry Apple Couscous with Leeks and Pecans

Preparation time: 15 minutes
Cooking time: 8 minutes
Servings: 4
INGREDIENTS:

*   2 teaspoons extra-virgin olive oil
*   2 leeks, white parts only, sliced
*   1 apple, diced
*   2 cups cooked couscous
*   2 tablespoons curry powder
*   ½ cup chopped pecans

DIRECTIONS:

1. Heat the olive oil in a skillet over medium heat until shimmering. Add the leeks and sauté for 5 minutes or until soft.
2. Add the diced apple and cook for 3 more minutes until tender. Add the couscous and curry powder. Stir to combine. Transfer them in a large serving bowl, then mix in the pecans and serve.

NUTRITION: Calories: 254 Fat: 11.9g Protein: 5.4g Carbs: 34.3g

472. Lebanese Flavor Broken Thin Noodles

Preparation time: 15 minutes
Cooking time: 25 minutes
Servings: 6
INGREDIENTS:

*   1 tablespoon extra-virgin olive oil
*   1 (3-ounce / 85-g) cup vermicelli, broken into 1- to 1½-inch pieces
*   3 cups shredded cabbage
*   1 cup brown rice
*   3 cups low-sodium vegetable soup
*   ½ cup water
*   2 garlic cloves, mashed
*   ¼ teaspoon sea salt
*   1/8 teaspoon crushed red pepper flakes
*   ½ cup coarsely chopped cilantro
*   Fresh lemon slices, for serving

DIRECTIONS:

1. Heat the olive oil in a saucepan over medium-high heat until shimmering. Add the vermicelli and sauté for 3 minutes or until toasted. Add the cabbage and sauté for 4 minutes or until tender.
2. Pour in the brown rice, vegetable soup, and water. Add the garlic and sprinkle with salt and red pepper flakes.
3. Bring to a boil over high heat. Reduce the heat to medium low. Put the lid on and simmer for another 10 minutes. Turn off the heat, then let sit for 5 minutes without opening the lid.
4. Pour them on a large serving platter and spread with cilantro. Squeeze the lemon slices over and serve warm.

NUTRITION: Calories: 127 Fat: 3.1g Protein: 4.2g Carbs: 22.9g

473. Lemony Farro and Avocado Bowl

Preparation time: 15 minutes
Cooking time: 25 minutes
Servings: 4
INGREDIENTS:

*   1 tablespoon plus 2 teaspoons extra-virgin olive oil, divided
*   ½ medium onion, chopped
*   1 carrot, shredded
*   2 garlic cloves, minced
*   1 (6-ounce / 170-g) cup pearled farro
*   2 cups low-sodium vegetable soup
*   2 avocados, peeled, pitted, and sliced
*   Zest and juice of 1 small lemon
*   ¼ teaspoon sea salt

DIRECTIONS:

1. Heat 1 tablespoon of olive oil in a saucepan over medium-high heat until shimmering. Add the onion and sauté for 5 minutes or until translucent. Add the carrot and garlic and sauté for 1 minute or until fragrant.
2. Add the farro and pour in the vegetable soup. Bring to a boil over high heat. Reduce the heat to low. Put the lid on and simmer for 20 minutes or until the farro is al dente.
3. Transfer the farro in a large serving bowl, then fold in the avocado slices. Sprinkle with lemon zest and salt, then drizzle

with lemon juice and 2 teaspoons of olive oil. Stir to mix well and serve immediately.

NUTRITION: Calories: 210 Fat: 11.1g Protein: 4.2g Carbs: 27.9g

474. Rice and Blueberry Stuffed Sweet Potatoes

Preparation time: 15 minutes
Cooking time: 20 minutes
Servings: 4
INGREDIENTS:

- 2 cups cooked wild rice
- ½ cup dried blueberries
- ½ cup chopped hazelnuts
- ½ cup shredded Swiss chard
- 1 teaspoon chopped fresh thyme
- 1 scallion, white and green parts, peeled and thinly sliced
- Sea salt and freshly ground black pepper, to taste
- 4 sweet potatoes, baked in the skin until tender

DIRECTIONS:

1. Preheat the oven to 400°f (205°c). Combine all the ingredients, except for the sweet potatoes, in a large bowl. Stir to mix well.
2. Cut the top third of the sweet potato off length wire, then scoop most of the sweet potato flesh out. Fill the potato with the wild rice mixture, then set the sweet potato on a greased baking sheet.
3. Bake in the preheated oven for 20 minutes or until the sweet potato skin is lightly charred. Serve immediately.

NUTRITION: Calories: 393 Fat: 7.1g Protein: 10.2g Carbs: 76.9g

475. Farro Salad Mix

Preparation time: 15 minutes
Cooking time: 33 minutes
Servings: 4-6
INGREDIENTS:

- 1 teaspoon Dijon mustard
- 1½ cups whole farro
- 2 ounces' feta cheese, crumbled (½ cup)
- 2 tablespoons lemon juice
- 2 tablespoons minced shallot
- 3 tablespoons chopped fresh dill
- 3 tablespoons extra-virgin olive oil
- 6 ounces' asparagus, trimmed and cut into 1-inch lengths
- 6 ounces' cherry tomatoes, halved
- 6 ounces' sugar snap peas, strings removed, cut into 1-inch lengths
- Salt and pepper

DIRECTIONS:

1. Bring 4 quarts' water to boil in a Dutch oven. Put in asparagus, snap peas, and 1 tablespoon salt and cook until crisp-tender, approximately 3 minutes.
2. Use a slotted spoon to move vegetables to large plate and allow to cool completely, about 15 minutes. Put in farro to water, return to boil, and cook until grains are soft with slight chew, 15 to 30 minutes.
3. Drain farro, spread in rimmed baking sheet, and allow to cool completely, about 15 minutes.

4. Beat oil, lemon juice, shallot, mustard, ¼ teaspoon salt, and ¼ teaspoon pepper together in a big container.
5. Put in vegetables, farro, tomatoes, dill, and ¼ cup feta and toss gently to combine. Sprinkle with salt and pepper to taste. Move to serving platter and drizzle with remaining ¼ cup feta. Serve.

NUTRITION: Calories: 240 Carbs: 26g Fat: 12g Protein: 9g

476. Farrotto Mix

Preparation time: 15 minutes
Cooking time: 40 minutes
Servings: 6
INGREDIENTS:

- ½ onion, chopped fine
- 1 cup frozen peas, thawed
- 1 garlic clove, minced
- 1 tablespoon minced fresh chives
- 1 teaspoon grated lemon zest plus 1 teaspoon juice
- 1½ cups whole farro
- 2 tablespoons extra-virgin olive oil
- 2 teaspoons minced fresh tarragon
- 3 cups chicken broth
- 3 cups water
- 4 ounces' asparagus, trimmed and cut on bias into 1-inch lengths
- 4 ounces' pancetta, cut into ¼-inch pieces
- Salt and pepper

DIRECTIONS:

1. Pulse farro using a blender until about half of grains are broken into smaller pieces, about 6 pulses.
2. Bring broth and water to boil in moderate-sized saucepan on high heat. Put in asparagus and cook until crisp-tender, 2 to 3 minutes.
3. Use a slotted spoon to move asparagus to a container and set aside. Decrease heat to low, cover broth mixture, and keep warm.
4. Cook pancetta in a Dutch oven on moderate heat until lightly browned and fat has rendered, approximately 5 minutes.
5. Put in 1 tablespoon oil and onion and cook till they become tender, approximately 5 minutes. Mix in garlic and cook until aromatic, approximately half a minute.
6. Put in farro and cook, stirring often, until grains are lightly toasted, approximately three minutes.
7. Stir 5 cups warm broth mixture into farro mixture, decrease the heat to low, cover, and cook until almost all liquid has been absorbed and farro is just al dente, about 25 minutes, stirring twice during cooking.
8. Put in peas, tarragon, ¾ teaspoon salt, and ½ teaspoon pepper and cook, stirring continuously, until farro becomes creamy, approximately 5 minutes.
9. Remove from the heat, mix in cheese, chives, lemon zest and juice, remaining 1 tablespoon oil, and reserved asparagus.
10. Adjust consistency with remaining warm broth mixture as required (you may have broth left over). Sprinkle with salt and pepper to taste. Serve.

NUTRITION: Calories: 218 Carbs: 41g Fat: 2g Protein: 7g

477. Fennel-thyme Farro

Preparation time: 15 minutes
Cooking time: 50 minutes
Servings: 4-6
INGREDIENTS:

- ¼ cup minced fresh parsley
- 1 onion, chopped fine
- 1 small fennel bulb, stalks discarded, bulb halved, cored, and chopped fine
- 1 teaspoon minced fresh thyme or ¼ teaspoon dried
- 1½ cups whole farro
- 2 teaspoons sherry vinegar
- 3 garlic cloves, minced
- 3 tablespoons extra-virgin olive oil
- Salt and pepper

DIRECTIONS:

1. Bring 4 quarts' water to boil in a Dutch oven. Put in farro and 1 tablespoon salt, return to boil, and cook until grains are soft with slight chew, 15 to 30 minutes.
2. Drain farro, return to now-empty pot, and cover to keep warm. Heat 2 tablespoons oil in 12-inch frying pan on moderate heat until it starts to shimmer.
3. Put in onion, fennel, and ¼ teaspoon salt and cook, stirring intermittently, till they become tender, 8 to 10 minutes. Put in garlic and thyme and cook until aromatic, approximately half a minute.
4. Put in residual 1 tablespoon oil and farro and cook, stirring often, until heated through, approximately 2 minutes.
5. Remove from the heat, mix in, parsley, and vinegar. Sprinkle with salt and pepper to taste. Serve.

NUTRITION: Calories: 338 Carbs: 56g Fat: 10g Protein: 11g

478. Feta-Grape-Bulgur Salad with Grapes and Feta

Preparation time: 15 minutes
Cooking time: 1 hour & 30 minutes
Servings: 4-6
INGREDIENTS:

- ¼ cup chopped fresh mint
- ¼ cup extra-virgin olive oil
- ¼ teaspoon ground cumin
- ½ cup slivered almonds, toasted
- 1 cup water
- 1½ cups medium-grind bulgur, rinsed
- 2 ounces' feta cheese, crumbled (½ cup)
- 2 scallions, sliced thin
- 5 tablespoons lemon juice (2 lemons)
- 6 ounces seedless red grapes, quartered (1 cup)
- Pinch cayenne pepper
- Salt and pepper

DIRECTIONS:

1. Mix bulgur, water, ¼ cup lemon juice, and ¼ teaspoon salt in a container. Cover and allow to sit at room temperature until grains are softened and liquid is fully absorbed, about 1½ hours.
2. Beat remaining 1 tablespoon lemon juice, oil, cumin, cayenne, and ¼ teaspoon salt together in a big container.

3. Put in bulgur, grapes, 1/3 cup almonds, 1/3 cup feta, scallions, and mint and gently toss to combine. Sprinkle with salt and pepper to taste. Sprinkle with remaining almonds and remaining feta before you serve.

NUTRITION: Calories: 500 Carbs: 45g Fat: 14g Protein: 50g

479. Greek Style Meaty Bulgur

Preparation time: 15 minutes
Cooking time: 30 minutes
Servings: 4-6
INGREDIENTS:

- ½ cup jarred roasted red peppers, rinsed, patted dry, and chopped
- 1 bay leaf
- 1 cup medium-grind bulgur, rinsed
- 1 onion, chopped fine
- 1 tablespoon chopped fresh dill
- 1 teaspoon extra-virgin olive oil
- 1 1/3 cups vegetable broth
- 2 teaspoons minced fresh marjoram or ½ teaspoon dried
- 3 garlic cloves, minced
- 8 ounces ground lamb
- Lemon wedges
- Salt and pepper

DIRECTIONS:

1. Heat oil in a big saucepan on moderate to high heat until just smoking. Put in lamb, ½ teaspoon salt, and ¼ teaspoon pepper and cook, breaking up meat with wooden spoon, until browned, 3 to 5 minutes.
2. Mix in onion and red peppers and cook until onion is softened, 5 to 7 minutes. Mix in garlic and marjoram and cook until aromatic, approximately half a minute.
3. Mix in bulgur, broth, and bay leaf and bring to simmer. Decrease heat to low, cover, and simmer gently until bulgur is tender, 16 to 18 minutes.
4. Remove from the heat, lay clean dish towel underneath lid and let bulgur sit for about 10 minutes.
5. Put in dill and fluff gently with fork to combine. Sprinkle with salt and pepper to taste. Serve with lemon wedges.

NUTRITION: Calories: 137 Carbs: 16g Fat: 5g Protein: 7g

480. Hearty Barley Mix

Preparation time: 15 minutes
Cooking time: 50 minutes
Servings: 4
INGREDIENTS:

- 1/8 teaspoon ground cardamom
- ½ cup plain yogurt
- ½ teaspoon ground cumin
- 2/3 cup raw sunflower seeds
- ¾ teaspoon ground coriander
- 1 cup pearl barley
- 1½ tablespoons minced fresh mint
- 1½ teaspoons grated lemon zest plus 1½ tablespoons juice
- 3 tablespoons extra-virgin olive oil
- 5 carrots, peeled
- 8 ounces' snow peas, strings removed, halved along the length
- Salt and pepper

DIRECTIONS:

1. Beat yogurt, ½ teaspoon lemon zest and 1½ teaspoons juice, 1½ teaspoons mint, ¼ teaspoon salt, and 1/8 teaspoon pepper together in a small-sized container; cover put inside your fridge until ready to serve.
2. Bring 4 quarts' water to boil in a Dutch oven. Put in barley and 1 tablespoon salt, return to boil, and cook until tender, 20 to 40 minutes. Drain barley, return to now-empty pot, and cover to keep warm.
3. In the meantime, halve carrots crosswise, then halve or quarter along the length to create uniformly sized pieces.
4. Heat 1 tablespoon oil in 12-inch frying pan on moderate to high heat until just smoking. Put in carrots and ½ teaspoon coriander and cook, stirring intermittently, until mildly charred and just tender, 5 to 7 minutes.
5. Put in snow peas and cook, stirring intermittently, until spotty brown, 3 to 5 minutes; move to plate.
6. Heat 1½ teaspoons oil in now-empty frying pan on moderate heat until it starts to shimmer. Put in sunflower seeds, cumin, cardamom, remaining ¼ teaspoon coriander, and ¼ teaspoon salt.
7. Cook, stirring continuously, until seeds are toasted, approximately 2 minutes; move to small-sized container.
8. Beat remaining 1 teaspoon lemon zest and 1 tablespoon juice, remaining 1 tablespoon mint, and remaining 1½ tablespoons oil together in a big container.
9. Put in barley and carrot–snow pea mixture and gently toss to combine. Sprinkle with salt and pepper to taste. Serve, topping individual portions with spiced sunflower seeds and drizzling with yogurt sauce.

NUTRITION: Calories: 193 Carbs: 44g Fat: 1g Protein: 4g

481. Hearty Barley Risotto

Preparation time: 15 minutes
Cooking time: 60 minutes
Servings: 4-6

INGREDIENTS:

- 1 carrot, peeled and chopped fine
- 1 cup dry white wine
- 1 onion, chopped fine
- 1 teaspoon minced fresh thyme or ¼ teaspoon dried
- 1½ cups pearl barley
- 2 tablespoons extra-virgin olive oil
- 4 cups chicken or vegetable broth
- 4 cups water
- Salt and pepper

DIRECTIONS:

1. Bring broth and water to simmer in moderate-sized saucepan. Decrease heat to low and cover to keep warm.
2. Heat 1 tablespoon oil in a Dutch oven on moderate heat until it starts to shimmer. Put in onion and carrot and cook till they become tender, 5 to 7 minutes.
3. Put in barley and cook, stirring frequently, until lightly toasted and aromatic, about 4 minutes. Put in wine and cook, stirring often, until fully absorbed, approximately two minutes.
4. Mix in 3 cups warm broth and thyme, bring to simmer, and cook, stirring intermittently, until liquid is absorbed and bottom of pot is dry, 22 to 25 minutes.

5. Mix in 2 cups warm broth, bring to simmer, and cook, stirring intermittently, until liquid is absorbed and bottom of pot is dry, fifteen to twenty minutes.
6. Carry on cooking risotto, stirring frequently and adding warm broth as required to stop pot bottom from becoming dry, until barley is cooked through, 15 to 20 minutes.
7. Remove from the heat, adjust consistency with remaining warm broth as required. Mix in cheese and residual 1 tablespoon oil and sprinkle with salt and pepper to taste. Serve.

NUTRITION: Calories: 222 Carbs: 33g Fat: 5g Protein: 6g

482. Hearty Freekeh Pilaf

Preparation time: 15 minutes
Cooking time: 60 minutes
Servings: 4-6

INGREDIENTS:

- ¼ cup chopped fresh mint
- ¼ cup extra-virgin olive oil, plus extra for serving
- ¼ cup shelled pistachios, toasted and coarsely chopped
- ¼ teaspoon ground coriander
- ¼ teaspoon ground cumin
- 1 head cauliflower (2 pounds), cored and cut into ½-inch florets
- 1 shallot, minced
- 1½ cups whole freekeh
- 1½ tablespoons lemon juice
- 1½ teaspoons grated fresh ginger
- 3 ounces pitted dates, chopped (½ cup)
- Salt and pepper

DIRECTIONS:

1. Bring 4 quarts' water to boil in a Dutch oven. Put in freekeh and 1 tablespoon salt, return to boil, and cook until grains are tender, 30 to 45 minutes. Drain freekeh, return to now-empty pot, and cover to keep warm.
2. Heat 2 tablespoons oil in 12-inch non-stick frying pan on moderate to high heat until it starts to shimmer.
3. Put in cauliflower, ½ teaspoon salt, and ¼ teaspoon pepper, cover, and cook until florets are softened and start to brown, approximately five minutes.
4. Remove lid and continue to cook, stirring intermittently, until florets turn spotty brown, about 10 minutes.
5. Put in remaining 2 tablespoons oil, dates, shallot, ginger, coriander, and cumin and cook, stirring often, until dates and shallot are softened and aromatic, approximately 3 minutes.
6. Decrease heat to low, put in freekeh, and cook, stirring often, until heated through, about 1 minute. Remove from the heat, mix in pistachios, mint, and lemon juice.
7. Sprinkle with salt and pepper to taste and drizzle with extra oil. Serve.

NUTRITION: Calories: 520 Carbs: 54g Fat: 14g Protein: 36g

483. Herby-Lemony Farro

Preparation time: 15 minutes
Cooking time: 40 minutes
Servings: 4-6

INGREDIENTS:

- ¼ cup chopped fresh mint
- ¼ cup chopped fresh parsley
- 1 garlic clove, minced
- 1 onion, chopped fine
- 1 tablespoon lemon juice
- 1½ cups whole farro
- 3 tablespoons extra-virgin olive oil
- Salt and pepper

DIRECTIONS:

1. Bring 4 quarts' water to boil in a Dutch oven. Put in farro and 1 tablespoon salt, return to boil, and cook until grains are soft with slight chew, 15 to 30 minutes. Drain farro, return to now-empty pot, and cover to keep warm.
2. Heat 2 tablespoons oil in 12-inch frying pan on moderate heat until it starts to shimmer. Put in onion and ¼ teaspoon salt and cook till they become tender, approximately five minutes.
3. Mix in garlic and cook until aromatic, approximately half a minute. Put in residual 1 tablespoon oil and farro and cook, stirring often, until heated through, approximately two minutes.
4. Remove from the heat, mix in parsley, mint, and lemon juice. Sprinkle with salt and pepper to taste. Serve.

NUTRITION: Calories: 243 Carbs: 22g Fat: 14g Protein: 10g

484. Mushroom-Bulgur Pilaf

Preparation time: 15 minutes
Cooking time: 30 minutes
Servings: 4

INGREDIENTS:

- ¼ cup minced fresh parsley
- ¼ ounce dried porcini mushrooms, rinsed and minced
- ¾ cup chicken or vegetable broth
- ¾ cup water
- 1 cup medium-grind bulgur, rinsed
- 1 onion, chopped fine
- 2 garlic cloves, minced
- 2 tablespoons extra-virgin olive oil
- 8 ounces cremini mushrooms, trimmed, halved if small or quartered if large
- Salt and pepper

DIRECTIONS:

1. Heat oil in a big saucepan on moderate heat until it starts to shimmer. Put in onion, porcini mushrooms, and ½ teaspoon salt and cook until onion is softened, approximately 5 minutes.
2. Mix in cremini mushrooms, increase heat to medium-high, cover, and cook until cremini release their liquid and begin to brown, about 4 minutes.
3. Mix in garlic and cook until aromatic, approximately half a minute. Mix in bulgur, broth, and water and bring to simmer.
4. Decrease heat to low, cover, and simmer gently until bulgur is tender, 16 to 18 minutes. Remove from the heat, lay clean dish towel underneath lid and let pilaf sit for about ten minutes.

5. Put in parsley to pilaf and fluff gently with fork to combine. Sprinkle with salt and pepper to taste. Serve.

NUTRITION: Calories: 259 Carbs: 50g Fat: 3g Protein: 11g

485. Baked Brown Rice

Preparation time: 15 minutes
Cooking time: 1 hour & 25 minutes
Servings: 4-6

INGREDIENTS:

- ½ cup minced fresh parsley
- ¾ cup jarred roasted red peppers, rinsed, patted dry, and chopped
- 1 cup chicken or vegetable broth
- 1½ cups long-grain brown rice, rinsed
- 2 onions, chopped fine
- 2¼ cups water
- 4 teaspoons extra-virgin olive oil
- Lemon wedges
- Salt and pepper

DIRECTIONS:

1. Place the oven rack in the center of the oven and pre-heat your oven to 375 degrees. Heat oil in a Dutch oven on moderate heat until it starts to shimmer.
2. Put in onions and 1 teaspoon salt and cook, stirring intermittently, till they become tender and well browned, 12 to 14 minutes.
3. Mix in water and broth and bring to boil. Mix in rice, cover, and move pot to oven. Bake until rice becomes soft and liquid is absorbed, 65 to 70 minutes.
4. Remove pot from oven. Sprinkle red peppers over rice, cover, and allow to sit for about five minutes.
5. Put in parsley to rice and fluff gently with fork to combine. Sprinkle with salt and pepper to taste. Serve with lemon wedges.

NUTRITION: Calories: 100 Carbs: 27g Fat: 21g Protein: 2g

486. Barley Pilaf

Preparation time: 15 minutes
Cooking time: 45 minutes
Servings: 4-6

INGREDIENTS:

- ¼ cup minced fresh parsley
- 1 small onion, chopped fine
- 1½ cups pearl barley, rinsed
- 1½ teaspoons lemon juice
- 1½ teaspoons minced fresh thyme or ½ teaspoon dried
- 2 garlic cloves, minced
- 2 tablespoons minced fresh chives
- 2½ cups water
- 3 tablespoons extra-virgin olive oil
- Salt and pepper

DIRECTIONS:

1. Heat oil in a big saucepan on moderate heat until it starts to shimmer. Put in onion and ½ teaspoon salt and cook till they become tender, approximately 5 minutes.
2. Mix in barley, garlic, and thyme and cook, stirring often, until barley is lightly toasted and aromatic, approximately three minutes.

3. Mix in water and bring to simmer. Decrease heat to low, cover, and simmer until barley becomes soft and water is absorbed, 20 to 40 minutes.

4. Remove from the heat, lay clean dish towel underneath lid and let pilaf sit for about ten minutes. Put in parsley, chives, and lemon juice to pilaf and fluff gently with fork to combine. Sprinkle with salt and pepper to taste. Serve.

NUTRITION: Calories: 39 Carbs: 8g Fat: 1g Protein: 1g

487. Basmati Rice Pilaf Mix

Preparation time: 15 minutes
Cooking time: 25 minutes
Servings: 4-6
INGREDIENTS:

- ¼ cup currants
- ¼ cup sliced almonds, toasted
- ¼ teaspoon ground cinnamon
- ½ teaspoon ground turmeric
- 1 small onion, chopped fine
- 1 tablespoon extra-virgin olive oil
- 1½ cups basmati rice, rinsed
- 2 garlic cloves, minced
- 2¼ cups water
- Salt and pepper

DIRECTIONS:

1. Heat oil in a big saucepan on moderate heat until it starts to shimmer. Put in onion and ¼ teaspoon salt and cook till they become tender, approximately 5 minutes.

2. Put in rice, garlic, turmeric, and cinnamon and cook, stirring often, until grain edges begin to turn translucent, approximately three minutes.

3. Mix in water and bring to simmer. Decrease heat to low, cover, and simmer gently until rice becomes soft and water is absorbed, 16 to 18 minutes.

4. Remove from the heat, drizzle currants over pilaf. Cover, laying clean dish towel underneath lid, and let pilaf sit for about ten minutes.

5. Put in almonds to pilaf and fluff gently with fork to combine. Sprinkle with salt and pepper to taste. Serve.

NUTRITION: Calories: 180 Carbs: 36g Fat: 2g Protein: 4g

488. Brown Rice Salad with Asparagus, Goat Cheese, and Lemon

Preparation time: 15 minutes
Cooking time: 35 minutes
Servings: 4-6
INGREDIENTS:

- ¼ cup minced fresh parsley
- ¼ cup slivered almonds, toasted
- 1-pound asparagus, trimmed and cut into 1-inch lengths
- 1 shallot, minced
- 1 teaspoon grated lemon zest plus 3 tablespoons juice
- 1½ cups long-grain brown rice
- 2 ounces' goat cheese, crumbled (½ cup)
- 3½ tablespoons extra-virgin olive oil
- Salt and pepper

DIRECTIONS:

1. Bring 4 quarts' water to boil in a Dutch oven. Put in rice and 1½ teaspoons salt and cook, stirring intermittently, until rice is tender, about half an hour.

2. Drain rice, spread onto rimmed baking sheet, and drizzle with 1 tablespoon lemon juice. Allow it to cool completely, about 15 minutes.

3. Heat 1 tablespoon oil in 12-inch frying pan on high heat until just smoking. Put in asparagus, ¼ teaspoon salt, and ¼ teaspoon pepper and cook, stirring intermittently, until asparagus is browned and crisp-tender, about 4 minutes; move to plate and allow to cool slightly.

4. Beat remaining 2½ tablespoons oil, lemon zest and remaining 2 tablespoons juice, shallot, ½ teaspoon salt, and ½ teaspoon pepper together in a big container.

5. Put in rice, asparagus, 2 tablespoons goat cheese, 3 tablespoons almonds, and 3 tablespoons parsley. Gently toss to combine and allow to sit for about 10 minutes.

6. Sprinkle with salt and pepper to taste. Move to serving platter and drizzle with remaining 2 tablespoons goat cheese, remaining 1 tablespoon almonds, and remaining 1 tablespoon parsley. Serve.

NUTRITION: Calories: 197 Carbs: 6g Fat: 16g Protein: 7g

489. Carrot-Almond-Bulgur Salad

Preparation time: 1 hour & 45 minutes
Cooking time: 0 minutes
Servings: 4-6
INGREDIENTS:

- 1/8 teaspoon cayenne pepper
- 1/3 cup chopped fresh cilantro
- 1/3 cup chopped fresh mint
- 1/3 cup extra-virgin olive oil
- ½ cup sliced almonds, toasted
- ½ teaspoon ground cumin
- 1 cup water
- 1½ cups medium-grind bulgur, rinsed
- 3 scallions, sliced thin
- 4 carrots, peeled and shredded
- 6 tablespoons lemon juice (2 lemons)
- Salt and pepper

DIRECTIONS:

1. Mix bulgur, water, ¼ cup lemon juice, and ¼ teaspoon salt in a container. Cover and allow to sit at room temperature until grains are softened and liquid is fully absorbed, about 1½ hours.

2. Beat remaining 2 tablespoons lemon juice, oil, cumin, cayenne, and ½ teaspoon salt together in a big container.

3. Put in bulgur, carrots, scallions, almonds, mint, and cilantro and gently toss to combine. Sprinkle with salt and pepper to taste. Serve.

NUTRITION: Calories: 240 Carbs: 54g Fat: 2g Protein: 7g

490. Chickpea-Spinach-Bulgur

Preparation time: 15 minutes
Cooking time: 23 minutes
Servings: 4-6

INGREDIENTS:

- ¾ cup chicken or vegetable broth
- ¾ cup water
- 1 (15-ounce) can chickpeas, rinsed
- 1 cup medium-grind bulgur, rinsed
- 1 onion, chopped fine
- 1 tablespoon lemon juice
- 2 tablespoons za'atar
- 3 garlic cloves, minced
- 3 ounces (3 cups) baby spinach, chopped
- 3 tablespoons extra-virgin olive oil
- Salt and pepper

DIRECTIONS:

1. Heat 2 tablespoons oil in a big saucepan on moderate heat until it starts to shimmer. Put in onion and ½ teaspoon salt and cook till they become tender, approximately 5 minutes.
2. Mix in garlic and 1 tablespoon za'atar and cook until aromatic, approximately half a minute. Mix in bulgur, chickpeas, broth, and water and bring to simmer. Decrease heat to low, cover, and simmer gently until bulgur is tender, 16 to 18 minutes.
3. Remove from the heat, lay clean dish towel underneath lid and let bulgur sit for about ten minutes.
4. Put in spinach, lemon juice, remaining 1 tablespoon za'atar, and residual 1 tablespoon oil and fluff gently with fork to combine. Sprinkle with salt and pepper to taste. Serve.

NUTRITION: Calories: 319 Carbs: 43g Fat: 12g Protein: 10g

491. Italian Seafood Risotto

Preparation time: 15 minutes
Cooking time: 60 minutes
Servings: 4-6

INGREDIENTS:

- 1/8 teaspoon saffron threads, crumbled
- 1 (14.5-ounce) can diced tomatoes, drained
- 1 cup dry white wine
- 1 onion, chopped fine
- 1 tablespoon lemon juice
- 1 teaspoon minced fresh thyme or ¼ teaspoon dried
- 12 ounces' large shrimp (26 to 30 per pound), peeled and deveined, shells reserved
- 12 ounces' small bay scallops
- 2 bay leaves
- 2 cups Arborio rice
- 2 cups chicken broth
- 2 tablespoons minced fresh parsley
- 2½ cups water
- 4 (8-ounce) bottles clam juice
- 5 garlic cloves, minced
- 5 tablespoons extra-virgin olive oil
- Salt and pepper

DIRECTIONS:

1. Bring shrimp shells, broth, water, clam juice, tomatoes, and bay leaves to boil in a big saucepan on moderate to high heat. Decrease the heat to a simmer and cook for 20 minutes.
2. Strain mixture through fine-mesh strainer into big container, pressing on solids to extract as much liquid as possible; discard solids. Return broth to now-empty saucepan, cover, and keep warm on low heat.
3. Heat 2 tablespoons oil in a Dutch oven on moderate heat until it starts to shimmer. Put in onion and cook till they become tender, approximately 5 minutes.
4. Put in rice, garlic, thyme, and saffron and cook, stirring often, until grain edges begin to turn translucent, approximately 3 minutes.
5. Put in wine and cook, stirring often, until fully absorbed, approximately three minutes. Mix in 3½ cups warm broth, bring to simmer, and cook, stirring intermittently, until almost fully absorbed, about 15 minutes.
6. Carry on cooking rice, stirring often and adding warm broth, 1 cup at a time, every few minutes as liquid is absorbed, until rice is creamy and cooked through but still somewhat firm in center, about 15 minutes.
7. Mix in shrimp and scallops and cook, stirring often, until opaque throughout, approximately three minutes. Remove pot from heat, cover, and allow to sit for about 5 minutes.
8. Adjust consistency with remaining warm broth as required. Mix in remaining 3 tablespoons oil, parsley, and lemon juice and sprinkle with salt and pepper to taste. Serve.

NUTRITION: Calories: 450 Carbs: 12g Fat: 40g Protein: 31g

492. Classic Stovetop White Rice

Preparation time: 15 minutes
Cooking time: 22 minutes
Servings: 4-6

INGREDIENTS:

- 1 tablespoon extra-virgin olive oil
- 2 cups long-grain white rice, rinsed
- 3 cups water
- Basmati, jasmine, or Teammate rice can be substituted for the long-grain rice.
- Salt and pepper

DIRECTIONS:

1. Heat oil in a big saucepan on moderate heat until it starts to shimmer. Put in rice and cook, stirring frequently, until grain edges begin to turn translucent, approximately 2 minutes.
2. Put in water and 1 teaspoon salt and bring to simmer. Cover, decrease the heat to low, and simmer gently until rice becomes soft and water is absorbed, approximately 20 minutes.
3. Remove from the heat, lay clean dish towel underneath lid and let rice sit for about ten minutes. Gently fluff rice with fork. Sprinkle with salt and pepper to taste. Serve.

NUTRITION: Calories: 160 Carbs: 36g Fat: 0g Protein: 3g

493. Classic Tabbouleh

Preparation time: 2 hours
Cooking time: 0 minutes
Servings: 4-6

INGREDIENTS:

- 1/8 teaspoon cayenne pepper
- ¼ cup lemon juice (2 lemons)
- ½ cup medium-grind bulgur, rinsed
- ½ cup minced fresh mint
- 1½ cups minced fresh parsley
- 2 scallions, sliced thin
- 3 tomatoes, cored and cut into ½-inch pieces
- 6 tablespoons extra-virgin olive oil
- Salt and pepper

DIRECTIONS:

1. Toss tomatoes with ¼ teaspoon salt using a fine-mesh strainer set over bowl and let drain, tossing occasionally, for 30 minutes; reserve 2 tablespoons drained tomato juice.
2. Toss bulgur with 2 tablespoons lemon juice and reserved tomato juice in a container and allow to sit until grains start to become tender, 30 to 40 minutes.
3. Beat remaining 2 tablespoons lemon juice, oil, cayenne, and ¼ teaspoon salt together in a big container. Put in tomatoes, bulgur, parsley, mint, and scallions and toss gently to combine.
4. Cover and allow to sit at room temperature until flavors have blended and bulgur is tender, about 1 hour. Before serving, toss salad to recombine and sprinkle with salt and pepper to taste.

NUTRITION: Calories: 150 Carbs: 8g Fat: 12g Protein: 4g

494. Farro Cucumber-Mint Salad

Preparation time: 15 minutes
Cooking time: 30 minutes
Servings: 4-6

INGREDIENTS:

- 1 cup baby arugula
- 1 English cucumber, halved along the length, seeded, and cut into ¼-inch pieces
- 1½ cups whole farro
- 2 tablespoons lemon juice
- 2 tablespoons minced shallot
- 2 tablespoons plain Greek yogurt
- 3 tablespoons chopped fresh mint
- 3 tablespoons extra-virgin olive oil
- 6 ounces' cherry tomatoes, halved
- Salt and pepper

DIRECTIONS:

1. Bring 4 quarts' water to boil in a Dutch oven. Put in farro and 1 tablespoon salt, return to boil, and cook until grains are soft with slight chew, 15 to 30 minutes.
2. Drain farro, spread in rimmed baking sheet, and allow to cool completely, about fifteen minutes.
3. Beat oil, lemon juice, shallot, yogurt, ¼ teaspoon salt, and ¼ teaspoon pepper together in a big container.
4. Put in farro, cucumber, tomatoes, arugula, and mint and toss gently to combine. Sprinkle with salt and pepper to taste. Serve.

NUTRITION: Calories: 97 Carbs: 15g Fat: 4g Protein: 2g

495. Chorizo-Kidney Beans Quinoa Pilaf

Preparation time: 15 minutes
Cooking time: 37 minutes
Servings: 4

INGREDIENTS:

- ¼ pound dried Spanish chorizo diced (about 2/3 cup)
- ¼ teaspoon red pepper flakes
- ¼ teaspoon smoked paprika
- ½ teaspoon cumin
- ½ teaspoon sea salt
- 1 3/4 cups water
- 1 cup quinoa
- 1 large clove garlic minced
- 1 small red bell pepper finely diced
- 1 small red onion finely diced
- 1 tablespoon tomato paste
- 1 15-ounce can kidney beans rinsed and drained

DIRECTIONS:

1. Place a nonstick pot on medium high fire and heat for 2 minutes. Add chorizo and sauté for 5 minutes until lightly browned. Stir in peppers and onion. Sauté for 5 minutes.
2. Add tomato paste, red pepper flakes, salt, paprika, cumin, and garlic. Sauté for 2 minutes. Stir in quinoa and mix well. Sauté for 2 minutes.
3. Add water and beans. Mix well. Cover and simmer for 20 minutes or until liquid is fully absorbed. Turn off fire and fluff quinoa. Let it sit for 5 minutes more while uncovered. Serve and enjoy.

NUTRITION: Calories: 260 Protein: 9.6g Carbs: 40.9g Fat: 6.8g

496. Goat Cheese 'N Red Beans Salad

Preparation time: 15 minutes
Cooking time: 0 minutes
Servings: 6

INGREDIENTS:

- 2 cans of Red Kidney Beans, drained and rinsed well
- Water or vegetable broth to cover beans
- 1 bunch parsley, chopped
- 1 1/2 cups red grape tomatoes, halved
- 3 cloves garlic, minced
- 3 tablespoons olive oil
- 3 tablespoons lemon juice
- 1/2 teaspoon salt
- 1/2 teaspoon white pepper
- 6 ounces' goat cheese, crumbled

DIRECTIONS:

1. In a large bowl, combine beans, parsley, tomatoes and garlic. Add olive oil, lemon juice, salt and pepper.
2. Mix well and refrigerate until ready to serve. Spoon into individual dishes topped with crumbled goat cheese.

NUTRITION: Calories: 385 Protein: 22.5g Carbs: 44.0g Fat: 15.0g

497. Greek Farro Salad

Preparation time: 15 minutes
Cooking time: 20 minutes
Servings: 4

INGREDIENTS:

- Farro:
- ½ teaspoon fine-grain sea salt
- 1 cup farro, rinsed
- 1 tablespoon olive oil
- 2 garlic cloves, pressed or minced
- Salad:
- ½ small red onion, chopped and then rinsed under water to mellow the flavor
- 1 avocado, sliced into strips
- 1 cucumber, sliced into thin rounds
- 15 pitted Kalamata olives, sliced into rounds
- 1-pint cherry tomatoes, sliced into rounds
- 2 cups cooked chickpeas (or one 14-ounce can, rinsed and drained)
- 5 ounces mixed greens
- Lemon wedges
- Herbed Yogurt INGREDIENTS:
- 1/8 teaspoon salt
- 1 ¼ cups plain Greek yogurt
- 1 ½ tablespoon lightly packed fresh dill, roughly chopped
- 1 ½ tablespoon lightly packed fresh mint, torn into pieces
- 1 tablespoon lemon juice (about ½ lemon)
- 1 tablespoon olive oil

DIRECTIONS:

1. In a blender, blend and puree all herbed yogurt ingredients and set aside. Then cook the farro by placing in a pot filled halfway with water.
2. Bring to a boil, reduce fire to a simmer and cook for 15 minutes or until farro is tender. Drain well. Mix in salt, garlic, and olive oil and fluff to coat.
3. Evenly divide the cooled farro into 4 bowls. Evenly divide the salad ingredients on the 4 farro bowl. Top with ¼ of the yogurt dressing. Serve and enjoy.

NUTRITION: Calories: 428 Protein: 17.7g Carbs: 47.6g Fat: 24.5g

498. White Bean and Tuna Salad

Preparation time: 15 minutes
Cooking time: 8 minutes
Servings: 4

INGREDIENTS:

- 1 (12 ounce) can solid white albacore tuna, drained
- 1 (16 ounce) can Great Northern beans, drained and rinsed
- 1 (2.25 ounce) can sliced black olives, drained
- 1 teaspoon dried oregano
- 1/2 teaspoon finely grated lemon zest
- 1/4 medium red onion, thinly sliced
- 3 tablespoons lemon juice
- 3/4-pound pinto beans, trimmed and snapped in half
- 4 large hard-cooked eggs, peeled and quartered
- 6 tablespoons extra-virgin olive oil
- Salt and ground black pepper, to taste

DIRECTIONS:

1. Place a saucepan on medium high fire. Add a cup of water and the pinto beans. Cover and cook for 8 minutes. Drain immediately once tender.
2. In a salad bowl, whisk well oregano, olive oil, lemon juice, and lemon zest. Season generously with pepper and salt and mix until salt is dissolved.
3. Stir in drained pinto beans, tuna, beans, olives, and red onion. Mix thoroughly to coat. Adjust seasoning to taste. Spread eggs on top. Serve and enjoy.

NUTRITION: Calories: 551 Protein: 36.3g Carbs: 33.4g Fat: 30.3g

499. Spicy Sweet Red Hummus

Preparation time: 15 minutes
Cooking time: 0 minutes
Servings: 8

INGREDIENTS:

- 1 (15 ounce) can garbanzo beans, drained
- 1 (4 ounce) jar roasted red peppers
- 1 1/2 tablespoons tahini
- 1 clove garlic, minced
- 1 tablespoon chopped fresh parsley
- 1/2 teaspoon cayenne pepper
- 1/2 teaspoon ground cumin
- 1/4 teaspoon salt
- 3 tablespoons lemon juice

DIRECTIONS:

1. In a blender, add all ingredients and process until smooth and creamy. Adjust seasoning to taste if needed. Can be stored in an airtight container for up to 5 days.

NUTRITION: Calories: 64 Protein: 2.5g Carbs: 9.6g Fat: 2.2g

500. Black Bean Chili with Mangoes

Preparation time: 15 minutes
Cooking time: 10 minutes
Servings: 4

INGREDIENTS:

- 2 tablespoons coconut oil
- 1 onion, chopped
- 2 (15-ounce / 425-g) cans black beans, drained and rinsed
- 1 tablespoon chili powder
- 1 teaspoon sea salt
- ¼ teaspoon freshly ground black pepper
- 1 cup water
- 2 ripe mangoes, sliced thinly
- ¼ cup chopped fresh cilantro, divided
- ¼ cup sliced scallions, divided

DIRECTIONS:

1. Heat the coconut oil in a pot over high heat until melted. Put the onion in the pot and sauté for 5 minutes or until translucent.
2. Add the black beans to the pot. Sprinkle with chili powder, salt, and ground black pepper. Pour in the water. Stir to mix well.
3. Bring to a boil. Reduce the heat to low, then simmering for 5 minutes or until the beans are tender. Turn off the heat and mix in the mangoes, then garnish with scallions and cilantro before serving.

NUTRITION: Calories: 430 Fat: 9.1g Protein: 20.2g Carbs: 71.9g

501. Israeli Style Eggplant and Chickpea Salad

Preparation time: 5 minutes
Cooking time: 20 minutes
Servings: 6

INGREDIENTS:

- 2 tablespoons balsamic vinegar
- 2 tablespoons freshly squeezed lemon juice
- 1 teaspoon ground cumin
- ¼ teaspoon sea salt
- 2 tablespoons olive oil, divided
- 1 (1-pound / 454-g) medium globe eggplant, stem removed, cut into flat cubes (about ½ inch thick)
- 1 (15-ounce / 425-g) can chickpeas, drained and rinsed
- ¼ cup chopped mint leaves
- 1 cup sliced sweet onion
- 1 garlic clove, finely minced
- 1 tablespoon sesame seeds, toasted

DIRECTIONS:

1. Preheat the oven to 550°f (288°c) or the highest level of your oven or broiler. Grease a baking sheet with 1 tablespoon of olive oil.
2. Combine the balsamic vinegar, lemon juice, cumin, salt, and 1 tablespoon of olive oil in a small bowl. Stir to mix well.
3. Arrange the eggplant cubes on the baking sheet, then brush with 2 tablespoons of the balsamic vinegar mixture on both sides.
4. Broil in the preheated oven for 8 minutes or until lightly browned. Flip the cubes halfway through the cooking time.
5. Meanwhile, combine the chickpeas, mint, onion, garlic, and sesame seeds in a large serving bowl. Drizzle with remaining balsamic vinegar mixture. Stir to mix well.
6. Remove the eggplant from the oven. Allow to cool for 5 minutes, then slice them into ½-inch strips on a clean work surface.
7. Add the eggplant strips in the serving bowl, then toss to combine well before serving.

NUTRITION: Calories: 125 Fat: 2.9g Protein: 5.2g Carbs: 20.9g

502. Italian Sautéed Cannellini Beans

Preparation time: 15 minutes
Cooking time: 15 minutes
Servings: 6

INGREDIENTS:

- 2 teaspoons extra-virgin olive oil
- ½ cup minced onion
- ¼ cup red wine vinegar
- 1 (12-ounce / 340-g) can no-salt-added tomato paste
- 2 tablespoons raw honey
- ½ cup water
- ¼ teaspoon ground cinnamon
- 2 (15-ounce / 425-g) cans cannellini beans

DIRECTIONS:

1. Heat the olive oil in a saucepan over medium heat until shimmering. Add the onion and sauté for 5 minutes or until translucent.

2. Pour in the red wine vinegar, tomato paste, honey, and water. Sprinkle with cinnamon. Stir to mix well.
3. Reduce the heat to low, then pour all the beans into the saucepan. Cook for 10 more minutes. Stir constantly. Serve immediately.

NUTRITION: Calories: 435 Fat: 2.1g Protein: 26.2g Carbs: 80.3g

503. Lentil and Vegetable Curry Stew

Preparation time: 15 minutes
Cooking time: 4 hours & 7 minutes
Servings: 8

INGREDIENTS:

- 1 tablespoon coconut oil
- 1 yellow onion, diced
- ¼ cup yellow Thai curry paste
- 2 cups unsweetened coconut milk
- 2 cups dry red lentils, rinsed well and drained
- 3 cups bite-sized cauliflower florets
- 2 golden potatoes, cut into chunks
- 2 carrots, peeled and diced
- 8 cups low-sodium vegetable soup, divided
- 1 bunch kale, stems removed and roughly chopped
- Sea salt, to taste
- ½ cup fresh cilantro, chopped
- Pinch crushed red pepper flakes

DIRECTIONS:

1. Heat the coconut oil in a nonstick skillet over medium-high heat until melted. Add the onion and sauté for 5 minutes or until translucent.
2. Pour in the curry paste and sauté for another 2 minutes, then fold in the coconut milk and stir to combine well. Bring to a simmer and turn off the heat.
3. Put the lentils, cauliflower, potatoes, and carrot in the slow cooker. Pour in 6 cups of vegetable soup and the curry mixture. Stir to combine well.
4. Cover and cook on high for 4 hours or until the lentils and vegetables are soft. Stir periodically.
5. During the last 30 minutes, fold the kale in the slow cooker and pour in the remaining vegetable soup. Sprinkle with salt.
6. Pour the stew in a large serving bowl and spread the cilantro and red pepper flakes on top before serving hot.

NUTRITION: Calories: 530 Fat: 19.2g Protein: 20.3g Carbs: 75.2g

504. Lush Moroccan Chickpea, Vegetable, and Fruit Stew

Preparation time: 15 minutes
Cooking time: 6 hours & 4 minutes
Servings: 6

INGREDIENTS:

- 1 large bell pepper, any color, chopped
- 6 ounces (170 g) pinto beans, trimmed and cut into bite-size pieces
- 3 cups canned chickpeas, rinsed and drained
- 1 (15-ounce / 425-g) can diced tomatoes, with the juice
- 1 large carrot, cut into ¼-inch rounds
- 2 large potatoes, peeled and cubed
- 1 large yellow onion, chopped

- 1 teaspoon grated fresh ginger
- 2 garlic cloves, minced
- 1¾ cups low-sodium vegetable soup
- 1 teaspoon ground cumin
- 1 tablespoon ground coriander
- ¼ teaspoon ground red pepper flakes
- Sea salt and ground black pepper, to taste
- 8 ounces (227 g) fresh baby spinach
- ¼ cup diced dried figs
- ¼ cup diced dried apricots
- 1 cup plain Greek yogurt

DIRECTIONS:

1. Place the bell peppers, pinto beans, chicken peas, tomatoes and juice, carrot, potatoes, onion, ginger, and garlic in the slow cooker.
2. Pour in the vegetable soup and sprinkle with cumin, coriander, red pepper flakes, salt, and ground black pepper. Stir to mix well.
3. Put the slow cooker lid on and cook on high for 6 hours or until the vegetables are soft. Stir periodically. Open the lid and fold in the spinach, figs, apricots, and yogurt. Stir to mix well.
4. Cook for 4 minutes or until the spinach is wilted. Pour them in a large serving bowl. Allow to cool for at least 20 minutes, then serve warm.

NUTRITION: Calories: 611 Fat: 9.0g Protein: 30.7g Carbs: 107.4g

505. Smoked Salmon Goat Cheese Endive Bites

Preparation time: 15 minutes
Cooking time: 0 minutes
Servings: 4
INGREDIENTS:

- 1 package herbed goat cheese
- 3 endive heads
- 1 package smoked wild salmon

DIRECTIONS:

1. Pull the leaves apart from endives and cut the ends off of them. Add goat cheese to endive leaves. Add salmon slices on top of the goat cheese. Serve.

NUTRITION: Calories: 46 Carbs: 1g Fat: 3g Protein: 3g

506. Baked tofu

Preparation time: 10 Minutes
Cooking time: 10 minutes
Servings: 4
Ingredients:

- 250 g Japanese tofu
- 100 g of wheat flour
- 2 tablespoons oil
- 100g Daikon radish (Japanese radish)
- 1 piece of fresh ginger
- Japanese soy sauce

Directions:

1. Dip the tofu briefly in cold water.
2. Drain, dab thoroughly and carefully cut into 8 equal cubes.
3. Turn the tofu pieces in flour and bake in hot oil in a pan on each side for about 1 minute over medium heat until golden brown.
4. Peel the radish and ginger and finely grate each separately. Squeeze out the radish and form four equal portions out of it by hand.
5. Arrange 2 pieces of tofu on each plate. Place a portion of radish next to each and decorate the top with ginger. Serve with a bowl of Japanese soy sauce.

Nutrition: Calories: 149 Fat: 11.5g Carbs: 8.9g Protein: 2.4g

507. Cheesy Cauliflower Frittata

Preparation time: 10 minutes
Cooking time: 30 minutes
Servings: 4
Ingredients:

- 2 tbsp. olive oil
- 1/2 lb. cauliflower florets
- 1/2 cup skimmed milk
- 6 eggs
- 1 red bell pepper, seeded and chopped
- 1/2 cup Fontina cheese, grated
- 1/2 tsp. red pepper

- 1/2 tsp. turmeric
- Salt and black pepper to taste

Directions

1. Preheat oven to 360 F. In a bowl, beat the eggs with milk. Add in Fontina cheese, red pepper, turmeric, salt, and pepper. Mix in red bell pepper. Warmth olive oil in a skillet and pours in the egg mixture; cook for 4-5 minutes. Set aside.
2. Blanch the cauliflower florets in a pot for 5 minutes until tender. Spread over the egg mixture. Set the skillet and bake for 15 minutes or until it is set and golden brown. Allow cooling before slicing. Serve sliced.

Nutrition: Calories 123 Fat 11 g Total Carbs 7 gTotal Sugars 1 g Protein 14 g Potassium 245 mg

508. Cilantro Mozzarella and Olive Cakes

Preparation time: 10 minutes
Cooking time: 25 minutes
Servings: 6
Ingredients:

- 1/4 cup black olives
- 1/2 cup low-fat milk
- 4 tbsp. coconut oil, softened
- 1 egg, beaten
- 1 cup corn flour
- 1 tsp. baking powder
- 3 sun-dried tomatoes, finely chopped
- 2 tbsp. fresh parsley, chopped
- 2 tbsp. fresh cilantro, chopped
- 1/4 tsp. kosher salt

Directions

1. Preheat oven to 360 F. In a bowl, whisk the egg with milk and coconut oil. In a separate bowl, mix the salt, corn flour, cilantro, and baking powder.
2. Combine the wet ingredients with the dry mixture. Stir in black olives, tomatoes and herbs. Set the mixture into greased ramekins and bake for around 18-20 minutes or until cooked and golden.

Nutrition: Calories: 323 Fat: 11 g Carbs: 6 g Protein: 14.3 g

509. Mushroom and Quinoa Cups

Preparation time: 10 minutes
Cooking time: 30 minutes
Servings: 6
Ingredients:

- 6 eggs
- 1 cup quinoa, cooked
- Salt and black pepper to taste
- 1 cup Gruyere cheese, grated
- 1 small yellow onion, chopped
- 1 cup mushrooms, sliced
- 1/2 cup green olives, chopped

Directions

1. Beat the eggs, salt, pepper, Gruyere cheese, onion, mushrooms, and green olives in a bowl.
2. Set into a silicone muffin tray and bake for 30 minutes at 360 F. Serve warm.

Nutrition: Calories 233 Fat 12 g Total Carbs 4 g Total Sugars 2 g Protein 21 g Potassium 213 mg

510. Zucchini and Mushroom Egg Cakes

Preparation time: 10 minutes
Cooking time: 15 minutes
Servings: 4
Ingredients:

- 1 onion, chopped
- 1 cup mushrooms, sliced
- 1 red bell pepper, chopped
- 1 zucchini, chopped
- Salt and black pepper to taste
- 8 eggs, whisked
- 1 tbsp. olive oil
- 2 tbsp. chives, chopped

Directions

1. Preheat the oven to 360 F. Warm the olive oil in a skillet over medium heat and sauté onion, zucchini, mushrooms, salt, and pepper for 5 minutes until tender. Distribute the mixture across muffin cups and top with the eggs.
2. Sprinkle with salt, pepper, and chives and bake for 10 minutes. Serve immediately.

Nutrition: Calories: 245 Fat: 12 g Carbs: 2 g Protein: 12.8 g

511. Cinnamon and Coconut Porridge

Preparation time: 5 minutes
Cooking time: 5 minutes
Servings: 4
Ingredients:

- 1 cup water
- 1/2 cup 36-percent low-fat cream
- 1/2 cup unsweetened dried coconut, shredded
- 1 tablespoon oat bran
- 1 tablespoon flaxseed meal
- 1/2 tablespoon almond butter
- 1 1/2 teaspoons stevia
- 1/2 teaspoon cinnamon
- Toppings, such as blueberries or banana slices

Directions:

1. Add the ingredients to a small pot and mix well until fully incorporated. Transfer the pot to your stove over medium-low heat and bring the mix to a slow boil.
2. Stir well and remove from the heat. Divide the mixture into equal servings and let them sit for 10 minutes. Top with your desired toppings and enjoy!

Nutrition: Calories 276 Fat 21 Total Carbs 3 g Total Sugars 1.5g Protein 13.9g Potassium 342 mg

512. Banana Steel Oats

Preparation time: 10 minutes
Cooking time: 10 minutes
Servings: 3
Ingredients:

- 1 small banana
- 1 cup almond milk
- 1/4 teaspoon cinnamon, ground
- 1/2 cup rolled oats
- 1 tablespoon honey

Directions:

1. Take a saucepan and add half the banana, whisk in almond milk, ground cinnamon. Season with sunflower seeds.
2. Stir until the banana is mashed well, bring the mixture to a boil and stir in oats. Set heat to medium-low and simmer for 5-7 minutes until the oats are tender. Dice the remaining half of banana and put on the top of the oatmeal. Enjoy!

Nutrition: Calories 244 Fat 11 Total Carbs 2 gTotal Sugars 2 g Protein 13 g

513. Crunchy Flax and Almond Crackers

Preparation time: 15 minutes
Cooking time: 60 minutes
Servings: 12
Ingredients:

- 1/2 cup ground flaxseeds
- 1/2 cup almond flour
- 1 tablespoon coconut flour
- 2 tablespoons shelled hemp seeds
- 1/4 teaspoon sunflower seeds
- 1 egg white
- 2 tablespoons unsalted almond butter, melted

Directions:

1. Warmth your oven to 300 degrees F. Line a baking sheet with parchment paper, keep it on the side. Add flax, almond, coconut flour, hemp seed, seeds to a bowl and mix. Add egg white and melted almond butter, mix until combined.
2. Set dough to a sheet of parchment paper and cover with another sheet of paper. Roll out dough. Cut into crackers and bake for 60 minutes. Let them cool and enjoy!

Nutrition: Calories 143 Fat 11 g Total Carbs 3 g Total Sugars 1.7 g Protein 11 g

514. Quinoa and Cinnamon Bowl

Preparation time: 10 minutes
Cooking time: 15 minutes
Servings: 2
Ingredients:

- 1 cup uncooked quinoa
- 11/2 cups water
- 1/2 teaspoon ground cinnamon
- 1/2 teaspoon sunflower seeds
- A drizzle of almond/coconut milk for serving

Directions:

1. Rinse quinoa thoroughly underwater. Take a medium-sized saucepan and add quinoa, water, cinnamon, and seeds. Stir and

place it over medium-high heat. Bring the mix to a boil. Set heat to low and simmer.

2. Once cooked, detach from the heat and let it cool. Serve with a drizzle of almond or coconut milk. Enjoy!

Nutrition: Calories: 165 Fat: 9 g Carbs: 3 g Protein: 9 g

515. Quinoa and Date Bowl

Preparation time: 10 minutes
Cooking time: 15 minutes
Servings: 2
Ingredients:

- 1 date, pitted and chopped finely
- 1/2 cup red quinoa, dried
- 1 cup unsweetened almond milk
- 1/8 teaspoon vanilla extract
- 1/4 cup fresh strawberries
- 1/8 teaspoon ground cinnamon

Directions:

1. Take a pan and place it over low heat. Add quinoa, almond milk, cinnamon, vanilla, and cook for about 15 minutes, making sure to keep stirring from time to time.
2. Garnish with strawberries and enjoy!

Nutrition: Calories: 323 Fat: 11 g Carbs: 6 g Protein: 14.3 g

516. Chickpea Snack Mix

Preparation time: 10 minutes
Cooking time: 30 minutes
Servings: 8
Ingredients:

- 1 cup roasted chickpeas, drained
- 2 tablespoons coconut oil, melted
- 1/4 cup raw pumpkin seeds
- 1/4 cup raw pecan halves
- 1/3 cup dried cherries

Directions

1. Pat the chickpeas dry using paper towels. Drizzle coconut oil over the chickpeas.
2. Roast the chickpeas in the preheated oven at 380 degrees F for about 20 minutes, tossing them once or twice.
3. Toss your chickpeas with the pumpkin seeds and pecan halves. Continue baking until the nuts are fragrant about 8 minutes; let cool completely.
4. Add in the dried cherries and stir to combine. Bon appétit!

Nutrition: Calories: 109 Fat: 7.9g; Carbs: 7.4g; Protein: 3.4g

517. Muhammara Dip with a Twist

Preparation time: 10 minutes
Cooking time: 35 minutes
Servings: 9
Ingredients:

- 3 red bell peppers
- 5 tablespoons olive oil
- 2 garlic cloves, chopped
- 1 tomato, chopped
- 3/4 cup bread crumbs
- 2 tablespoons molasses
- 1 teaspoon ground cumin

- 1/4 sunflower seeds, toasted
- 1 Maras pepper, minced
- 2 tablespoons tahini
- Sea salt and red pepper, to taste

Directions

1. Set by preheating your oven to 400 degrees F.
2. Set the peppers on a parchment-lined baking pan. Bake for about 30 minutes; peel the peppers and transfer them to your food processor.
3. Meanwhile, heat 2 tablespoons of the olive oil in a frying pan over medium-high heat. Sauté the garlic and tomatoes for about 5 minutes or until they've softened.
4. Add the sautéed vegetables to your food processor. Attach in the remaining ingredients and process until creamy and smooth.
5. Bon appétit!

Nutrition: Calories: 149 Fat: 11.5g Carbs: 8.9g Protein: 2.4g

518. Spinach, Chickpea and Garlic Crostini

Preparation time: 10 minutes
Cooking time: 10 minutes
Servings: 6
Ingredients:

- 1 baguette, cut into slices
- 4 tablespoons extra-virgin olive oil
- Sea salt and red pepper, to season
- 3 garlic cloves, minced
- 1 cup boiled chickpeas, drained
- 2 cups spinach
- 1 tablespoon fresh lemon juice

Directions

1. Preheat your broiler.
2. Brush the slices of bread with 2 tablespoons of the olive oil and sprinkle with sea salt and red pepper. Place under the preheated broiler for about 2 minutes or until lightly toasted.
3. In a mixing bowl, thoroughly combine the garlic, chickpeas, spinach, lemon juice and the remaining 2 tablespoons of the olive oil.
4. Spoon the chickpea mixture onto each toast. Bon appétit!

Nutrition: Calories: 242 Fat: 6.1g Carbs: 38.5g Protein: 8.9g

519. Mushroom and Cannellini Bean "Meatballs"

Preparation time: 10 minutes
Cooking time: 15 minutes
Servings: 4
Ingredients:

- 4 tablespoons olive oil
- 1 cup button mushrooms, chopped
- 1 shallot, chopped
- 2 garlic cloves, crushed
- 1 cup canned or boiled cannellini beans, drained
- 1 cup quinoa, cooked
- Sea salt and ground black pepper, to flavor
- 1 teaspoon smoked paprika

- 1/2 teaspoon red pepper flakes
- 1 teaspoon mustard seeds
- 1/2 teaspoon dried dill

Directions
1. Set 2 tablespoons of the olive oil in a nonstick skillet. Once hot, cook the mushrooms and shallot for 3 minutes or until just tender.
2. Add in the garlic, beans, quinoa and spices. Mix to combine well and then, shape the mixture into equal balls using oiled hands.
3. Then, heat the remaining 2 tablespoons of the olive oil in a nonstick skillet over medium heat. Once hot, fry the meatballs for about 10 minutes until golden brown on all sides.
4. Serve with cocktail sticks. Bon appétit!

Nutrition: Calories: 195 Fat: 14.1g Carbs: 13.2g Protein: 3.9g

520. Cucumber Rounds with Hummus

Preparation time: 10 minutes
Cooking time: 0 minutes
Servings: 6
Ingredients:

- 1 cup hummus, preferably homemade
- 2 large tomatoes, diced
- 1/2 teaspoon red pepper flakes
- Sea salt and ground black pepper, to flavor
- 2 English cucumbers, sliced into rounds

Directions
1. Divide the hummus dip between the cucumber rounds.
2. Top them with tomatoes; sprinkle red pepper flakes, salt and black pepper over each cucumber.
3. Serve well chilled and enjoy!

Nutrition: Calories: 88 Fat: 3.6g Carbs: 11.3g Protein: 2.6g

521. Stuffed Jalapeño Bites

Preparation time: 10 minutes
Cooking time: 15 minutes
Servings: 6
Ingredients:

- 1/2 cup raw sunflower seeds, soaked overnight and drained
- 4 tablespoons scallions, chopped
- 1 teaspoon garlic, minced
- 3 tablespoons nutritional yeast
- 1/2 cup cream of onion soup
- 1/2 teaspoon cayenne pepper
- 1/2 teaspoon mustard seeds
- 12 jalapeños, halved and seeded
- 1/2 cup breadcrumbs

Directions
1. In your food processor or high-speed blender, blitz raw sunflower seeds, scallions, garlic, nutritional yeast, soup, cayenne pepper and mustard seeds until well combined.
2. Spoon the mixture into the jalapeños and top them with the breadcrumbs.
3. Bake in the preheated oven. Serve warm.
4. Bon appétit!

Nutrition: Calories: 108 Fat: 6.6g Carbs: 7.3g Protein: 5.3g

522. Mexican-Style Onion Rings

Preparation time: 10 minutes
Cooking time: 35 minutes
Servings: 6
Ingredients:

- 2 medium onions, cut into rings
- 1/4 cup all-purpose flour
- 1/4 cup spelt flour
- 1/3 cup rice milk, unsweetened
- 1/3 cup ale beer
- Sea salt and ground black pepper, to flavor
- 1/2 teaspoon cayenne pepper
- 1/2 teaspoon mustard seeds
- 1 cup tortilla chips, crushed
- 1 tablespoon olive oil

Directions
1. Start by preheating your oven to 420 degrees F.
2. In a shallow bowl, mix the flour, milk and beer.
3. In another shallow bowl, mix the spices with the crushed tortilla chips. Set the onion rings in the flour mixture.
4. Then, roll them over the spiced mixture, pressing down to coat well.
5. Arrange the onion rings on a parchment-lined baking pan. Brush them with olive oil and bake for approximately 30 minutes. Bon appétit!

Nutrition: Calories: 213 Fat: 10.6g Carbs: 26.2g Protein: 4.3g

523. Roasted Root Vegetables

Preparation time: 10 minutes
Cooking time: 35 minutes
Servings: 6
Ingredients:

- 1/4 cup olive oil
- 2 carrots, peeled and cut
- 2 parsnips, peeled and cut
- 1 celery stalk, peeled and cut
- 1 pound sweet potatoes, peeled and cut
- 1/4 cup olive oil
- 1 teaspoon mustard seeds
- 1/2 teaspoon basil
- 1/2 teaspoon oregano
- 1 teaspoon red pepper flakes
- 1 teaspoon dried thyme
- Sea salt and ground black pepper, to flavor

Directions
1. Toss the vegetables with the remaining ingredients until well coated.
2. Roast the vegetables in the preheated oven at 400 degrees F for about 35 minutes, stirring halfway through the cooking time.
3. Taste, adjust the seasonings and serve warm. Bon appétit!

Nutrition: Calories: 261 Fat: 18.2g Carbs: 23.3g Protein: 2.3g

524. Indian-Style Hummus Dip

Preparation time: 10 minutes
Cooking time: 0 minutes
Servings: 6

Ingredients:

- 20 ounces canned or boiled chickpeas, drained
- 1 teaspoon garlic, sliced
- 1/4 cup tahini
- 1/4 cup olive oil
- 1 lime, freshly squeezed
- 1/4 teaspoon turmeric
- 1/2 teaspoon cumin powder
- 1 teaspoon curry powder
- 1 teaspoon coriander seeds
- 1/4 cup chickpea liquid, or more, as needed
- 2 tablespoons fresh cilantro, roughly chopped

Directions

1. Blitz the chickpeas, garlic, tahini, olive oil, lime, turmeric, cumin, curry powder and coriander seeds in your blender or food processor.
2. Blend until your desired consistency is reached, gradually adding the chickpea liquid.
3. Place in your refrigerator until ready to serve. Garnish with fresh cilantro.
4. Serve with naan bread or veggie sticks, if desired. Bon appétit!

Nutrition: Calories: 171 Fat: 10.4g Carbs: 15.3g; Protein: 5.4g

525. Roasted Carrot and Bean Dip

Preparation time: 10 minutes
Cooking time: 50 minutes
Servings: 10

Ingredients:

- 1 1/2 pounds carrots, trimmed
- 2 tablespoons olive oil
- 4 tablespoons tahini
- 8 ounces canned cannellini beans, drained
- 1 teaspoon garlic, chopped
- 2 tablespoons lemon juice
- 2 tablespoons soy sauce
- Sea salt and ground black pepper, to flavor
- 1/2 teaspoon paprika
- 1/2 teaspoon dried dill
- 1/4 cup pepitas, toasted

Directions

1. Set by preheating your oven to 390 degrees F. Line a roasting pans with parchment paper.
2. Now, toss the carrots with the olive oil and arrange them on the prepared roasting pan.
3. Roast the carrots for about 50 minutes or until tender. Transfer the roasted carrots to the bowl of your food processor.
4. Add in the tahini, beans, garlic, lemon juice, soy sauce, salt, black pepper, paprika and dill. Process until your dip is creamy and uniform.
5. Garnish with toasted pepitas and serve with dippers of choice. Bon appétit!

Nutrition: Calories: 121 Fat: 8.3g Carbs: 11.2g Protein: 2.8g

SNACK & DESSERT

526. Nacho Cheese

Preparation time: 10 minutes
Cooking time: 15 minutes
Servings: 4

Ingredients:

- 2 cups peeled chopped russet potatoes
- 1 cup chopped carrots
- 1/2 to 3/4 cup water
- 1 tablespoon freshly squeezed lemon juice
- 1/2 cup nutritional yeast
- 1/2 teaspoon onion powder
- 1/2 teaspoon garlic powder
- 1 teaspoon salt
- 1/4 cup Super-Simple Salsa (here) or store bought (optional)

Directions:

1. Stew the potatoes and carrots until soft, about 15 minutes.
2. Put 1/2 cup of water into a blender, followed by the lemon juice, nutritional yeast, onion powder, garlic powder, salt, and salsa (if using). Blend until completely smooth. If the consistency is too thick, add the remaining 1/4 cup of water to thin it out.

Nutrition: Calories: 237 Fat: 1g Protein: 13g Sodium: 724mg Fiber: 11g

527. Mushroom Gravy

Preparation time: 10 minutes
Cooking time: 10 minutes
Servings: 4

Ingredients:

- 1 tablespoon oil
- 1 small yellow onion, diced
- 1 cup finely chopped button mushrooms
- 11/2 teaspoons minced garlic (3 cloves)
- 4 tablespoons flour
- 11/4 cups water
- 1 tablespoon soy sauce
- 1/2 teaspoon dried oregano
- 2 bay leaves
- Freshly ground black pepper

Directions:

1. Warmth the oil in a saucepan, then attach the onion, mushrooms, and garlic. Sauté until the onions are translucent.
2. Attach the flour and mix to form a thick paste.
3. Add the water, soy sauce, oregano, and bay leaves, and bring to a simmer over medium heat. Season with pepper.
4. Remove the bay leaves. Use a whisk to gently merge the gravy until it thickens. Add more water if you prefer thinner gravy.

Nutrition: Calories: 79 Fat: 4g Protein: 2g Sodium: 230mg Fiber: 1g

528. The Greatest Guacamole

Preparation time: 10 minutes
Cooking time: 0 minutes
Servings: 4

Ingredients:

- 2 large avocados, halved, peeled, and roughly chopped
- Juice of 1/2 lime
- 2 teaspoons olive oil
- 1/4 red onion, finely diced
- 1/2 teaspoon minced garlic (1 clove)
- 1/2 teaspoon ground cumin
- 1 tablespoon freshly chopped cilantro
- 1/2 Roma tomato, diced
- Pinch salt
- Freshly ground black pepper

Directions:

1. Mash the avocados to the desired consistency in a medium-size bowl.
2. Add the lime juice and oil. Stir in the red onion, garlic, cumin, cilantro, and tomato, then season with salt and pepper.

Nutrition: Calories: 233 Fat: 22g Protein: 2g Sodium: 48mg Fiber: 7g

529. Super Simple Salsa

Preparation time: 10 minutes
Cooking time: 0 minutes
Servings: 4

Ingredients:

- 2 cups chopped tomatoes
- 1/2 cup diced yellow onion
- 2 tablespoons minced cilantro
- Juice of 1/2 lime, plus more for seasoning (optional)
- 1 jalapeño pepper, seeded and chopped
- 1/2 teaspoon ground cumin
- Pinch salt
- Freshly ground black pepper

Directions:

1. Combine the tomatoes, onion, cilantro, lime juice, jalapeño, and cumin in a bowl; mix well.
2. Flavor with salt and pepper, and add more lime juice (if using).

Nutrition: Calories: 25 Fat: 1g Protein: 1g Sodium: 46mg Fiber: 2g

530. Cashew Cream

Preparation time: 5 minutes
Cooking time: 0 minutes
Servings: 4

Ingredients:

- 1 cup raw cashews,
- 1/2 cup water
- 1/4 teaspoon salt
- Freshly ground black pepper

Directions:
1. Place the soaked cashews, water, and salt in a high-speed blender or food processor; blend until completely smooth.
2. Season with pepper.

Nutrition: Calories: 197 Fat: 16g Protein: 5g Sodium: 154mg Fiber: 1g

531. Spinach Dip

Preparation Time: 20 Minutes
Cooking Time: 5 Minutes
Servings: 8
Ingredients:
- ¾ cup cashews
- 3.5 ounces' soft tofu
- 6 ounces of spinach leaves
- 1 medium white onion, peeled, diced
- 2 teaspoons minced garlic
- ½ teaspoon salt
- 3 tablespoons olive oil

Directions:
1. Place cashews in a bowl, cover with hot water, and then let them soak for 15 minutes.
2. After 15 minutes, drain the cashews and then set aside until required.
3. Take a medium skillet pan, add oil to it and then place the pan over medium heat.
4. Add onion, cook for 3 to 5 minutes until tender, stir in garlic and then continue cooking for 30 seconds until fragrant.
5. Spoon the onion mixture into a blender, add remaining ingredients and then pulse until smooth.
6. Tip the dip into a bowl and then serve with chips.

Nutrition: Calories: 134.6 Cal;Fat: 8.6 g; Protein: 10 g; Carbs: 6.3 g; Fiber: 1.4 g

532. Tomatillo Salsa

Preparation Time: 5 Minutes
Cooking Time: 15 Minutes
Servings: 8
Ingredients:
- 5 medium tomatillos, chopped
- 3 cloves of garlic, peeled, chopped
- 3 Roma tomatoes, chopped
- 1 jalapeno, chopped
- ½ of a medium red onion, peeled, chopped
- 1 Anaheim chili
- 2 teaspoons salt
- 1 teaspoon ground cumin
- 1 lime, juiced
- ¼ cup cilantro leaves
- ¾ cup of water

Directions:
1. Take a medium pot, place it over medium heat, pour in water, and then add onion, tomatoes, tomatillo, jalapeno, and Anaheim chili.
2. Sauté the vegetables for 15 minutes, remove the pot from heat, add cilantro and lime juice and then stir in salt.
3. Remove pot from heat and then pulse by using an immersion blender until smooth.
4. Serve the salsa with chips.

Nutrition: Calories: 317.4 Cal; Fat: 0 g; Protein: 16 g; Carbs: 64 g; Fiber: 16 g

533. Arugula Pesto Couscous

Preparation Time: 10 Minutes
Cooking Time: 20 Minutes
Servings: 4
Ingredients:
- 8 ounces' Israeli couscous
- 3 large tomatoes, chopped
- 3 cups arugula leaves
- ½ cup parsley leaves
- 6 cloves of garlic, peeled
- ½ cup walnuts
- ¾ teaspoon salt
- 1 cup and 1 tablespoon olive oil
- 2 cups vegetable broth

Directions:
1. Take a medium saucepan, place it over medium-high heat, add 1 tablespoon oil and then let it heat.
2. Add couscous, stir until mixed, and then cook for 4 minutes until fragrant and toasted.
3. Pour in the broth, stir until mixed, bring it to a boil, switch heat to medium level and then simmer for 12 minutes until the couscous has absorbed all the liquid and turn tender.
4. When done, remove the pan from heat, fluff it with a fork, and then set aside until required.
5. While couscous cooks, prepare the pesto, and for this, place walnuts in a blender, add garlic, and then pulse until nuts have broken.
6. Add arugula, parsley, and salt, pulse until well combined, and then blend in oil until smooth.
7. Transfer couscous to a salad bowl, add tomatoes and prepared pesto, and then toss until mixed.
8. Serve straight away.

Nutrition: Calories: 73 Cal; Fat: 4 g; Protein: 2 g; Carbs: 8 g; Fiber: 2 g

534. Pico de Gallo

Preparation Time: 5 Minutes
Cooking Time: 0 Minutes
Servings: 6
Ingredients:
- ½ of a medium red onion, peeled, chopped
- 2 cups diced tomato
- ½ cup chopped cilantro
- 1 jalapeno pepper, minced
- 1/8 teaspoon salt
- ¼ teaspoon ground black pepper
- ½ of a lime, juiced
- 1 teaspoon olive oil

Directions:
1. Take a large bowl, place all the ingredients in it and then stir until well mixed.
2. Serve the Pico de Gallo with chips.

Nutrition: Calories: 790 Cal; Fat: 6.4 g; Protein: 25.6 g; Carbs: 195.2 g; Fiber: 35.2 g

535. Beet Balls

Preparation Time: 10 Minutes
Cooking Time: 0 Minutes
Servings: 6

Ingredients:

- ½ cup oats
- 1 medium beet, cooked
- ½ cup almond flour
- 1/3 cup shredded coconut and more for coating
- ¾ cup Medjool dates, pitted
- 1 tablespoon cocoa powder
- ¼ cup chocolate chips, unsweetened

Directions:

1. Place cooked beets in a blender and then pulse until chopped into very small pieces.
2. Add remaining ingredients and then pulse until the dough comes together.
3. Shape the dough into eighteen balls, coat them in some more coconut and then serve.

Nutrition: Calories: 114.2 Cal; Fat: 2.4 g; Protein: 5 g; Carbs: 19.6 g; Fiber: 4.9 g

536. Cheesy Crackers

Preparation Time: 10 Minutes
Cooking Time: 20 Minutes
Servings: 3

Ingredients:

- 1 ¾ cup almond meal
- 3 tablespoons nutritional yeast
- ½ teaspoon of sea salt
- 2 tablespoons lemon juice
- 1 tablespoon melted coconut oil
- 1 tablespoon ground flaxseed
- 2 ½ tablespoons water

Directions:

1. Switch on the oven, then set it to 350 degrees F and let it preheat.
2. Meanwhile, take a medium bowl, place flaxseed in it, stir in water, and then let the mixture rest for 5 minutes until thickened.
3. Place almond meal in a medium bowl, add salt and yeast and then stir until mixed.
4. Add lemon juice and oil into the flaxseed mixture and then whisk until mixed.
5. Pour the flaxseed mixture into the almond meal mixture and then stir until dough comes together.
6. Place a piece of a wax paper on a clean working space, place the dough on it, cover with another piece of wax paper, and then roll dough into a 1/8-inch-thick crust.
7. Cut the dough into a square shape, sprinkle salt over the top and then bake for 15 to 20 minutes until done. Serve straight away.

Nutrition: Calories: 30 Cal; Fat: 1 g; Protein: 1 g; Carbs: 5 g; Fiber: 0 g

537. Tomato Soup

Preparation Time: 10 Minutes
Cooking Time: 10 Minutes
Servings: 2

Ingredients:

- 56 ounces stewed tomatoes
- ¼ teaspoon salt
- ¼ teaspoon ground black pepper
- 1 medium red bell pepper, cored, diced
- ¼ teaspoon dried thyme
- 6 leaves of basil, chopped
- ¼ teaspoon dried oregano
- 1 teaspoon olive oil

Directions:

1. Take a medium pot, place it over medium heat, add oil, and when hot, add bell pepper and then cook for 4 minutes.
2. Add remaining ingredients into the pot, stir until mixed, switch heat to medium-high heat, and bring the mixture to simmer.
3. Remove pot from the heat and then puree the soup until smooth.
4. Taste to adjust seasoning, ladle soup into bowls and then serve.

Nutrition: Calories: 170 Cal; Fat: 1.1 g; Protein: 3.5 g; Carbs: 36 g; Fiber: 2.6 g

538. Meatballs Platter

Preparation Time: 10 Minutes
Cooking Time: 15 Minutes
Servings: 4

Ingredients:

- 1-pound beef meat, ground
- ¼ cup panko breadcrumbs
- A pinch of salt and black pepper
- 3 tablespoons red onion, grated
- ¼ cup parsley, chopped
- 2 garlic cloves, minced
- 2 tablespoons lemon juice
- Zest of 1 lemon, grated
- 1 egg
- ½ teaspoon cumin, ground
- ½ teaspoon coriander, ground
- ¼ teaspoon cinnamon powder
- 2 ounces' feta cheese, crumbled
- Cooking spray

Directions:

1. In a bowl, blend the beef with the breadcrumbs, salt, pepper and the rest of the ingredients except the cooking spray, stir well and shape medium balls out of this mix.
2. Arrange the meatballs on a baking sheet lined with parchment paper, grease them with cooking spray and bake at 450 degrees F for 15 minutes.
3. Position the meatballs on a platter and serve as a snack.

Nutrition: Calories: 300, Fat: 15.4, Fiber: 6.4, Carbs: 22.4, Protein: 35

539. Yogurt Dip

Preparation Time: 10 Minutes
Cooking Time: 0 Minutes
Servings: 6
Ingredients:
- 2 cups Greek yogurt
- 2 tablespoons pistachios, toasted and chopped
- A pinch of salt and white pepper
- 2 tablespoons mint, chopped
- 1 tablespoon kalamata olives, pitted and chopped
- ¼ cup za'atar spice
- ¼ cup pomegranate seeds
- 1/3 cup olive oil

Directions:
1. In a bowl, blend the yogurt with the pistachios and the rest of the ingredients, whisk well.
2. Divide into small cups and serve with pita chips on the side.

Nutrition: Calories: 294, Fat: 18, Fiber: 1, Carbs: 21, Protein: 10

540. Tomato Bruschetta

Preparation Time: 10 Minutes
Cooking Time: 10 Minutes
Servings: 6
Ingredients:
- 1 baguette, sliced
- 1/3 cup basil, chopped
- 6 tomatoes, cubed
- 2 garlic cloves, minced
- A pinch of salt and black pepper
- 1 teaspoon olive oil
- 1 tablespoon balsamic vinegar
- ½ teaspoon garlic powder
- Cooking spray

Directions:
1. Arrange the baguette slices in the baking sheet lined with parchment paper, grease them with cooking spray and bake at 400 degrees F for 10 minutes.
2. In a bowl, mix the tomatoes with the basil and the remaining ingredients, toss well and leave aside for 10 minutes.
3. Divide the tomato mix on each baguette slice, arrange them all on a platter and serve.

Nutrition: Calories: 162, Fat: 4, Fiber: 7, Carbs: 29, Protein: 4

541. Artichoke Flatbread

Preparation Time: 10 Minutes
Cooking Time: 15 Minutes
Servings: 4
Ingredients:
- 5 tablespoons olive oil
- 2 garlic cloves, minced
- 2 tablespoons parsley, chopped
- 2 round whole wheat flatbreads
- ½ cup mozzarella cheese, grated
- 14 ounces canned artichokes, drained and quartered
- 1 cup baby spinach, chopped
- ½ cup cherry tomatoes, halved
- ½ teaspoon basil, dried
- Salt and black pepper to the taste

Directions:
1. In a bowl, mix the parsley with the garlic and 4 tablespoons oil, whisk well and spread this over the flatbreads.
2. Sprinkle the mozzarella.

3. In a bowl, mix the artichokes with the spinach, tomatoes, basil, salt, pepper and the rest of the oil, toss and divide over the flatbreads as well.
4. Arrange the flatbreads on a baking sheet lined with parchment paper and bake at 425 degrees F for 15 minutes.
5. Serve a snack.

Nutrition: Calories: 223, Fat: 11.2, Fiber: 5.34, Carbs: 15.5, Protein: 7.4

542. Red Pepper Tapenade

Preparation Time: 10 Minutes
Cooking Time: 0 Minutes
Servings: 4
Ingredients:
- 7 ounces roasted red peppers, chopped
- 1/3 cup parsley, chopped
- 14 ounces canned artichokes, drained and chopped
- 3 tablespoons olive oil
- ¼ cup capers, drained
- 1 and ½ tablespoons lemon juice
- 2 garlic cloves, minced

Directions:
1. In your blender, combine the red peppers and the rest of the ingredients and pulse well.
2. Divide into cups and serve as a snack.

Nutrition: Calories: 200, Fat: 5.6, Fiber: 4.5, Carbs: 12.4, Protein: 4.6

543. Coriander Falafel

Preparation Time: 10 Minutes
Cooking Time: 10 Minutes
Servings: 8
Ingredients:
- 1 cup canned garbanzo beans, drained and rinsed
- 1 bunch parsley leaves
- 1 yellow onion, chopped
- 5 garlic cloves, minced
- 1 teaspoon coriander, ground
- A pinch of salt and black pepper
- ¼ teaspoon cayenne pepper
- ¼ teaspoon baking soda
- ¼ teaspoon cumin powder
- 1 teaspoon lemon juice
- 3 tablespoons tapioca flour
- Olive oil for frying

Directions:
1. In your food processor, combine the beans with the parsley, onion and the rest the ingredients except the oil and the flour and pulse well.
2. Transfer the mix to a bowl, add the flour, stir well, shape 16 balls out of this mix and flatten them a bit.
3. Heat up a pan with some oil over medium-high heat, add the falafels, cook them for 5 minutes on each side, transfer to paper towels, drain excess grease, arrange them on a platter and serve as an appetizer.

Nutrition: Calories: 112, Fat: 6.2, Fiber: 2, Carbs: 12.3, Protein: 3.1

544. Red Pepper Hummus

Preparation Time: 10 Minutes
Cooking Time: 0 Minutes
Servings: 6
Ingredients:

- 6 ounces roasted red peppers, peeled and chopped
- 16 ounces canned chickpeas, drained and rinsed
- ¼ cup Greek yogurt
- 3 tablespoons tahini paste
- Juice of 1 lemon
- 3 garlic cloves, minced
- 1 tablespoon olive oil
- A pinch of salt and black pepper
- 1 tablespoon parsley, chopped

Directions:

1. In your food processor, combine the red peppers with the rest of the ingredients except the oil and the parsley and pulse well.
2. Add the oil, pulse again, divide into cups, sprinkle the parsley on top and serve as a party spread.

Nutrition: Calories: 255, Fat: 11.4, Fiber: 4.5, Carbs: 17.4, Protein: 6.5

545. White Bean Dip

Preparation Time: 10 Minutes
Cooking Time: 0 Minutes
Servings: 4
Ingredients:

- 15 ounces canned white beans
- 6 ounces canned artichoke hearts, drained and quartered
- 4 garlic cloves, minced
- 1 tablespoon basil, chopped
- 2 tablespoons olive oil
- Juice of ½ lemon
- Zest of ½ lemon, grated
- Salt and black pepper to the taste

Directions:

1. In your food processor, combine the beans with the artichokes and the rest of the ingredients except the oil and pulse well.
2. Add the oil gradually, pulse the mix again, divide into cups and serve as a party dip.

Nutrition: Calories: 274, Fat: 11.7, Fiber: 6.5, Carbs: 18.5, Protein: 16.5

546. Hummus with Ground Lamb

Preparation Time: 10 Minutes
Cooking Time: 15 Minutes
Servings: 8
Ingredients:

- 10 ounces hummus
- 12 ounces' lamb meat, ground
- ½ cup pomegranate seeds
- ¼ cup parsley, chopped
- 1 tablespoon olive oil
- Pita chips for serving

Directions:

1. Heat up a pan with the oil over medium-high heat, add the meat, and brown for 15 minutes stirring often.
2. Spread the hummus on a platter, spread the ground lamb all over, also spread the pomegranate seeds and the parsley and serve with pita chips as a snack.

Nutrition: Calories: 133, Fat: 9.7, Fiber: 1.7, Carbs: 6.4, Protein: 5.4

547. Bulgur Lamb Meatballs

Preparation Time: 10 Minutes
Cooking Time: 15 Minutes
Servings: 6
Ingredients:

- 1 and ½ cups Greek yogurt
- ½ teaspoon cumin, ground
- 1 cup cucumber, shredded
- ½ teaspoon garlic, minced
- A pinch of salt and black pepper
- 1 cup bulgur
- 2 cups water
- 1-pound lamb, ground
- ¼ cup parsley, chopped
- ¼ cup shallots, chopped
- ½ teaspoon allspice, ground
- ½ teaspoon cinnamon powder
- 1 tablespoon olive oil

Directions:

1. In a bowl, blend the bulgur with the water, cover the bowl, leave aside for 10 minutes, drain and transfer to a bowl.
2. Add the meat, the yogurt and the rest of the ingredients except the oil, stir well and shape medium meatballs out of this mix.
3. Heat up a pan with the oil over medium-high heat, add the meatballs, cook them for 7 minutes on each side, arrange them all on a platter and serve as a snack.

Nutrition: Calories: 300, Fat: 9.6, Fiber: 4.6, Carbs: 22.6, Protein: 6.6

548. Eggplant Dip

Preparation Time: 10 Minutes
Cooking Time: 40 Minutes
Servings: 4
Ingredients:

- 1 eggplant, poked with a fork
- 2 tablespoons tahini paste
- 2 tablespoons lemon juice
- 2 garlic cloves, minced
- 1 tablespoon olive oil
- Salt and black pepper to the taste
- 1 tablespoon parsley, chopped

Directions:

1. Put the eggplant in a roasting pan, bake at 400 degrees F for 40 minutes, cool down, peel and transfer to your food processor.
2. Add the rest of the fixings excluding the parsley, pulse well, divide into small bowls and serve as a snack with the parsley sprinkled on top.

Nutrition: Calories: 121, Fat: 4.3, Fiber: 1, Carbs: 1.4, Protein: 4.3

549. Veggie Fritters

Preparation Time: 10 Minutes
Cooking Time: 10 Minutes
Servings: 8
Ingredients:

- 2 garlic cloves, minced
- 2 yellow onions, chopped
- 4 scallions, chopped
- 2 carrots, grated
- 2 teaspoons cumin, ground
- ½ teaspoon turmeric powder
- Salt and black pepper to the taste
- ¼ teaspoon coriander, ground
- 2 tablespoons parsley, chopped
- ¼ teaspoon lemon juice

- ½ cup almond flour
- 2 beets, peeled and grated
- 2 eggs, whisked
- ¼ cup tapioca flour
- 3 tablespoons olive oil

Directions:
1. In a bowl, combine the garlic with the onions, scallions and the rest of the ingredients except the oil, stir well and shape medium fritters out of this mix.
2. Heat up a pan with the oil on medium-high heat, add the fritters, cook for 5 minutes on each side, arrange on a platter and serve.

Nutrition: Calories: 209, Fat: 11.2, Fiber: 3, Carbs: 4.4, Protein: 4.8

550. Vinegar Beet Bites

Preparation Time: 10 Minutes
Cooking Time: 30 Minutes
Servings: 4
Ingredients:
- 2 beets, sliced
- Sea salt and black pepper
- 1/3 cup balsamic vinegar
- 1 cup olive oil

Directions:
1. Spread the beet slices on a baking sheet lined with parchment paper, add the rest of the ingredients, toss and bake at 350 degrees F for 30 minutes.
2. Serve the beet bites cold as a snack.

Nutrition: Calories: 199, Fat: 5.4, Fiber: 3.5, Protein: 3.5

551. Lentils Stuffed Potato Skins

Preparation Time: 10 Minutes
Cooking Time: 30 Minutes
Servings: 8
Ingredients:
- 16 red baby potatoes
- ¾ cup red lentils, cooked and drained
- 2 tablespoons olive oil
- 2 garlic cloves, minced
- 1 tablespoon chives, chopped
- ½ teaspoon hot chili sauce
- Salt and black pepper to the taste

Directions:
1. Put potatoes in a pot, add water to cover them, bring to a boil over medium low heat, cook for 15 minutes, drain, cool them down, cut in halves, remove the pulp, transfer it to a blender and pulse it a bit.
2. Add the rest of the ingredients to the blender, pulse again well and stuff the potato skins with this mix.
3. Arrange the stuffed potatoes on a baking sheet lined with parchment paper, introduce them in the oven at 375 degrees F and bake for 15 minutes.
4. Arrange on a platter and serve as an appetizer.

Nutrition: Calories: 300, Fat: 9.3, Fiber: 14.5, Carbs: 22.5, Protein: 8.5

552. Hot Chocolate

Preparation time: 5 minutes
Cooking time: 10 minutes
Servings: 4
Ingredients:
- ¼ cup of cocoa powder
- 1/8 teaspoon salt
- ½ teaspoon vanilla extract, unsweetened
- ¼ cup of coconut sugar

- 3 cups almond milk, unsweetened

Directions:
1. Take a medium saucepan, add salt, sugar, and cocoa powder in it, whisk until combined, and then whisk in milk.
2. Place the pan over medium-high heat and then bring the milk mixture to a simmer and turn hot, continue whisking.
3. Divide the hot chocolate evenly into four mugs and then serve.

Nutrition: Calories: 137 Cal; Fat: 3 g; Protein: 6 g; Carbs: 21 g; Fiber: 2 g

553. Stuffed Dried Figs

Preparation time: 20 minutes
Cooking time: 0 minutes
Servings: 4
Ingredients:
- 12 dried figs
- 2 tbsps. Thyme honey
- 2 tbsps. Sesame seeds
- 24 walnut halves

Directions:
1. Cut off the tough stalk ends of the figs.
2. Slice open each fig.
3. Stuff the fig openings with two walnut halves and close
4. Arrange the figs on a plate, drizzle with honey, and sprinkle the sesame seeds on it.
5. Serve.

Nutrition: Calories: 110 Carbs: 26 Fat: 3g, Protein: 1g

554. Feta Cheesecake

Preparation time: 30 minutes
Cooking time: 90 minutes
Servings: 12
Ingredients:
- 2 cups graham cracker crumbs (about 30 crackers)
- ½ tsp ground cinnamon
- 6 tbsps. Unsalted butter, melted
- ½ cup sesame seeds, toasted
- 12 ounces' cream cheese, softened
- 1 cup crumbled feta cheese
- 1 cup of sugar
- 2 cups plain yogurt
- 2 tbsps. Grated lemon zest
- 1 tsp vanilla

Directions:
1. Set the oven to 350°f.
2. Mix the cracker crumbs, butter, cinnamon, and sesame seeds with a fork. Move the combination to a springform pan and spread until it is even. Refrigerate.
3. In a separate bowl, mix the cream cheese and feta. With an electric mixer, beat both kinds of cheese together., beating the mixture with each new addition. Add sugar, then keep beating until creamy. Mix in yogurt, vanilla, and lemon zest.
4. Bring out the refrigerated springform and spread the batter on it. Then place it in a baking pan. Pour water in the pan till it is halfway full.
5. Bake for about 50 minutes. Remove cheesecake and allow it to cool. Refrigerate for at least 4 hours.
6. It is done. Serve when ready.

Nutrition: Calories: 98 Carbs: 7g Fat: 7g Protein: 3g

555. Pear Croustade

Preparation time: 30 minutes
Cooking time: 60 minutes
Servings: 10
Ingredients:

- 1 cup plus 1 tbsp. All-purpose flour, divided
- 4 ½ tbsps. Sugar, divided
- 1/8 tsp salt
- 6 tbsps. Unsalted butter, chilled, cut into ½ inch cubes
- 1 large-sized egg, separated
- 1 1/2 tbsps. Ice-cold water
- 3 firm, ripe pears (bosc), peeled, cored, sliced into ¼ inch slices
  1 tbsp. Fresh lemon juice
- 1/3 tsp ground allspice
- 1 tsp anise seeds

Directions:

1. Pour 1 cup of flour, 1 ½ tbsps. Of sugar, butter, and salt into a food processor and combine the ingredients by pulsing.
2. Whisk the yolk of the egg and ice water in a separate bowl. Mix the egg mixture with the flour mixture. It will form a dough, wrap it, and set aside for an hour.
3. Set the oven to 400°f.
4. Mix the pear, sugar, leftover flour, allspice, anise seed, and lemon juice in a large bowl to make a filling.
5. Arrange the filling on the center of the dough.
6. Bake for about 40 minutes. Cool for about 15 minutes before serving.

Nutrition: Calories: 498 Carbs: 32g Fat: 32g Protein: 18g

556. Melomakarona

Preparation time: 20 minutes
Cooking time: 45 minutes
Servings: 20
Ingredients:

- 4 cups of sugar, divided
- 4 cups of water
- 1 cup plus 1 tbsp. Honey, divided
- 1 (2-inch) strip orange peel, pith removed
- 1 cinnamon stick
- ½ cup extra-virgin olive oil
- ¼ cup unsalted butter,
- ¼ cup metaxa brandy or any other brandy
- 1 tbsp. Grated
- Orange zest
- ¾ cup of orange juice
- ¼ tsp baking soda
- 3 cups pastry flour
- ¾ cup fine semolina flour
- 1 ½ tsp baking powder
- 4 tsp ground cinnamon, divided
- 1 tsp ground cloves, divided
- 1 cup finely chopped walnut
- 1/3 cup brown sugar

Directions:

1. Mix 3 ½ cups of sugar, 1 cup honey, orange peel, cinnamon stick, and water in a pot and heat it for about 10 minutes.
2. Mix the sugar, oil, and butter for about minutes, then add the brandy, leftover honey, and zest. Then add a mixture of baking soda and orange juice. Mix thoroughly.
3. In a distinct bowl, blend the pastry flour, baking powder, semolina, 2 tsp of cinnamon, and ½ tsp. Of cloves. Add the mixture to the mixer slowly. Run the mixer until the ingredients form a dough. Cover and set aside for 30 minutes.
4. Set the oven to 350°f

5. With your palms, form small oval balls from the dough. Make a total of forty balls.
6. Bake the cookie balls for 30 minutes, then drop them in the prepared syrup.
7. Create a mixture with the walnuts, leftover cinnamon, and cloves. Spread the mixture on the top of the baked cookies.
8. Serve the cookies or store them in a closed-lid container.

Nutrition: Calories: 294 Carbs: 44g Fat: 12g Protein: 3g

557. Loukoumades (Fried Honey Balls)

Preparation time: 20 minutes
Cooking time: 45 minutes
Servings: 10
Ingredients:

- 2 cups of sugar
- 1 cup of water
- 1 cup honey
- 1 ½ cups tepid water
- 1 tbsp. Brown sugar
- ¼ cup of vegetable oil
- 1 tbsp. Active dry yeast
- 1 ½ cups all-purpose flour, 1 cup cornstarch, ½ tsp salt
- Vegetable oil for frying
- 1 ½ cups chopped walnuts
- ¼ cup ground cinnamon

Directions:

1. Boil the sugar and water on medium heat. Add honey after 10 minutes. Cool and set aside.
2. Mix the tepid water, oil, brown sugar,' and yeast in a large bowl. Allow it to sit for 10 minutes. In a distinct bowl, blend the flour, salt, and cornstarch. With your hands mix the yeast and the flour to make a wet dough. Cover and set aside for 2 hours.
3. Fry in oil at 350°f. Use your palm to measure the sizes of the dough as they are dropped in the frying pan. Fry each batch for about 3-4 minutes.
4. Immediately the loukoumades are done frying, drop them in the prepared syrup.
5. Serve with cinnamon and walnuts.

Nutrition: Calories: 355 Carbs: 64g Fat: 7g Protein: 6g

558. Crème Caramel

Preparation time: 60 minutes
Cooking time: 60 minutes
Servings: 12
Ingredients:

- 5 cups of whole milk
- 2 tsp vanilla extract
- 8 large egg yolks
- 4 large-sized eggs
- 2 cups sugar, divided
- ¼ cup 0f water

Directions:

1. Preheat the oven to 350°f
2. Heat the milk with medium heat wait for it to be scalded.
3. Mix 1 cup of sugar and eggs in a bowl and add it to the eggs.
4. With a nonstick pan on high heat, boil the water and remaining sugar. Do not stir, instead whirl the pan. When the sugar forms caramel, divide it into ramekins.
5. Divide the egg mixture into the ramekins and place in a baking pan. Increase water to the pan until it is half full. Bake for 30 minutes.
6. Remove the ramekins from the baking pan, cool, then refrigerate for at least 8 hours. Serve.

Nutrition: Calories: 110 Carbs: 21g Fat: 1g Protein: 2g

559. Raspberry Muffins

Preparation time: 10 minutes
Cooking time: 25 minutes
Servings: 12
Ingredients:

- ½ cup and 2 tablespoons whole-wheat flour
- 1 ½ cup raspberries, fresh and more for decorating
- 1 cup white whole-wheat flour
- 1/8 teaspoon salt
- ¾ cup of coconut sugar
- 2 teaspoons baking powder
- 1 teaspoon apple cider vinegar
- 1 ¼ cups water
- ½ cup olive oil

Directions:

1. Switch on the oven, then set it to 400 degrees' f and let it preheat.
2. Meanwhile, take a large bowl, place both flours in it, add salt and baking powder and then stir until combined.
3. Take a medium bowl, add oil to it, and then whisk in the sugar until dissolved.
4. Whisk in vinegar and water until blended, slowly stir in flour mixture until smooth batter comes together, and then fold in berries.
5. Take a 12-cups muffin pan, grease it with oil, fill evenly with the prepared mixture and then put a raspberry on top of each muffin.
6. Bake the muffins for 25 minutes until the top golden brown, and then serve.

Nutrition: Calories: 109; Fat: 3.4 g; Protein: 2.g; Carbs: 17.6 g; Fiber: 1 g

560. Chocolate Chip Cake

Preparation time: 10 minutes
Cooking time: 50 minutes
Servings: 10
Ingredients:

- 2 cups white whole-wheat flour
- ¼ teaspoon baking soda
- 1/3 cup coconut sugar
- 2 teaspoons baking powder
- ½ teaspoon salt
- ½ cup chocolate chips, vegan
- 1 teaspoon vanilla extract, unsweetened
- 1 tablespoon applesauce
- 1 teaspoon apple cider vinegar
- ¼ cup melted coconut oil
- ½ teaspoon almond extract, unsweetened
- 1 cup almond milk, unsweetened

Directions:

1. Switch on the oven, then set it to 360 degrees' f and let it preheat.
2. Meanwhile, take a 9-by-5 inches' loaf pan, grease it with oil, and then set aside until required.
3. Take a large bowl, add sugar to it, pour in oil, vanilla and almond extract, vinegar, apple sauce, and milk, and then whisk until well combined.
4. Take a large bowl, place flour in it, add salt, baking powder, and soda, and then stir until mixed.
5. Stir the flour mixture into the milk mixture until smooth batter comes together, and then fold in 1/3 cup of chocolate chips.
6. Spoon the batter into the loaf pan, scatter remaining chocolate chips on top and then bake for 50 minutes.
7. When done, let the bread cool for 10 minutes and then cut it into slices.
8. Serve straight away.

Nutrition: Calories: 218; Fat: 8 g; Protein: 3.4 g; Carbs: 32 g; Fiber: 2 g

561. Coffee Cake

Preparation time: 10 minutes
Cooking time: 45 minutes
Servings: 9
Ingredients:
For the cake:

- 1/3 cup coconut sugar
- 1 teaspoon vanilla extract, unsweetened
- ¼ cup olive oil
- 1/8 teaspoon almond extract, unsweetened
- 1 ¾ cup white whole-wheat flour
- 2 teaspoons baking powder
- ½ teaspoon salt
- ¼ teaspoon baking soda
- 1 teaspoon apple cider vinegar
- 1 tablespoon applesauce
- 1 cup almond milk, unsweetened

For the streusel:

- ½ cup white whole-wheat flour
- 2 teaspoons cinnamon
- 1/3 cup coconut sugar
- ½ teaspoon salt
- 2 tablespoons olive oil
- 1 tablespoon coconut butter

Directions:

1. Switch on the oven, then set it to 350 degrees' f and let it preheat.
2. Meanwhile, take a large bowl, pour in milk, add applesauce, vinegar, sugar, oil, vanilla, and almond extract and then whisk until blended.
3. Take a medium bowl, place flour in it, add salt, baking powder, and soda and then stir until mixed.
4. Stir the flour mixture into the milk mixture until smooth batter comes together, and then spoon the mixture into a loaf pan lined with parchment paper.
5. Prepare streusel and for this, take a medium bowl, place flour in it, and then add sugar, salt, and cinnamon.
6. Stir until mixed, and then mix butter and oil with fingers until the crumble mixture comes together.
7. Spread the prepared streusel on top of the batter of the cake and then bake for 45 minutes until the top turn golden brown and cake have thoroughly cooked.
8. When done, let the cake rest in its pan for 10 minutes, remove it to cool completely and then cut it into slices.
9. Serve straight away.

Nutrition: Calories: 259; Fat: 10 g; Protein: 3 g; Carbs: 37 g; Fiber: 1 g

562. Chocolate Marble Cake

Preparation time: 15 minutes
Cooking time: 50 minutes
Servings: 8
Ingredients:

- 1 ½ cup white whole-wheat flour
- 1 tablespoon flaxseed meal
- 2 ½ tablespoons cocoa powder
- ¼ teaspoon salt
- 4 tablespoons chopped walnuts

- 1 teaspoon baking powder
- 2/3 cup coconut sugar
- ¼ teaspoon baking soda
- 1 teaspoon vanilla extract, unsweetened
- ¼ cup olive oil
- 1 cup almond milk, unsweetened

Directions:

1. Switch on the oven, then set it to 350 degrees' f and let it preheat.
2. Meanwhile, take a medium bowl, place flour in it, add salt, baking powder, and soda in it and then stir until mixed.
3. Take a large bowl, pour in milk, add sugar, flaxseed, oil, and vanilla, whisk until sugar has dissolved, and then whisk in flour mixture until smooth batter comes together.
4. Spoon half of the prepared batter in a medium bowl, add cocoa powder and then stir until combined.
5. Take a loaf pan, line it with a parchment sheet, spoon half of the chocolate batter in it, and then spread it evenly.
6. Layer the chocolate batter cover with the remaining chocolate batter
7. Make swirls into the batter with a toothpick, smooth the top with a spatula, sprinkle walnuts on top, and then bake for 50 minutes until done.
8. When done, let the cake rest in its pan for 10 minutes, then remove it to cool completely and cut it into slices. Serve straight away.

Nutrition: Calories: 299; Fat: 14 g; Protein: 6 g; Carbs: 39 g; Fiber: 3 g

563. Sweet Chocolate Cookies

Preparation time: 10 minutes
Cooking time: 10 minutes
Servings: 11
Ingredients:

- 1 ¼ cups white whole-wheat flour
- 1 ½ tablespoon flax seeds
- ½ teaspoon baking soda
- ½ cup of coconut sugar
- ¼ teaspoon of sea salt
- ¼ cup powdered coconut sugar
- 1 teaspoon baking powder
- 2 teaspoons vanilla extract, unsweetened
- 4 ½ tablespoons water
- ½ cup of coconut oil
- 1 cup chocolate chips, vegan

Directions:

1. Take a large bowl, place flax seeds in it, stir in water and then let the mixture rest for 5 minutes until creamy.
2. Then add remaining ingredients into the flax seed's mixture except for flour and chocolate chips and then beat until light batter comes together.
3. Beat in flour, ¼ cup at a time, until smooth batter comes together, and then fold in chocolate chips.
4. Use an ice cream scoop to scoop the batter onto a baking sheet lined with parchment sheet with some distance between cookies and then bake for 10 minutes until cookies turn golden brown.

5. When done, let the cookies cool on the baking sheet for 3 minutes and then cool completely on the wire rack for 5 minutes.
6. Serve straight away.

Nutrition: Calories: 141; Fat: 7 g; Protein: 1 g; Carbs: 17 g; Fiber: 2 g

564. Lemon Cake

Preparation time: 10 minutes
Cooking time: 50 minutes
Servings: 9
Ingredients:

- 1 ½ cup white whole-wheat flour
- 1 ½ teaspoon baking powder
- 2 tablespoons almond flour
- 1 lemon, zested
- ¼ teaspoon baking soda
- 1/8 teaspoon turmeric powder
- 1/3 teaspoon salt
- ¼ teaspoon vanilla extract, unsweetened
- 1/3 cup lemon juice
- ½ cup maple syrup
- ¼ cup olive oil
- ¼ cup of water

For the frosting:

- 1 tablespoon lemon juice
- 1/8 teaspoon salt
- ¼ cup maple syrup
- 2 tablespoons powdered sugar
- 6 ounces' vegan cream cheese, softened

Directions:

1. Switch on the oven, then set it to 350 degrees' f and let it preheat.
2. Take a large bowl, pour in water, lemon juice, and oil, add vanilla extract and maple syrup, and whisk until blended.
3. Whisk in flour, ¼ cup at a time, until smooth, and then whisk in almond flour, salt, turmeric, lemon zest, baking soda, and powder until well combined.
4. Take a loaf pan, grease it with oil, spoon prepared batter in it, and then bake for 50 minutes.
5. Meanwhile, prepare the frosting and for this, take a small bowl, place all of its ingredients in it, whisk until smooth, and then let it chill until required.
6. When the cake has cooked, let it cool for 10 minutes in its pan and then let it cool completely on the wire rack.
7. Spread the prepared frosting on top of the cake, slice the cake, and then serve.

Nutrition: Calories: 275; Fat: 12 g; Protein: 3 g; Carbs: 38 g; Fiber: 1 g

565. Banana Muffins

Preparation time: 10 minutes
Cooking time: 30 minutes
Servings: 12
Ingredients:

- 1 ½ cups mashed banana
- 1 ½ cups and 2 tablespoons white whole-wheat flour, divided
- ¼ cup of coconut sugar
- ¾ cup rolled oats, divided
- 1 teaspoon ginger powder
- 1 tablespoon ground cinnamon, divided
- 2 teaspoons baking powder
- ½ teaspoon salt
- 1 teaspoon baking soda
- 1 tablespoon vanilla extract, unsweetened
- ½ cup maple syrup
- 1 tablespoon rum
- ½ cup of coconut oil

Directions:

1. Switch on the oven, then set it to 350 degrees' f and let it preheat.
2. Meanwhile, take a medium bowl, place 1 ½ cup flour in it, add ½ cup oars, ginger, baking powder and soda, salt, and 2 teaspoons cinnamon and then stir until mixed.
3. Place ¼ cup of coconut oil in a heatproof bowl, melt it in the microwave oven and then whisk in maple syrup until combined.
4. Add mashed banana along with rum and vanilla, stir until combined, and then whisk this mixture into the flour mixture until smooth batter comes together.
5. Take a separate medium bowl, place remaining oats and flour in it, add cinnamon, coconut sugar, and coconut oil and then stir with a fork until crumbly mixture comes together.
6. Take a 12-cups muffin pan, fill evenly with prepared batter, top with oats mixture, and then bake for 30 minutes until firm and the top turn golden brown.
7. When done, let the muffins cool for 5 minutes in its pan and then cool the muffins completely before serving.

Nutrition: Cal: 240; Fat: 9.3 g; Protein: 2.6 g; Carbs: 35.4 g; Fiber: 2 g

566. Baked Apples

Preparation time: 5 minutes
Cooking time: 20 minutes
Servings: 4
Ingredients:

- 6 medium apples, peeled, cut into chunks
- 1 teaspoon ground cinnamon
- 2 tablespoons melted coconut oil

Directions:

1. Switch on the oven, then set it to 350 degrees' f and let it preheat.
2. Take a medium baking dish, and then spread apple pieces in it.
3. Take a small bowl, place coconut oil in it, stir in cinnamon, drizzle this mixture over apples and then toss until coated.
4. Place the baking dish into the oven and then bake for 20 minutes or more until apples turn soft, stirring halfway.
5. Serve straight away.

Nutrition: Calories: 170 Cal; Fat: 3.8 g; Protein: 0.5 g; Carbs: 31 g; Fiber: 5.5 g

567. Chocolate Strawberry Shake

Preparation time: 5 minutes
Cooking time: 0 minutes
Servings: 2
Ingredients:

- 2 cups almond milk, unsweetened
- 4 bananas, peeled, frozen
- 4 tablespoons cocoa powder
- 2 cups strawberries, frozen

Directions:

1. Place all the ingredients into the jar of a high-speed food processor or blender in the order stated in the ingredients list and then cover it with the lid.
2. Pulse for 1 minute until smooth, and then serve.

Nutrition: Calories: 208 Cal; Fat: 0.2 g; Protein: 12.4 g; Carbs: 26.2 g; Fiber: 1.4 g

568. Chocolate Clusters

Preparation time: 15 minutes
Cooking time: 10 minutes
Servings: 12
Ingredients:

- 1 cup chopped dark chocolate, vegan
- 1 cup cashews, roasted, salt
- 1 teaspoon sea salt flakes

Directions:

1. Take a large baking sheet, line it with wax paper, and then set aside until required.
2. Take a medium bowl, place chocolate in it, and then microwave for 1 minute.
3. Stir the chocolate and then continue microwaving it at 1-minute intervals until chocolate melts completely, stirring at every interval.
4. When melted, stir the chocolate to bring it to 90 degrees' f and then stir in cashews.
5. Scoop the walnut-chocolate mixture on the prepared baking sheet, ½ tablespoons per cluster, and then sprinkle with salt.
6. Let the clusters stand at room temperature until harden and then serve.

Nutrition: Calories: 79.4 Cal; Fat: 6.6 g; Protein: 1 g; Carbs: 5.8 g; Fiber: 1.1 g

569. Banana Coconut Cookies

Preparation time: 5 minutes
Cooking time: 20 minutes
Servings: 9
Ingredients:

- 1 ½ cup shredded coconut, unsweetened
- 1 cup mashed banana

Directions:

1. Switch on the oven, then set it to 350 degrees' f and let it preheat.
2. Take a medium bowl, place the mashed banana in it and then stir in coconut until well combined.
3. Take a large baking sheet, line it with a parchment sheet, and then scoop the prepared mixture on it, 2 tablespoons of mixture per cookie.
4. Cook cookies about 17-20 minutes, or until edges are browned and surface is dry.
5. Allow the cookies to cool completely before removing from baking sheet.

6. The bottoms of the cookies can stick a little, so use a spatula when removing cookies from sheet.

Nutrition: Calories: 51 Cal; Fat: 3 g; Protein: 0.2 g; Carbs: 4 g; Fiber: 1 g

570. Chocolate Pots

Preparation time: 4 hours 10 minutes
Cooking time: 3 minutes
Servings: 4

Ingredients:

- 6 ounces' chocolate, unsweetened
- 1 cup medjool dates, pitted
- 1 ¾ cups almond milk, unsweetened

Directions:

1. Cut the chocolate into small pieces, place them in a heatproof bowl and then microwave for 2 to 3 minutes until melt completely, stirring every minute.
2. Place dates in a blender, pour in the milk, and then pulse until smooth.
3. Add chocolate into the blender and then pulse until combined.
4. Divide the mixture into the small mason jars and then let them rest for 4 hours until set.
5. Serve straight away.

Nutrition: Cal: 321 Cal; Fat: 19 g; Protein: 6 g; Carbs: 34 g; Fiber: 4 g

571. Maple and Tahini Fudge

Preparation time: 2 hours
Cooking time: 3 minutes
Servings: 15

Ingredients:

- 1 cup dark chocolate chips, vegan
- ¼ cup maple syrup
- ½ cup tahini

Directions:

1. Take a heatproof bowl, place chocolate chips in it and then microwave for 2 to 3 minutes until melt completely, stirring every minute.
2. When melted, remove the chocolate bowl from the oven and then whisk in maple syrup and tahini until smooth.
3. Take a 4-by-8 inches baking dish, line it with wax paper, spoon the chocolate mixture in it and then press it into the baking dish.
4. Cover with another sheet with wax paper, press it down until smooth, and then let the fudge rest for 1 hour in the freezer until set.
5. Then cut the fudge into 15 squares and serve.

Nutrition: Calories: 110.7; Fat: 5.3 g; Protein: 2.2 g; Carbs: 15.1 g; Fiber: 1.6 g

572. Creaseless

Preparation time: 4 hours
Cooking time: 0 minutes
Servings: 5

Ingredients:

- 3 tablespoons agave syrup
- 1 cup coconut milk, unsweetened
- ½ teaspoon vanilla extract, unsweetened
- 1 cup of orange juice

Directions:

1. Place all the ingredients in a food processor or blender and then pulse until combined.

2. Pour the mixture into five molds of popsicle pan, insert a stick into each mold and then let it freeze for a minimum of 4 hours until hard.
3. Serve when ready.

Nutrition: Calories: 152 ; Fat: 10 g; Protein: 1 g; Carbs: 16 g; Fiber: 1 g

573. Kourabiedes Almond Cookies

Preparation time: 20 minutes
Cooking time: 25 minutes
Servings: 20

Ingredients:

- 1 ½ cups unsalted butter, clarified, at room temperature 2 cups
- Confectioners' sugar, divided
- 1 large egg yolk
- 2 tbsps. Brandy
- 1 1/2 tsp baking powder
- 1 tsp vanilla extract
- 5 cups all-purpose flour, sifted
- 1 cup roasted almonds, chopped

Directions:

1. Preheat the oven to 350°f
2. Thoroughly mix butter and ½ cup of sugar in a bowl. Add in the egg after a while. Create a brandy mixture by mixing the brandy and baking powder. Add the mixture to the egg, add vanilla, then keep beating until the ingredients are properly blended
3. Add flour and almonds to make a dough.
4. Roll the dough to form crescent shapes. You should be able to get about 40 pieces. Place the pieces on a baking sheet, then bake in the oven for 25 minutes.
5. Allow the cookies to cool, then coat them with the remaining confectioner's sugar.
6. Serve.

Nutrition: Calories: 102 Carbs: 10g Fat: 7g Protein: 2g

574. Ekmek Kataifi

Preparation time: 8 hours & 30 minutes
Cooking time: 25 minutes
Servings: 10

Ingredients:

- 1 cup of sugar
- 1 cup of water
- 2 (2-inch) strips lemon peel, pith removed
- 1 tbsp. Fresh lemon juice
- ½ cup plus 1 tbsp. Unsalted butter, melted
- ½lbs. Frozen kataifi pastry, thawed, at room temperature
- 2 ½ cups whole milk
- ½ tsp. Ground mastiha
- 2 large eggs
- ¼ cup fine semolina
- 1 tsp. Of cornstarch
- ¼ cup of sugar
- ½ cup sweetened coconut flakes
- 1 cup whipping cream
- 1 tsp. Vanilla extract
- 1 tsp. Powdered milk
- 3 tbsps. Of confectioners' sugar
- ½ cup chopped unsalted pistachios

Directions:

1. Set the oven to 350°f. Grease the baking pan with 1. Tbsp of butter.
2. Put a pot on medium heat, then add water, sugar, lemon juice, lemon peel. Leave to boil for about 10 minutes. Reserve.
3. Untangle the kataifi, coat with the leftover butter, then place in the baking pan.
4. Mix the milk and mastiha, then place it on medium heat. Remove from heat when the milk is scalded, then cool the mixture.
5. Mix the eggs, cornstarch, semolina, and sugar in a bowl, stir thoroughly, then whisk the cooled milk mixture into the bowl.
6. Transfer the egg and milk mixture to a pot and place on heat. Wait for it to thicken like custard, then add the coconut flakes and cover it with a plastic wrap. Cool.
7. Spread the cooled custard-like material over the kataifi. Place in the refrigerator for at least 8 hours.
8. Strategically remove the kataifi from the pan with a knife. Take it away in such a way that the mold faces up.
9. Whip a cup of cream, add 1 tsp. Vanilla, 1tsp. Powdered milk, and 3 tbsps. Of sugar. Spread the mixture all over the custard, wait for it to harden, then flip and add the leftover cream mixture to the kataifi side.

Nutrition: Calories: 649 Carbs: 37g Fat: 52g Protein: 11g

575. Lemon-lime sherbet

Preparation time: 5 minutes, plus 3 hours chilling time
Cooking time: 15 minutes
servings: 2

Ingredients:

- 2 cups of water
- 1 cup granulated sugar
- 3 tablespoons lemon zest, divided
- ½ cup freshly squeezed lemon juice
- Zest of 1 lime
- Juice of 1 lime
- ½ cup heavy (whipping) cream

Directions:

1. Place a large saucepan over medium-high heat and add the water, sugar, and two tablespoons of the lemon zest.
2. Bring the mixture to a boil and then reduce the heat and simmer for 15 minutes.
3. Transfer the mixture to a large bowl and add the remaining 1 tablespoon lemon zest, the lemon juice, lime zest, and lime juice.
4. Chill the mixture in the fridge until completely cold, about 3 hours.
5. Whisk in the heavy cream and transfer the mixture to an ice cream maker.
6. Freeze according to the manufacturer's instructions.

Nutrition: Calories: 151; Fat: 6g; Carbs: 26g; Phosphorus: 10mg; Potassium: 27mg; Sodium: 6mg;

576. Chocolate Covered Dates

Preparation time: 1 hours & 10 minutes
Cooking time: 3 minutes
Servings: 8

Ingredients:

- 16 medjool dates, pitted
- ½ teaspoon of sea salt
- ¾ cup almonds
- 1 teaspoon coconut oil

- 8 ounces' chocolate chips, vegan

Directions:

1. Take a medium baking sheet, line it with parchment paper, and then set aside until required.
2. Place an almond into the pit of each date and then wrap the date tightly around it.
3. Place chocolate chips in a heatproof bowl, add oil, and then microwave for 2 to 3 minutes until chocolate melts, stirring every minute.
4. Working on one date at a time, dip each date into the chocolate mixture and then place it onto the prepared baking sheet.
5. Sprinkle salt over the prepared dates and then let them rest in the refrigerator for 1 hour until chocolate is firm.
6. Serve straight away.

Nutrition: Calories: 179; Fat: 7.7 g; Protein: 3 g; Carbs: 28.5 g; Fiber: 3 g

577. Tart Apple Granita

Preparation time: 15 minutes, plus 4 hours freezing time
Cooking time: 20 minutes
Servings: 4

Ingredients:

- ½ cup granulated sugar
- ½ cup of water
- 2 cups unsweetened apple juice
- ¼ cup freshly squeezed lemon juice

Directions:

1. In a small saucepan over medium-high heat, heat the sugar and water.
2. Bring the mixture to a boil and then reduce the heat to low. Let it simmer for about 15 minutes or until the liquid has reduced by half.
3. Remove the pan from the heat and pour the liquid into a large shallow metal pan.
4. Let the liquid cool for about 30 minutes, and then stir in the apple juice and lemon juice.
5. Place the pan in the freezer.
6. After 1 hour, run a fork through the liquid to break up any ice crystals that have formed. Scrape down the sides as well.
7. Place the pan back in the freezer and repeat the stirring and scraping every 20 minutes, creating slush.
8. Serve when the mixture is completely frozen and looks like crushed ice, after about 3 hours.

Nutrition: Calories: 157; Fat: 0g; Carbs: 0g; Phosphorus: 10mg; Potassium: 141mg; Sodium: 5mg;

578. Lemon-Lime Sherbet

Preparation time: 5 minutes, plus 3 hours chilling time
Cooking time: 15 minutes
Servings: 2

Ingredients:

- 2 cups of water
- 1 cup granulated sugar
- 3 tablespoons lemon zest, divided
- ½ cup freshly squeezed lemon juice
- Zest of 1 lime
- Juice of 1 lime
- ½ cup heavy (whipping) cream

Directions:

1. Place a large saucepan over medium-high heat and add the water, sugar, and two tablespoons of the lemon zest.
2. Bring the mixture to a boil and then reduce the heat and simmer for 15 minutes.
3. Transfer the mixture to a large bowl and add the remaining 1 tablespoon lemon zest, the lemon juice, lime zest, and lime juice.
4. Chill the mixture in the fridge until completely cold, about 3 hours.
5. Whisk in the heavy cream and transfer the mixture to an ice cream maker.
6. Freeze according to the manufacturer's instructions.

Nutrition: Calories: 151; Fat: 6g; Carbs: 26g; Phosphorus: 10mg; Potassium: 27mg; Sodium: 6mg;

579. Tropical Vanilla Snow Cone

Preparation time: 15 minutes, plus freezing time
Cooking time: 15 minutes
Servings: 2
ingredients:

- 1 cup pineapple
- 1 cup of frozen strawberries
- 6 tablespoons water
- 2 tablespoons granulated sugar
- 1 tablespoon vanilla extract

Directions:

1. In a large saucepan, mix together the peaches, pineapple, strawberries, water, and sugar over medium-high heat and bring to a boil.
2. Reduce the heat to low and simmer the mixture, occasionally stirring, for 15 minutes.
3. Remove from the heat and let the mixture cool completely, for about 1 hour.
4. Stir in the vanilla and transfer the fruit mixture to a food processor or blender.
5. Purée until smooth, and pour the purée into a 9-by-13-inch glass baking dish.
6. Cover and place the dish in the freezer overnight.
7. When the fruit mixture is completely frozen, use a fork to scrape the sorbet until you have flaked flavored ice. Scoop the ice flakes into four serving dishes.

Nutrition: Calories: 92; Fat: 0g; Carbs: 22g; Phosphorus: 17mg; Potassium: 145mg; Sodium: 4mg; Protein: 1g

580. Vanilla Cupcakes

Preparation time: 10 minutes
Cooking time: 20 minutes
Servings: 18
Ingredients:

- 2 cups white whole-wheat flour
- 1 cup of coconut sugar
- ½ teaspoon salt
- 2 teaspoons baking powder
- 1 ¼ teaspoons vanilla extract, unsweetened
- ½ teaspoon baking soda
- 1 tablespoon apple cider vinegar
- ½ cup coconut oil, melted

- 1 ½ cups almond milk, unsweetened

Directions:

1. Switch on the oven, then set it to 350 degrees f, and then let it preheat.
2. Meanwhile, take a medium bowl, place vinegar in it, stir in milk, and then let it stand for 5 minutes until curdled.
3. Take a large bowl, place flour in it, add salt, baking soda and powder, and sugar and then stir until mixed.
4. Take a separate large bowl, pour in curdled milk mixture, add vanilla and coconut oil and then whisk until combined.
5. Whisk almond milk mixture into the flour mixture until smooth batter comes together, and then spoon the mixture into two 12-cups muffin pans lined with muffin cups.
6. Bake the muffins for 15 to 20 minutes until firm and the top turn golden brown, and then let them cool on the wire rack completely.
7. Serve straight away.

Nutrition: Calories: 152.4 Cal; Fat: 6.4 g; Protein: 1.5 g; Carbs: 22.6 g; Fiber: 0.5 g

581. Garlic and Herb Oodles

Preparation Time: 5minutes
Cooking time: 2 minutes
Servings: 3
Ingredients:

- 1 teaspoon extra-virgin olive oil or 2 tablespoons vegetable broth
- 1 teaspoon minced garlic (about 1 clove)
- 4 medium zucchinis, spiraled
- 1/2 teaspoon dried basil
- 1/2 teaspoon dried oregano
- 1/41/4 to 1/2 teaspoon red pepper flakes, to taste
- 1/4 teaspoon salt (optional)
- 1/4 teaspoon freshly ground black pepper

Directions:

1. Heat the olive oil. Add the garlic, zucchini, basil, oregano, red pepper flakes, salt (if using), and black pepper. Sauté for 1 to 2 minutes, until barely tender.
2. Divide the oodles evenly among 4 storage containers. Let cool before sealing the lids.

Nutrition: Calories: 120 Protein: 10g Fat: 44g Carbs: 32g Fibers: 5g

582. Feta Cheesecake

Preparation time: 30 minutes + 4 hours chilling time
Cooking time: 90 minutes
Servings: 12
Ingredients:

- 2 cups graham cracker crumbs (about 30 crackers)
- ½ tsp ground cinnamon
- 6 tbsps. Unsalted butter, melted
- ½ cup sesame seeds, toasted
- 12 ounces' cream cheese, softened
- 1 cup crumbled feta cheese
- 1 cup of sugar
- 2 cups plain yogurt
- 2 tbsps. Grated lemon zest
- 1 tsp vanilla

Directions:

1. Set the oven to 350°f.
2. Mix the cracker crumbs, butter, cinnamon, and sesame seeds with a fork. Move the combination to a springform pan and spread until it is even. Refrigerate.

3. In a separate bowl, mix the cream cheese and feta. With an electric mixer, beat both kinds of cheese together., beating the mixture with each new addition. Add sugar, then keep beating until creamy. Mix in yogurt, vanilla, and lemon zest.
4. Bring out the refrigerated springform and spread the batter on it. Then place it in a baking pan. Pour water in the pan till it is halfway full.
5. Bake for about 50 minutes. Remove cheesecake and allow it to cool. Refrigerate for at least 4 hours.
6. It is done. Serve when ready.

Nutrition: Calories: 98   Carbs: 7g   Fat: 7g   Protein: 3g

583. Almonds and Oats Pudding

Preparation time: 10 minutes
Cooking time: 15 minutes
Servings: 4
Ingredients:

- 1 tablespoon lemon juice
- Zest of 1 lime
- 1 and ½ cups of almond milk
- 1 teaspoon almond extract
- ½ cup oats
- 2 tablespoons stevia
- ½ cup silver almonds, chopped

Directions:
1. In a pan, blend the almond milk plus the lime zest and the other ingredients, whisk, bring to a simmer and cook over medium heat for 15 minutes.
2. Split the mix into bowls then serve cold.

Nutrition: Calories 174 Fat 12.1 Fiber 3.2 Carbs 3.9 Protein 4.8

584. Chocolate Cups

Preparation time: 2 hours
Cooking time: 0 minutes
Servings: 6
Ingredients:

- ½ cup avocado oil
- 1 cup, chocolate, melted
- 1 teaspoon matcha powder
- 3 tablespoons stevia

Directions:
1. In a bowl, mix the chocolate with the oil and the rest of the ingredients.
2. Whisk well and divide into cups.
3. Keep in the freezer for 2 hours before serving.

Nutrition: Calories 174 Fat 9.1 Fiber 2.2 Carbs 3.9 Protein 2.8

585. Mango Bowls

Preparation time: 10 minutes
Cooking time: 0 minutes
Servings: 4
Ingredients:

- 3 cups mango, cut into medium chunks
- ½ cup of coconut water
- ¼ cup stevia
- 1 teaspoon vanilla extract

Directions:
1. In a blender, blend the mango plus the rest of the ingredients, pulse well.
2. Divide into bowls and serve cold.

Nutrition: Calories 122 Fat 4 Fiber 5.3 Carbs 6.6 Protein 4.5

586. Cocoa and Pears Cream

Preparation time: 10 minutes
Cooking time: 0 minutes
Servings: 4
Ingredients:

- 2 cups heavy creamy
- 1/3 cup stevia
- ¾ cup cocoa powder
- 6 ounces' dark chocolate, chopped
- Zest of 1 lemon
- 2 pears, chopped

Directions:
1. In a blender, blend the cream plus the stevia and the rest of the ingredients.
2. Blend well.
3. Divide into cups and serve cold.

Nutrition: Calories 172 Fat 5.6 Fiber 3.5 Carbs 7.6 Protein 4

587. Pineapple Pudding

Preparation time: 10 minutes
Cooking time: 40 minutes
Servings: 4
Ingredients:

- 3 cups almond flour
- ¼ cup olive oil
- 1 teaspoon vanilla extract
- 2 and ¼ cups stevia
- 1 and ¼ cup natural apple sauce
- 2 teaspoons baking powder
- 1 and ¼ cups of almond milk
- 2 cups pineapple, chopped
- Cooking spray

Directions:
1. In a bowl, blend the almond flour plus the oil and the rest of the ingredients except the cooking spray and stir well.
2. Grease a cake pan with the cooking spray, pour the pudding mix inside, introduce in the oven and bake at 370 degrees' f for 40 minutes.
3. Serve the pudding cold.

Nutrition: Calories 223 Fat 8.1 Fiber 3.4 Carbs 7.6 Protein 3.4

588. Lime Vanilla Fudge

Preparation time: 3 hours
Cooking time: 0 minutes
Servings: 6
Ingredients:

- 1/3 cup cashew butter
- 5 tablespoons lime juice
- ½ teaspoon lime zest, grated
- 1 tablespoons stevia

Directions:
1. In a bowl, mix the cashew butter with the other ingredients and whisk well.
2. Line a muffin tray with parchment paper, scoop 1 tablespoon of lime fudge mix in each of the muffin tins and keep in the freezer for 3 hours before serving.

Nutrition: Calories 200 Fat 4.5 Fiber 3.4 Carbs 13.5 Protein 5

589. Mixed Berries Stew

Preparation time: 10 minutes
Cooking time: 15 minutes
Servings: 6

Ingredients:

- Zest of 1 lemon, grated
- Juice of 1 lemon
- ½ pint blueberries
- 1-pint strawberries halved
- 2 cups of water
- 2 tablespoons stevia

Directions:

1. In a pan, blend the berries plus the water, stevia and the other ingredients.
2. Bring to a simmer, cook over medium heat for 15 minutes.
3. Divide into bowls and serve cold.

Nutrition: Calories 172 Fat 7 Fiber 3.4 Carbs 8 Protein 2.3

590. Orange and Apricots Cake

Preparation time: 10 minutes
Cooking time: 20 minutes
Servings: 8

Ingredients:

- ¾ cup stevia
- 2 cups almond flour
- ¼ cup olive oil
- ½ cup almond milk
- 1 teaspoon baking powder
- ½ teaspoon vanilla extract
- Juice and zest of 2 oranges
- 2 cups apricots, chopped

Directions:

1. In a bowl, blend the stevia plus the flour and the rest of the ingredients, whisk and pour into a cake pan lined with parchment paper.
2. Introduce in the oven at 375 degrees f, bake for 20 minutes.
3. Cool down, slice and serve.

Nutrition: Calories 221 Fat 8.3 Fiber 3.4 Carbs 14.5 Protein 5

591. Blueberry Cake

Preparation time: 10 minutes
Cooking time: 30 minutes
Servings: 6

Ingredients:

- 2 cups almond flour
- 3 cups blueberries
- 1 cup walnuts, chopped
- 3 tablespoons stevia
- 1 teaspoon vanilla extract
- 2 tablespoons avocado oil
- 1 teaspoon baking powder
- Cooking spray

Directions:

1. In a bowl, blend the flour plus the blueberries, walnuts and the other ingredients except for the cooking spray, and stir well.

2. Grease a cake pan with the cooking spray, pour the cake mix inside, introduce everything in the oven at 350 degrees' f and bake for 30 minutes.
3. Cool the cake down, slice and serve.

Nutrition: Calories 225 Fat 9 Fiber 4.5 Carbs 10.2 Protein 4.5

592. Almond Peaches Mix

Preparation time: 10 minutes
Cooking time: 10 minutes
Servings: 4

Ingredients:

- 1/3 cup almonds, toasted
- 1/3 cup pistachios, toasted
- 1 teaspoon mint, chopped
- ½ cup of coconut water
- 1 teaspoon lemon zest, grated
- 4 peaches, halved
- 2 tablespoons stevia

Directions:

1. In a pan, combine the peaches with the stevia and the rest of the ingredients.
2. Simmer over medium heat for 10 minutes.
3. Divide into bowls and serve cold.

Nutrition: Calories 135 Fat 4.1 Fiber 3.8 Carbs 4.1 Protein 2.3

593. Spiced Peaches

Preparation time: 5 minutes
Cooking time: 10 minutes
Servings: 2

Ingredients:

- Canned peaches with juices – 1 cup
- Cornstarch – ½ tsp.
- Ground cloves – 1 tsp.
- Ground cinnamon – 1 tsp.
- Ground nutmeg – 1 tsp.
- Zest of ½ lemon
- Water – ½ cup

Directions:

1. Drain peaches.
2. Combine cinnamon, cornstarch, nutmeg, ground cloves, and lemon zest in a pan on the stove.
3. Heat on medium heat and add peaches.
4. Bring to a boil, decrease the heat then simmer for 10 minutes.
5. Serve.

Nutrition: Calories: 70; Fat: 0g; Carb: 14g; Phosphorus: 23mg; Potassium: 176mg; Sodium: 3mg; Protein: 1g

594. Blueberry Mini Muffins

Preparation time: 10 minutes
Cooking time: 20 minutes
Servings: 4

Ingredients:

- All-purpose white flour – ¼ cup
- Coconut flour – 1 tbsp.
- Baking soda – 1 tsp.
- Nutmeg – 1 tbsp. Grated
- Vanilla extract – 1 tsp.

- Stevia – 1 tsp.
- Fresh blueberries – ¼ cup

Directions:
1. Preheat the oven to 325f.
2. Mix all the ingredients in a bowl.
3. Divide the batter into four and spoon into a lightly oiled muffin tin.
4. Bake in the oven for 15 to 20 minutes or until cooked through.
5. Cool and serve.

Nutrition: Calories: 62; Fat: 0g; Carb: 9g; Phosphorus: 103mg; Potassium: 65mg; Sodium: 62mg; Protein: 4g;

595. Baked Peaches with Cream Cheese

Preparation time: 10 minutes
Cooking time: 15 minutes
Servings: 4
Ingredients:
- Plain cream cheese – 1 cup
- Crushed meringue cookies – ½ cup
- Ground cinnamon – ¼ tsp.
- Pinch ground nutmeg
- Canned peach halves – 8, in juice
- Honey – 2 tbsp.

Directions:
1. Preheat the oven to 350f.
2. Line a baking sheet with parchment paper. Set aside.
3. In a small bowl, stir together the meringue cookies, cream cheese, cinnamon, and nutmeg.
4. Spoon the cream cheese mixture evenly into the cavities in the peach halves.
5. Place the peaches on the baking sheet and bake for 15 minutes or until the fruit is soft and the cheese is melted.
6. Remove the peaches from the baking sheet onto plates.
7. Drizzle with honey and serve.

Nutrition: Calories: 260; Fat: 20; Carb: 19g; Phosphorus: 74mg; Potassium: 198mg; Sodium: 216mg; Protein: 4g;

596. Strawberry Ice Cream

Preparation time: 5 minutes + frozen time
Cooking time: 0 minutes
Servings: 3
Ingredients:
- Stevia – ½ cup
- Lemon juice – 1 tbsp.
- Non-dairy coffee creamer – ¾ cup
- Strawberries – 10 oz.
- Crushed ice – 1 cup

Directions:
1. Blend everything in a blender until smooth.
2. Freeze until frozen.
3. Serve.

Nutrition: Calories: 94.4; Fat: 6g; Carb: 8.3g; Phosphorus: 25mg; Potassium: 108mg; Sodium: 25mg; Protein: 1.3g;

597. Raspberry Brule

Preparation time: 15 minutes
Cooking time: 10 minute
Servings: 4
Ingredients:
- Light sour cream – ½ cup
- Plain cream cheese – ½ cup
- Brown sugar – ¼ cup, divided
- Ground cinnamon – ¼ tsp.
- Fresh raspberries – 1 cup

Directions:
1. Preheat the oven to broil.
2. In a bowl, beat together the cream cheese, sour cream, 2 tbsp. Brown sugar and cinnamon for 4 minutes or until the mixture are very smooth and fluffy.
3. Evenly divide the raspberries among 4 (4-ounce) ramekins.
4. Spoon the cream cheese mixture over the berries and smooth the tops.
5. Sprinkle ½ tbsp. Brown sugar evenly over each ramekin.
6. Place the ramekins on a baking sheet and broil 4 inches from the heating element until the sugar is caramelized and golden brown.
7. Cool and serve.

Nutrition: Calories: 188; Fat: 13g; Carb: 16g; Phosphorus: 60mg; Potassium: 158mg; Sodium: 132mg;

598. Crazy Chocolate Cake

Preparation time: 1 hours
Cooking time: 35 minutes
Servings: 12
Ingredients:
For the cake:
- Cooking spray, for greasing
- 1½ cups all-purpose flour
- 1 cup granulated sugar
- ¼ cup Dutch process cocoa powder
- 1 teaspoon baking soda
- ½ teaspoon salt
- 1 teaspoon white vinegar
- 5 tablespoons vegetable oil
- 1 teaspoon vanilla extract
- 1 cup water

For the frosting:
- 6 cups powdered sugar
- 1 cup cocoa powder
- 2 cups vegan butter, softened
- 1 teaspoon vanilla extract
- 1 pinch salt

Directions:
1. For the cake, warm your oven to 350°F. Grease or spray an 8-inch square baking dish or a 9-inch round cake pan.
2. In a large bowl, combine the flour, sugar, cocoa powder, baking soda, and salt. Add the vinegar, vegetable oil, vanilla extract, and water directly to the dry ingredients. Stir the batter until no lumps remain.

3. Put the batter into the greased dish and bake for 35 minutes or until a toothpick inserted into the center comes out clean.
4. Once the cake is baked, cool it in the pan for 10 minutes. Transfer it to a plate and refrigerate for about 30 minutes, then frost.
5. For the frosting, mix the powdered sugar plus cocoa powder in a large bowl. Beat the vegan butter on medium-high speed until pale and creamy using an electric hand mixer or a stand mixer with the paddle attachment.
6. Reduce the mixer speed to medium and add the powdered sugar and cocoa mix, ½ cup at a time, mixing well between each addition (about 5 minutes total). Add the vanilla extract and salt and mix on high speed for 1 minute.

Nutrition: Calories: 831 Fat: 44 g Carbs: 111 g Protein: 5 g

599. Cranberry Orange Pound Cake

Preparation time: 25 minutes
Cooking time: 50 minutes
Servings: 6-8
Ingredients:
- 2 cups fresh cranberries
- 2 tablespoons, plus 1 1/3 cups sugar, divided
- 1 cup plain coconut yogurt
- 1 large banana, mashed
- 2 teaspoons grated orange zest
- 1 teaspoon vanilla extract
- ½ cup vegetable oil
- 1½ cups all-purpose flour
- 2 teaspoons baking powder
- ½ teaspoon salt
- 1/3 cup, plus 2 tablespoons freshly squeezed orange juice
- 1 cup powdered sugar

Directions:
1. Preheat the oven to 350°F. Grease a standard-size loaf pan. Line the bottom with parchment paper lengthwise, letting some hang over the edges. Set aside.
2. Mix the cranberries and 2 tablespoons of granulated sugar in a food processor or blender until coarsely chopped. Set aside.
3. In a large bowl, whisk together the yogurt, 1 cup of sugar, the banana, orange zest, vanilla extract, and oil. Stir in the cranberry mixture.
4. Mix the flour, baking powder, plus salt in a medium bowl. Incorporate the dry mixture into the wet mixture until smooth.
5. Pour the batter into the loaf pan and bake for 50 minutes, or until a toothpick inserted in the center comes out clean.
6. While the cake bakes, make the orange simple syrup. Mix the rest of the 1/3 cup of sugar plus 1/3 cup of orange juice in a small saucepan over medium heat. Simmer until your sugar dissolves and the syrup is clear. Set aside.
7. Remove the cake from oven and let cool for 10 minutes. Remove from the loaf pan and place on a wire rack on top of a rimmed baking sheet to catch the syrup. Pour the simple syrup over the cake. Let cool completely.
8. Make the orange glaze. Whisk the powdered sugar and the remaining 2 tablespoons of orange juice in a medium bowl until no lumps remain. Drizzle over the cooled cake. Serve and store leftovers in an airtight container.

Nutrition: Calories: 536 Fat: 15 g Carbs: 99 g Protein: 3 g

600. Strawberry Rhubarb Coffee Cake

Preparation time: 25 minutes
Cooking time: 55 minutes
Servings: 6-8
Ingredients:
For the filling:
- 2 cups rhubarb, thinly sliced
- 2 cups strawberries, sliced
- 1 tablespoon lemon juice
- 2/3 cup granulated sugar
- 3 tablespoons cornstarch

For the cake:
- 1½ cups all-purpose flour
- ¼ teaspoon baking soda
- 1 teaspoon baking powder
- ¼ teaspoon salt
- ¼ cup vegan butter, softened
- ¾ cup granulated sugar
- ½ cup coconut yogurt
- 1 banana, mashed
- 1 teaspoon vanilla extract

For the topping:
- ¾ cup all-purpose flour
- ½ cup granulated sugar
- ½ teaspoon ground cinnamon
- ¼ teaspoon ground nutmeg
- 5 tablespoons melted butter

Directions:
1. For the filling, set a medium saucepan over medium heat. Add the rhubarb, strawberries, lemon juice, sugar, and cornstarch and stir to combine.
2. Simmer, then adjust to low and continue simmering until thickened, stirring often, for 5 to 7 minutes. Remove the filling from heat and let cool.
3. For the cake, preheat the oven to 350°F. Mix the flour, baking soda, baking powder, plus salt in a small bowl. Set aside.
4. Combine the butter plus sugar using an electric hand mixer and a large bowl or a stand mixer with the paddle attachment and beat on high until light and fluffy, about 5 minutes.
5. Put the yogurt, banana, plus vanilla extract and beat until combined. Adjust the speed to low then slowly add the dry mixture until fully incorporated.
6. Pour the batter evenly into a prepared 9-inch springform pan. Top with cooled strawberry-rhubarb filling and set aside.
7. For the topping, combine the flour, sugar, cinnamon, nutmeg, and butter in a medium bowl. Stir to form a crumble topping. Sprinkle evenly over the filling.
8. Bake within 45 minutes or until a toothpick inserted in the center comes out clean and the topping is browned. Let cool for 10 minutes and serve or store in an airtight container.

Nutrition: Calories: 479 Fat: 14 g Carbs: 86 g Protein: 5 g

601. Apple Crumble

Preparation time: 15 minutes
Cooking time: 25 minutes
Servings: 6
Ingredients:
For the filling:

- 4 to 5 apples, cored and chopped (about 6 cups)
- ½ cup unsweetened applesauce, or ¼ cup water
- 2 to 3 tablespoons unrefined sugar (coconut, date, sucanat, maple syrup)
- 1 teaspoon ground cinnamon
- Pinch sea salt

For the crumble:

- 2 tablespoons almond butter, or cashew or sunflower seed butter
- 2 tablespoons maple syrup
- 1½ cups rolled oats
- ½ cup walnuts, finely chopped
- ½ teaspoon ground cinnamon
- 2 to 3 tablespoons unrefined granular sugar (coconut, date, sucanat)

Directions:

1. Preheat the oven to 350°F. Put the apples and applesauce in an 8-inch-square baking dish, and sprinkle with the sugar, cinnamon, and salt. Toss to combine.
2. In a medium bowl, mix together the nut butter and maple syrup until smooth and creamy. Add the oats, walnuts, cinnamon, and sugar and stir to coat, using your hands if necessary.
3. Sprinkle the topping over the apples, and put the dish in the oven. Bake for 20 to 25 minutes, or until the fruit is soft and the topping is lightly browned.

Nutrition: Calories: 356 Fat: 17g Carbs: 49g Protein: 7g

602. Tangy Heirloom Carrot

Preparation Time: 10 minutes
Cooking Time: 45 minutes
Servings: 6
Ingredients

- 1 bunch heirloom carrots
- 1 tablespoon fresh thyme leaves
- ½ tablespoon coconut oil
- 1 tablespoon date paste
- 1/8 cup freshly-squeezed orange juice
- 1/8 teaspoon salt
- Extra salt if needed

Directions:

1. Preheat your oven to 350 degrees Fahrenheit. Wash carrots and discard green pieces. Take a small-sized bowl and add coconut oil, orange juice, salt, and date paste.
2. Pour mixture over carrots and spread on a large baking sheet. Sprinkle thyme and roast for 45 minutes. Sprinkle salt on top and enjoy!

Nutrition: Calories: 105 Carbs: 8g Fat: 7g Protein: 3g

603. Just Apple Slices

Preparation Time: 10 minutes
Cooking Time: 10 minutes
Servings: 4
Ingredients:

- 1 cup of coconut oil
- ¼ cup date paste
- 2 tablespoons ground cinnamon
- 4 granny smith apples, peeled and sliced, cored

Directions:

1. Take a large-sized skillet and place it over medium heat. Add oil and allow the oil to heat up. Stir in cinnamon and date paste into the oil.
2. Add cut up apples and cook for 5-8 minutes until crispy. Serve and enjoy!

Nutrition: Calories: 50 Carbs: 12g Fat: 0g Protein: 0g

Conclusion

The Pegan diet is a hybrid diet that incorporates the best of both Paleo and Vegan diets. The Pegan diet is promoted by Dr Mark Hyman, who is a family doctor and director of the Cleveland Clinic's Centre for Functional Medicine. the pegan diet is a new fad diet that combines the paleo diet with veganism. The pegan diet requires you to eliminate all meat and animal products from your diet, while at the same time eating a large amount of vegetables and plants.

The vegan diet is very advantageous as it reduces the risk of developing obesity, certain cancers, and type II diabetes. However, the diet falls short of certain amino acids that are the building blocks for proteins, which can only be achieved through diet. Moreover, it is deficient in iron, calcium, zinc, and vitamin B12.

For some individuals, a strict Paleo diet is too heavy and expensive to follow. It is also problematic when you consider the health issues. Veganism, on the other hand, is equally restrictive and quite a challenge for people to stick to. Hence the integration of these two highly opposing diets, the Pegan diet, a perfect mixture of healthy benefits and few limitations makes a lot of sense for those of us who want to follow a healthy lifestyle and agree add a limited amount of animal-based proteins in their diet.   .

You should avoid processed foods like sodas and grains found in prepared foods – including breads and other baked goods. These substances simply don't benefit our bodies in any way whatsoever! You should focus on eating whole foods from all parts of the plant kingdom, including vegetables, fruits, nuts and seeds. You can consume unsaturated oils (e.g., olive oil) because these are good for our hearts rather than refined oils (e.g., fry oil). And be sure to avoid anything fried!

The time to cook the recipe can be something better. It makes you think about the meal before you start cooking as well as you needs to be patient about cooking. In the time of making, you can take time to relax, and you can make a portion of good food for others by the time. There will be no meal wasted.

Following the instruction, you will be able to cook well, and it will make your dinner more delicious and of higher quality. Some recipes can be fun and healthy, as well. You can make your dinner more special by making a different recipe on your own. In this case, there will be no other recipes that you can make the same things as yours. You can make different flavors and different food you can ever eat.

Simple instructions give you a bit more instruction about the ingredients, and you need to be patient to make vegan food. The steps of the recipe are well described, and if you want to better food, you can follow them carefully.

The time to be patient to make a portion of good food is one of the important ways to make a good recipe. You need to follow the instruction in the recipe below. Live a healthy life by following the recipe for better health.

I hope you have learned something!

Appendix 1 Measurement Conversions

Volume Equivalents (Liquid)

US STANDARD	US STANDARD (OUNCES)	METRIC (APPROXIMATE)
2 tablespoons	1 fl. oz.	30 mL
1/4 cup	2 fl. oz.	60 mL
1/2 cup	4 fl. oz.	120 mL
1 cup	8 fl. oz.	240 mL
1 1/2 cups	12 fl. oz.	355 mL
2 cups or 1 pint	16 fl. oz.	475 mL
4 cups or 1 quart	32 fl. oz.	1 L
1 gallon	128 fl. oz.	4 L

Volume Equivalents (Dry)

US STANDARD	METRIC (APPROXIMATE)
1/8 teaspoon	0.5 mL
1/4 teaspoon	1 mL
1/2 teaspoon	2 mL
3/4 teaspoon	4 mL
1 teaspoon	5 mL
1 tablespoon	15 mL
1/4 cup	59 mL
1/3 cup	79 mL
1/2 cup	118 mL
2/3 cup	156 mL
3/4 cup	177 mL
1 cup	235 mL
2 cups or 1 pint	475 mL
3 cups	700 mL
4 cups or 1 quart	1 L

Oven Temperatures

FAHRENHEIT	CELSIUS (APPROXIMATE)
250°F	120°C
300°F	150°C
325°F	165°C
350°F	180°C
375°F	190°C
400°F	200°C
425°F	220°C
450°F	230°C

Appendix 2 Recipe Index